"Sheehy is a top-notch reporter. . . . She does a service with what she herself would call 'pioneer' work in late adult development, a largely unexplored terrain."

—*The Boston Globe*

"There are gold nuggets of personal stories in the book that rival the best literature. . . . Consider it a sort of cosmic Thomas Guide with exquisite storytelling."

—*Los Angeles Daily News*

"A good book on the psychological and physical journey of aging . . . Sheehy has done her homework. . . . She conducted extensive surveys of professional and working-class Americans, developed statistical profiles of age groups with the U.S. Census Bureau, and consulted with top-notch researchers."

—*The Philadelphia Inquirer*

"Sheehy is out to rock the culture again."

—*New York Daily News*

"*New Passages* has a lot to interest the reader who wants to know how to live the rest of a life that may last much longer than in the past and that may have to be lived with fewer economic resources."

—*The Houston Chronicle*

"Sheehy turns out to be a good guide to lead us through this brave and sometimes slightly ridiculous world of what passes for adulthood today."

—*Newark Star-Ledger*

"The range and profound human interest of the material, and Sheehy's dynamic, optimistic presentation of it, are such that it is almost impossible to imagine who would not be able to draw encouragement and sustenance from this sweeping vision of our personal futures."

—*Publishers Weekly*

NEW PASSAGES

New Passages

MAPPING YOUR
LIFE ACROSS TIME

Gail Sheehy

BALLANTINE BOOKS
NEW YORK

Grateful acknowledgment is made to the following for permission to reprint previously
published material:
THE ESTATE OF THOMAS WOLFE: Eight lines from "For Brother, What Are We?" from *Of Time
and the River* by Thomas Wolfe. Copyright © 1935 by Thomas Wolfe. Copyright renewed
© 1963 by Paul Gitlin, Administrator, C.T.A., of the Estate of Thomas Wolfe.
WILLIAMSON MUSIC: Lyric excerpt on pages 367–368 from "If I Loved You" by Richard
Rodgers and Oscar Hammerstein II. Copyright © 1945 by Williamson Music. Copyright
renewed. International copyright secured. All rights reserved. Reprinted by permission.

http://www.randomhouse.com

Library of Congress Catalog Card Number: 95-96199

ISBN: 0-345-40445-9

Cover design and illustration by Nigel Holmes

Manufactured in the United States of America

First Ballantine Books Edition: June 1996

10 9 8 7

FOR CLAY, MAURA, AND MOHM

NOTE FROM THE AUTHOR

I first began research on the new passages of middle life for men and women about seven years ago. By *middle life* I refer to the mid-forties to mid-sixties, the most unrevealed portion of adult life. The idea was to map out the predictable crises of this territory—an extension of my long fascination with the adult life cycle—but after the first seventy-five interviews, I had to pull up short. I had come upon a black hole of ignorance and denial, the silence called menopause. Before I could hope to understand the larger issues of middle life for contemporary women and men, I had to try to confront the cultural taboo surrounding the Change of Life. So what was meant to be a chapter in this book took on a life of its own.[1]

No time to make a passage myself—or so I thought. People were ready to have the conversation about menopause, and *The Silent Passage* became a conversation piece. Suddenly I was in constant demand to make speeches to help spotlight the many new women's health centers sprouting up across the country. It was a thrill to feel that one was in the right place at the right time, engaging with one's culture. But my own life was overtaken by the full-time job of publicity and public speaking.

At the peak of this razzle-dazzle of pleasant activism, my publisher threw a book party to celebrate *The Silent Passage*'s reaching number one on *The New York Times* best-seller list. I felt almost like an impostor. This book wasn't even meant to be! (In fact, when my husband, Clay Felker, first suggested that I expand on the magazine article I had written about menopause for *Vanity Fair,* I scoffed, "Oh, really, who would want to read a whole *book* about menopause?")

On the night of the party we were swept up in a gala outdoor garden dinner at an Italian trattoria. It was a mild summer evening. New York's literati gabbed with health professionals at checkered tables beneath trees giddily strung with lights. The trees gave way in places to pale lavender sky and faint stars and the suspended evening of endless possibilities that is June. I was a hundred feet off the ground. A wise friend of mine caught me in midair and whispered a warning. She could see the breathless half-finished hellos and airborne kisses, the jittery dance of narcissism.

"Be careful, you're becoming stress-addicted," said Pat Allen.

She was right. I had been performing for the previous year as a Little Ms. Menopause. As satisfying as that time was, I had become caught up in the world of externals and increasingly disconnected from what was real and important. The more public the expectations, the more compulsive I tend to become about trying to do it all perfectly, and the easier it is to be thrown by the slightest criticism. All the effort goes into keeping the show going, twenty-four hours a day. Stress builds up; body and mind almost never completely rest. It's a swell antidepressant. But losing myself in hyperactivity is also a classical way to avoid engaging a necessary passage.

And there were now issues I very much wanted to avoid. For one, the news that the husband of a dear friend of mine was battling cancer. When we are on the threshold of a new stage, we are particularly vulnerable to twinges about aging, and 50 is certainly a threshold. When a friend around our own age stares back at the beast, it gives death a human face. The marker event that makes our mortality suddenly feel so real and frightening does not have to concern death or happen to us directly. It can be the abrupt independence of a last child, the enfeeblement of a vigorous parent, a friend who slips from what seemed an unassailable position of success into has-been status and despair.

Since ultimately death cannot be avoided, the real question then becomes: How shall we live the rest of our lives? A hundred years ago that question seldom came up for people beyond their mid-forties. Their proper expectation upon approaching age 50 was to be dead.[2] Today, even though we know intellectually that we can expect to live much longer, our view of life beyond the mid-forties is still colored by mental snapshots of our mothers or fathers at that age: "My mother looked tired and, yes, *old,* at fifty," or "My father had his first heart attack at fifty; he was never the same man."

The first glimpses of a midlife perspective usually begin to startle us in the middle of our thirties. Time starts to pinch. I was in my mid-thirties when I began the research for *Passages,* a book about the adult life cycle that was published twenty years ago (in 1976).[3] It proposed that we continue to develop by stages and to confront predictable crises, or passages, between each stage of adulthood. At that stage in my own life I saw the mid-thirties as the halfway mark, the prime of life. The years between 35 and 45 I called the Deadline Decade, as if we had only until our mid-forties to resolve the crisis of midlife.

I stopped before 50 in *Passages.* Frankly I found it impossible to picture myself at that age. Like so many others of my generation, I couldn't imagine life beyond 50, and I certainly couldn't bring myself to consider it as a time of special possibility or potential. It had always conjured up moms who slipped into depression or some slope-shouldered fellow sitting in a fishing boat while the world goes by. It was supposed to be a time of winding down. The midlife crisis had long since blown over, and if one hadn't confronted it by then, there wasn't much family or societal support for taking the risk at 50. Careers were settled; one was either coasting toward retirement, resigned to failure, or somewhat patronized as a has-been success. Children were launched. Idealism had faded. Learning was completed. Love was about cuddling or rocking grandchildren, certainly not associated with computer dating or uninhibited sex. Since there were no instructions for what a woman should be after she has finished making babies and getting by on her physical charms, it might just be a sudden Dorian Gray transformation. My own dark fantasy was I would go to sleep and wake up one morning to the *Today* show and there would be Willard Scott, saluting my picture: "What a beyootiful little lady, a hundred and one years young!"

Given Western societies' revulsion against middle age, the map of the youth culture leads us to the edge of the known world, whereupon it simply drops off. We have been as ignorant about what lies on the other side as were Columbus and the early explorers of the New World. It requires a leap of faith, we are told. But when we do take the leap, trusting in the possibility of a new beginning, we find ourselves hurtling along the edge. On the other side we will be something else, but we have no idea what. It may be too frightening to look over the edge. Just as the early explorers assumed the world was flat, we have assumed the other side of youth is a sheer drop or, even worse, a slow, wasting decline.

That's the way I thought it was; that's the way most of us thought it was. We would get old in much the same way our parents did. The conventional maps in our minds and the timetables that go with them can keep us imprisoned in old ways of thinking about life beyond youth.

During the research for this book I discovered a whole unexplored territory in the middle that does not fit at all within the confines of the old map of youth and age. Surprise! The second half of adult life is *not* the stagnant, depressing downward slide we have always assumed it to be.

Wonderfully zesty women in their forties, fifties, and sixties came up to talk to me after my lectures. I kept asking them how it felt to be here, now, on the cusp of radical changes in the life cycle. Whether they talked about the degrees they were studying for, or the daringness of launching new businesses or digging up fossils in China, or the alcoholism or anger or anxiety they had shed, or the live-out lovers they were enjoying instead of remarriage, they all seemed to be exhilarated about starting over.

The more I lectured on female menopause, the more I kept getting the same question: Is there a *male menopause?* So I turned it around to ask the women themselves, "What do *you* think?" Most thought there was. It was worth investigating. When men at this stage slip into chronic depression, or start desperately chasing after girls their daughters' ages, or throw over careers they have spent lifetimes building to start from scratch in businesses they know nothing about, wives and friends mutter, "He's just acting crazy." That is only because we haven't tracked what is really going on under the surface.

The only way to find out how men felt about being in their forties, fifties, and sixties was to get them to talk about it. Not easy, since most men over 40 were conditioned early by their fathers to cauterize their feelings. At first, when I tried to interview some of the same men who had eagerly contributed woeful tales of their wives' Change of Life, they swallowed their tongues. "You are now entering the *inner sanctum*," I was warned.

And so, whenever I was scheduled to make a speech in another city, I began asking the sponsoring institution to help me set up a group interview with eight to ten men of varied backgrounds. None of the men who agreed to join my focus group in Detroit, for example, would be caught dead on a weekend in the woods looking for his Wild Man. They were shaped by a tough industrial city and heavy ethnic conditioning to be "real" men—i.e., stubborn, cocky, hard to read, convinced that they must remain forever strong, perpetually virile, providers and protectors of their families, and without doubts or needs or fears that require expressing their feelings. To join any sort of men's group still held a stigma.

"There's no way I'm going to be able to get eight to ten men for this type of project," said Suzanne Schut, director of public relations for St. Joseph's Mercy Hospital in Macomb County, Michigan. Gamely she reached out for a varied group of men and sent each of them a Life History Survey I had developed along with a copy of the *Vanity Fair* article I had written titled "Is There a Male Menopause?" Overnight the men called back. "I was shocked," said Suzanne. "They really *want* to come." These were questions they had been asking themselves. Ray Kudzia, a high school music teacher, said candidly, "The lady author, I don't know her, but I'm looking forward to talking to the other *men*. They may be feeling the same way I'm feeling, but we don't talk about it."

I found the same hunger wherever I called together men's groups. From Orlando to Rochester to Seattle, regular guys were ready to strip away most of their pretenses to search together for ways to change the model of masculinity—to move beyond the stud or jock prototype of youth—in preparation for the new stages ahead. I read it as an unstated phenomenon, a consequence of all the focus on women. Men have become sensitized to *what they're missing* in middle life. And many I interviewed are excited about reinventing themselves.

As I read over the transcripts of the hundreds of life history interviews I had done with women and men in middle life, a new theme, one of surprise and rebirths, was recapitulated loud and clear. More and more people were beginning to see there was the possibility of a new life to live, one in which we could concentrate on becoming better, stronger, deeper, wiser, funnier, freer, sexier, and more attentive to living the privileged moments, even as we were also getting older, lumpier, bumpier, slower, and closer to the end.

Of course, for some of us time will run out before we can really engage or enjoy the second half. No one can predict catastrophic illness, accidents, financial crashes. You will find people in this book wrestling with all these maladies, along with Alzheimer's, widowhood, and cancer. Some of them jolt us with their resilience; they fight back. There is one whole chapter on facing the Mortality Crisis. But this is not a book about dealing with the debilities of aging. We are so accustomed to focusing on what goes wrong with us as we get older, it seemed to me important to focus on what goes right with us. Whatever the future holds, the boundaries of vital living are still vastly enlarged for those moving into the second half of life.

But how to write about it? How to *believe* it? I had my own private doubts and fears to overcome.

On my mind more or less constantly was the "sentence" passed on the friend I mentioned earlier. Up to the day her husband went into the hospital for "routine" exploratory surgery, Peggy Downes, a professor and avid mountain climber, had been enthusiastically planning a trip to Provence with her partner of eighteen years, Chuck, to celebrate the freedom of an empty nest. Instead, overnight, they became locked in a battle with prostate cancer. Their ordeal haunted me.

One night after a phone call to Peggy I had a horrible nightmare. I began to suspect that my intimate involvement with Peggy's ordeal wasn't just about empathy for a friend. Most of us face some crisis in our forties or fifties that will force us to rethink and reflect on how we are going to live the second half. The longer we put off that task of reflection, the more everything, even the mundane, begins to remind us of death. The private feelings I was having were spilling over into the intellectual questions I was trying to confront in my research. My fear was a shadowy thing, while up ahead I could faintly glimpse a lighter, brighter place, if only I could reach it. But I had to step to the precipice and deal with the reality of my own age, my own place in life, my own mortality.

I prayed that Peggy and Chuck would come out of their dark combat with the spiritual energy for a renewal of growth. But there was a signal here for me too—I recognized it now—that a new passage had to be made, a *conscious* shift to another stage of life.

Call Peggy, I commanded myself.

But I didn't want to know. My construct for incorporating her experience was still too fragile. Like most people in middle life, I was in the process of shifting from searching for answers in the concrete to searching in the transcendent. My subjective definition of success was changing as well. The arrogance of possibility and the fiery excitement that fueled my twenties through my early forties were best expressed in several bracing lines of poetry by Goethe that I used to keep pinned up over my typewriter in those years:

> What you can do, or dream you can, begin it,
> Boldness has genius, power, and magic in it.

It spoke to the coltish will that had always worked for me before. But now my goals were changing. I was coming to a plateau in the long dance of achievement that had begun in school and continued throughout my career.

I was no longer so eager to please or so willing to allow my sense of well-being to be determined by the world's evaluation of my performance. There was a yearning in me for a different sort of tempo, almost as if my personal journey and my professional curiosity were coming together naturally. Writing *The Silent Passage* had been only the beginning of that journey of integration.

Eventually a plan took shape: to tie up all the outstanding obligations and then drop out for the month of February. I felt pulled toward a wholly unfamiliar environment. Another friend, Ellen McGrath, generously invited me to share her office in a half-empty resort town in Southern California where I could watch the waves roll in. She provided a touchstone of affectionate support while I dropped the masks and rituals of my predictable and recently very public life.

All the journals I had kept over the past few years and notes I had made during a weekend seminar on "The New Older Woman" were in a little zippered suitcase, stuffed under the bed. In this unhurried place on the Pacific, where no one would know to call me, I could unzip it and open up the journals and notes—along with the fears stirred in my unconscious from sharing Peggy's experience—to see what Furies would fly out. What unfinished business did I need to digest, put to rest, draw from? I was expecting to brace myself to accept the inevitable decline at this time of life. It would be frightening and sad. I would probably cry a lot and come out the other side with the crisp, dispassionate composure of the Older Woman.

I ran on the beach every morning, as I have walked or run on winter beaches all my life, hoping to work up to a plunge in the Pacific. Why not? I have been comfortable in the water since I was a tadpole no more than two and a half, when my mother and father tossed me back and forth in the shallows of Long Island Sound until I learned to swim. But I felt a little tentative about these waves. At high tide they reached up to slap at the rock cliffs behind the strip of beach. I went back to reading over my journals.

In the third week of my retreat I got up the nerve to call Peggy again. A new tumor had been found. Chuck faced another operation, another phase of radiation, possible chemotherapy. But there was almost a lilt to Peggy's voice. Her husband had decided to forgo aggressive treatment. They would celebrate the life they had left and go to France anyway.

That morning my old nightmare turned into a daymare. I tried my usual technique. I would write the fear out of me. I sat down to start writing

Peggy's story—and froze. All the information was there, but I couldn't transform it to give her experience to others. Peggy's story paralleled the very psychic drama that I was living. I too was running along the edge. The structure of my own world—the world of still-youngness where we can take our health for granted and throw ourselves at life, unprepared for inconsolable losses—was disintegrating. Since the thought of our own death is too terrifying to confront head-on, it keeps coming back in various disguises.

When I watched the sea somersault in all its exuberant energy, instead of thinking what I used to when I was younger, which was *I can't wait to dive through the waves,* now I thought of drowning. Realistically, I was sure I could still run into the waves and tumble inside those watery barrels; hadn't I often done so as an adult? But now suddenly I wanted to take no chance of losing my footing.

Those waves represented everything that can overpower us and take away what we love. I thought of myself and my husband as among the lucky ones. *You think you made it,* those waves seemed to be saying, *but we are going to swallow you up, too.* In the face of the randomness of life and death, could I get away with asserting the promise of a rebirth in the second half?

One morning, while I was off guard, a wave caught me and knocked me down. I was startled but not frightened; that was the surprise. It had been a gentle shove, like that of a playmate. Soft soapy foam gurgled around me and I felt suddenly girlish. I looked back out at the big waves and saw them as inviting.

All at once I realized—no! this wasn't about decline! Our middle life is a progress story. A series of little victories over little deaths. Surprise! We *can* go ahead. There is resurrection in life—and it is alright to say so.

It was an *Aha!* moment. Virginia Woolf called such little epiphanies "moments of being," when a shock pulls the gauzy curtain off everyday existence and throws a sudden floodlight on what our lives are really about. There *is* another side to this mountain. It was time to go into training for the journey. But now I felt an inward trust. I could be creative again.

I dived into the cold waves and came up on the other side, laughing.

Millions of people entering their forties and fifties today are able to make dramatic changes in their lives and habits, to look forward to living decades more in adequately functioning bodies with agile minds—so long as they

remain open to new vistas of learning and imagination and anticipate experiences yet to be conquered and savored. So there it was. The challenge for
me, the anchor in this sea of Second Adulthood, is a rebellious purpose—
to redefine middle life and put out the word:

This is a gift.

Contents

PART TWO

THE FLOURISHING FORTIES

BOOK TWO: SECOND ADULTHOOD

BOOK ONE

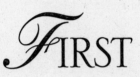

FIRST ADULTHOOD

Prologue

OH, PIONEERS!

Western culture from antiquity to the present has sought to divide human life into ages and stages. The need to find some order and predictability in the variousness of the human life cycle has inspired philosophers, poets, and playwrights from the Greeks and Hindus up through Shakespeare and on through the psychoanalysts Jung and Erikson to today's New Age bards.

From the beginning of this century to the middle of the 1970s the marker events of life—graduation, first job, marriage, first child, empty nest, retirement, widowhood, even death—always tended to occur for most people at predictable points in life. This was not a new notion. Back as far as the eighteenth century, chronological age has served as a uniform criterion for normalizing the roles and responsibilities that individuals assume over a lifetime. The ages 21 and 60 or 65 came to define the lower and upper boundaries of participation in the adult world.[1] But since the publication of *Passages* in 1976, age norms have shifted and are no longer normative.

Consider:

—9-year-old girls are developing breasts and pubic hair.
—9-year-old boys carry guns to school.
—16-year-olds can "divorce" a parent.
—30-year-old men still live at home with Mom.
—40-year-old women are just getting around to pregnancy.
—50-year-old men are forced into early retirement.

——55-year-old women can have egg donor babies.

——65-year-old women start first professional degrees.

——70-year-old men reverse aging by twenty years (with human growth hormone).

——80-year-olds move in together, enjoy sex, and scandalize their middle-aged children.

——90-year-olds have hip replacements.

——And every day the *Today* show's Willard Scott says "Happy birthday!" to more 100-year-old women.

What's going on?

There is a revolution in the life cycle. In the space of one short generation the whole shape of the life cycle has been fundamentally altered. People today are leaving childhood sooner, but they are taking longer to grow up and much longer to grow old. That shifts all the stages of adulthood ahead—by up to ten years.

Puberty arrives earlier by several years than it did at the turn of the century. Adolescence is now prolonged for the middle class until the end of the twenties and for blue-collar men and women until the mid-twenties, as more young adults live at home longer. True adulthood doesn't begin until 30. Most Baby Boomers, born after World War II, do not feel fully "grown up" until they are into their forties, and even then they resist. Unlike members of the previous generation, who almost universally had their children launched by that stage of life,[2] many late-baby couples or stepfamily parents will still be battling with rebellious children who are on the "catastrophic brink of *adolescence*"[3] while they themselves wrestle with the pronounced hormonal and psychic changes that come with the passage into middle life.

When our parents turned 50, we thought they were old. They thought they were old. Society told them they were old and they acted old. But today, women and men I have interviewed for *New Passages* routinely believe they are five to ten years younger than the age on their birth certificates—and in many ways, they are.

Middle age has already been pushed far into the fifties—if it is acknowledged at all today. The territory of the fifties, sixties, and beyond is changing so radically that it now opens up whole new passages leading to stages of life that are nothing like what our parents or grandparents experienced.

Fifty is now what 40 used to be.

Sixty is what 50 used to be.

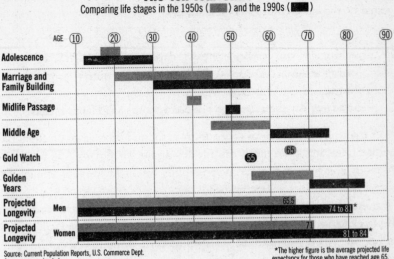

The Ten-Year Shift

Comparing life stages in the 1950s ( ) and the 1990s ( )

| | AGE ⑩ | ⑳ | ㉚ | ㊵ | ㊿ | ㉠ | ㉞ | ㉨ | ⑨⓪ |

Adolescence

Marriage and Family Building

Midlife Passage

Middle Age

Gold Watch — 55, 65

Golden Years

Projected Longevity — Men — 65.5, 74 to 81*

Projected Longevity — Women — 71, 81 to 84*

Source: Current Population Reports, U.S. Commerce Dept.
Ages are approximated.

*The higher figure is the average projected life expectancy for those who have reached age 65.

"Everything seems to be moved off by a decade," comedian-director David Steinberg observed in our interview.

"I don't know *how* to be fifty," admitted an Oregon psychotherapist when I was interviewing her in 1991, "but I do know I'm *not* going to be fifty like my mother." She was just getting ready to declare a moratorium on doing holiday meals and laundry for her thirtyish sons. This was *her* time for adventure.

A Louisville woman tried to convey to her adult son the dizzying sense of being out of sync with her age identity. "I'm sixty years old on paper, but in my head I'm forty-five. I can't begin to describe to you what that feels like."

Europeans, just like Americans, are marrying later, having fewer children, and living longer. A European Community study found that the number of Europeans over 60 has risen by half over the past thirty years, and their legions will swell by half again in the next thirty years.[4]

Certain pacesetters among the 45+ population are already eagerly remaking themselves to start again, sensing that they are probably going to live far longer than their parents. And they're right. For the first time in the history of the world most people in advanced societies can expect to live into the long late afternoon of life. Two thirds of the total gains in life expectancy accomplished since the human species emerged have been made in this century alone!

Midway through my speeches I often toss out a provocative figure suggested by the latest epidemiological studies:

> A woman who reaches age 50 today—and remains free of cancer and heart disease—can expect to see her ninety-second birthday.[5]

A tremendous buzz always goes up from the audience; gasps of euphoria and tentative applause quickly cascade downward into groans. And why not? Nobody ever prepared us for the possibility we might live long enough to forget the name of our first husband!

Even when all women, sickly or well, from every income group and every IQ level across the United States are averaged together, they can still expect *at least* thirty-two years and likely a span of forty or more years to fill with meaningful, gainful, and productive living—after reaching their fiftieth birthdays.[6] That amounts to a second adult lifetime.

Recent projections are almost as startling for men, who are living much longer than they expected. "If you get men through the thirty-five to sixty age period without their dying of heart disease, they are [in later decades] stronger and less frail than women," observed Ruth Kirschstein, then director of the National Institutes of Health's National Institute of General Medical Sciences.[7]

> Already the average healthy man who is 65 today—an age now reached by the great majority of the U.S. population—can expect to live until 81.[8]

Adult life of such quantity and quality has never before been experienced by a mass human civilization.[9] How does it alter the ages and stages of the adult life cycle?

The earlier stages—up to age 45—represent to me the Old Territories of the adult life cycle, ground that I have covered before. Nevertheless, I found radical alterations in those stages being encountered by newer generations. This book will briefly review and update the Tryout Twenties, Turbulent Thirties, and Flourishing Forties—in light of those refreshing and confusing changes. It is a necessary preparation for understanding the magnitude of changes that are taking place in *the new middle* of adult life today.

When I looked at midlife again, nearly two decades after writing about it for the first time, I was struck not by one but by a cascade of surprises. The territory of the Flourishing Forties, the Flaming Fifties, the Serene Sixties, and beyond is changing so fundamentally it now opens up whole new passages and stages of life.

Sadly, this is not an egalitarian phenomenon. The gap between the professional class and the poor seems to be widening inexorably. There is a whole new class of men who lack the skills and education to work in the postmodern economy and may never be able adequately to support a family and direct their own lives. And as America slides further into an ethic of self-indulgence, millions are killing themselves much earlier than they need to expire. Human behavior—diet, exercise, alcohol use, smoking, domestic violence, and failure to wear seatbelts—contributes to over 50 percent of all causes of death in America.

Nevertheless, the more fortunate in society will increasingly be faced with a new timetable for adult life. The life cycle will only get longer. The latest predictions by demographers are stunning:

> A girl born in the United States today has a one in three chance of living to 100.

Stop and recalculate. Imagine the day you turn 45 as the infancy of another life. That is what this book is about, an entirely new concept of the life cycle: a Second Adulthood in middle life.

Because the populations of developed countries are generally healthier today, people are entering old age in better shape than they used to. Thus life spans can be expected to continue to increase. Haven't you noticed? Older people don't seem to be dying off as quickly. During most of human history only one in ten people lived to the age of 65. In contemporary America eight in ten people sail past their sixty-fifth birthday.[10]

The fact that most middle-aged and "young-old" Americans today still have a living parent is a change in family dynamics with no precedent in history. The president of a nursing home, Nita Corré, reflected on the amazing changes she has seen just in her time at the Milwaukee Jewish Home: "Twenty years ago I'd see forty-year-olds bringing in their sixty-year-old parents. Now I'm seeing seventy-year-olds bringing in their ninety-year-old parents."

And contrary to expectations, the longer people live, the greater the extension of longevity they can anticipate.[11] Developed countries all over the world have been noting with some astonishment that their oldest old are not dying off. Sweden's statistics office gathered a gold-standard data set that produced a startling conclusion: Up until about 1950 the mortality rate among those over age 85 had remained about the same, but since then it has dropped, steadily, at a rate of about 2 percent a year. When a Finnish demographer collected mortality data for the oldest old from twenty-seven countries, he found that just like the elderly in Sweden, the oldest old elsewhere have shown a steady sustained increase in years of life since 1950.[12]

Yet another new stage, then, has been added to the average life span, inhabited by the young-old. Just as middle age has been pushed well into the fifties, one may not become "old" until very shortly before death.

These empirical facts alone throw off the predictable timetables around which industrialized societies have been organized and scramble the social roles that were linked to them. Whole new stages are springing up at several points along the route of adult life, like bright new cities, posing many new opportunities and discontinuities that simply have not been part of the maps in our minds. The old demarcation points we may still carry around—an adulthood that begins at 21 and ends at 65—are hopelessly out-of-date. Many of us feel a little lost. It's almost like being in a foreign country, where we don't know the language or the subway system. We need a new map.

The neurons in our brain are actually arranged into maps, according to recent scientific theory. Each map receives independent signals from the world. Gerald Edelman, the Nobel Prize–winning neuroscientist and author of *Bright Air, Brilliant Fire*, explains the process of thinking as "neuronal regrouping."[13] The brain extracts closely connected collections of cells, called a neuronal group, from a number of different maps and recombines them with neuronal groups from other maps to fit new stimuli. That is exactly the process I had in mind when I worked with designer Nigel Holmes to create the New Map of Adult Life you can consult on the inside front cover. It might help you redraw the maps in your own mind, change the lines of demarcation, and think about plotting your route across the vast new stretches of Second Adulthood.

In my view, we have a greater need than ever before to recognize the passages of our lives, not only because we are living longer but because the rapidity and complexity of changes taking place in the world are constantly reshaping the adult life cycle into something fundamentally different from what we have ever known. We are in the midst of an economic and electronic revolution. Everything—money, war, political change, the rise and fall of great corporations—moves faster while our attention spans grow shorter. Indeed, with our E-mail boxes and our fax and phone machines always "on," we have invaded our own solitude with an accelerated demand for immediate action and reaction. We seldom make time to process even the most meaningful experiences of our lives; we just speed through them.

Moreover, recent experiments have shattered our common notions about life expectancy. Scientists have uncovered the first evidence suggesting there may be no inborn limit to how old people can grow. The new research, led by James Carey of the University of California at Davis and James Vaupel of Duke University, suggests that given good health practices, the current life expectancy of about 75 years old may rise to 90 and 100 *in the foreseeable future.*[14]

With luck then, once Baby Boomers pass 45, another whole adult lifetime lies before them: thirty, forty, even fifty years. This reality does not easily compute with our old timetables. Along with any surprise, of course, come disorientation and a certain amount of anxiety. We now have not one but three adult lives to be anticipated, prepared for, mapped out. For clarity of discussion, I have given titles to these overarching periods:

Provisional Adulthood (18 to 30)
First Adulthood (30 to 45)
Second Adulthood (45 to 85+)

Each presents its own struggles and begs for a new dream. The ages we enter and leave each period will vary; it is the very presence and possibilities of these three different territories of the adult life cycle that are important. It is likely that we will share these three lives with different partners or journey through one or more of them alone. Young men are likely to have two marriages. Serial families will be the norm. A third partner, to share the mellow years after 55, is also increasingly common for a man, but he often doesn't marry her. And all along, we have new opportunities for development.

The leitmotif in the hundreds of life stories I have heard is surprise, astonishment even, that the middle years do not mean descent. On the contrary, this is the stage of greatest well-being in the lives of most healthy people today. This book will give you the life stories, the studies and statistics and latest surveys to prove it and to explain why.

My impression from talking to men and women all over the United States and in Britain is that this new perspective—only milliseconds old in evolutionary terms—has not caught up with most people. Once attention is called to it, this revolution in the life cycle is already quite observable in the social laboratory that is the United States, and in the near future it will reverberate through all modern countries. In Britain, for example, where social phenomena wash over the culture more slowly, the usual lag time is from five to ten years. But after the original publication of *New Passages* in the U.S., I did considerable cross-cultural research in the U.K., and it became apparent that there is already quite dramatic evidence of the ten-year delay in adult life stage development among Britons. In addition to its publication throughout the United Kingdom, *New Passages* has been deemed relevant by publishers in Europe, Japan, Israel, Brazil, and much of Latin America, as well as Taiwan.

Some receptivity to these ideas was found even in mainland China. During the International Conference on Women, delegates from Tulsa, Oklahoma, told me about discussing with their professional counterparts in Beijing the possibilities of leadership for women over 50. At first, the Chinese delegates parroted the old reality—life for women in China was over after 50—despite the blatant contradiction that the women speaking held powerful government positions and were all over 50 themselves. But when our American spokeswomen described the concept of *New Passages*, the Chinese women exclaimed, "Second Adulthood, yes! This is our new condition."

How do we find our way to this exciting Second Adulthood? I see a brand-new passage in the forties, when the transition from the end of First Adulthood to the beginning of Second Adulthood begins. The years between 45 and 55 constitute a bonus stage—truly new territory—and a central focus of this book. The vast New Territories of Second Adulthood, as I see it, break down into two major stages:

Age of Mastery (45 to 65)
Age of Integrity (65 to 85+)

Have you asked yourself: What can you make of your next life? Whom do you want to share it with, if anybody? What new ventures or adventures can you now dare try? What old shells can you slough off? Are there fatal traps you should avoid? What about those exploratory spiritual journeys you keep putting off? How can you best give back? What investments in learning and changes in lifestyle are you willing to undertake to make all these extra years ahead livable? How long do you *want* to live?

UPDATING THE PASSAGES CONCEPT

That there are new passages and stages beyond the mid-forties is only the most radical alteration in the life cycle. *All* of the life stages have shifted to some degree. Everybody likes to think of him or herself as unique. But there is comfort, too, in knowing that you are not the only one who is feeling less than grounded in a life cycle that today offers no clear boundaries or directional signals.

Passages helped to popularize an entirely new concept: that adulthood continues to proceed by stages of development throughout the life cycle. Unlike childhood stages, the stages of adult life are characterized not by physical growth but by steps in psychological and social growth. Marriage, childbirth, first job, empty nest are what we call *marker events,* the concrete happenings of our lives. A developmental stage, however, is not defined by marker events; it is defined by an underlying *impulse toward change* that signals us from the realm of mind or spirit. This inner realm is where we register the *meaning* of our participation in the external world: How do we *feel* about our job, family roles, social roles? In what ways are our values, goals, and aspirations being invigorated or violated by our present life structure? How many parts of our personality can we live out, and what parts are we leaving out?

It is discontent in the inner realm that signals the necessity to change and move on to the next stage of development. Erik Erikson, who died in 1994 having revolutionized our view of human growth and development, introduced the theory that each stage of life, from infancy through to advanced age, is associated with a specific psychological struggle that shapes a major aspect of our personalities.[15] Daniel J. Levinson elaborated on the theory in the lives of men.[16]

Passages was my word for those predictable "crises" or turning points that usher in a new stage, a crucial period of decision between progress and regression. In my book *Passages* I used the analogy of the lobster, which grows by developing and shedding a series of hard, protective shells. Each time it expands from within, the confining shell must be sloughed off, and it is left unprotected until a new covering grows. We, too, in each passage from one stage of human growth to the next, must shed a protective structure. We, too, are left exposed and vulnerable—but also yeasty and embryonic again. At such points we enjoy a *heightened potential* for making a real stretch of growth. But we can also fall back, lose ground, give up, or simply ignore the impulse to change and remain stuck in our shells. Whatever we do, the future will be rendered better or worse but, in any case, restructured.

That part of the concept continues to hold true and has been widely accepted.

Despite the recent shifts in the life cycle, there are still broad, general stages of adulthood with predictable passages between them. But the timetable is stretched out about five or ten years. Age norms for major life events have become highly elastic. Since we are all swimming around furiously in the fishbowl of daily life, we probably can't see the obvious: The bowl has gotten much bigger, and the water levels have all changed.

We are talking here about something that goes beyond any particular generation or social class or the details of private lives. Seven years ago I began work on comparing the life cycle as it has been expressed in different generational groups over the past fifty years. I soon found myself drawn into a subject infinitely more complex.

People who are today in their twenties, thirties, and early forties are also faced with drastically changed conditions, and that creates disequilibrium. Their private world is no longer a flat, linear progression, as it was for their parents. They are leading cyclical lives that demand they start over again and again. Three lives in one may sound like a bargain, but it comes at a price: The Age of Provisional Adulthood today is lived at a breathlessly accelerated pace, even though many of the responsibilities of full adulthood are delayed. The Age of Mastery cannot be about coasting until retirement or playing endless rounds of games. It must be a preparation for stages that in the past only the exceptional among us ever reached. Most people in the Age of Integrity (over 65) will continue to work in one way or another—part-time, or as consultants, contract teachers, community volunteers, or self-employed entrepreneurs—not only because they want to feel a sense of purpose or self-worth but because they will have to be prepared to support themselves for greatly elongated later lives. The psychotherapist who admitted she didn't know how to be 50 reflected a sentiment that could be voiced by a person of almost any age.

—Do you know how to be 30 and still living with Mom?
—Do you know how to be 40 and single and still fulfilled?
—Do you know how to be a forced retiree at 50?
—Do you know how to be a cancer survivor who seeks work and a new dream at 60?
—Do you know how to be a man today?

The women's movement and the globalization of economic competition have also contributed to the revolution in the life cycle. Most females over 30 feel an increasing comfort level in handling their multiple roles. Men, by contrast, are moving into greater disequilibrium. Many are wrestling with what it means to be a man and how to feel good about it without reverting to Neanderthal behavior or surrendering to what some complain is "the feminization of practically everything." Over the past twenty years, while women have enjoyed a continuous expansion of opportunities, many of the structures on which men depended have been crumbling. At the same time, most men have been working harder for less net income. Here is a sobering statistic.

> The median money income (in constant dollars from 1974 to 1992) either remained flat or declined for American men *in every age-group except those over 65.*[17]

In some age-groups men's incomes declined precipitously—down as much as 24 percent among young men. During the same two decades women *in every age-group* drove ahead from their formerly low wage levels; those between ages 35 and 54 were up by more than 25 percent. The overall gain in wages and salaries for women who worked year-round, full-time averaged 18 percent.[18]

Such facts are sure to provoke an outcry from many males: "You see, women are stealing our jobs!" But the reason for the 18 percent gain is the far greater numbers of women now participating in the work force, a much higher percentage of whom are working full-time, usually to make ends meet in families where the fathers are either nonexistent, absent, laid off, or underemployed. And as Susan Faludi points out in *Backlash*, "About a third of the new jobs [for women] were at or below the poverty level—jobs men turn down."[19]

WHAT TO DO WITH THIS LEFTOVER LIFE?

The more interviews I did and surveys I conducted, the more apparent it became that not only is this ongoing revolution in adulthood taking place in the second half—although that is the newest and most uncharted frontier—but every age and stage are affected. Some of the social roles and developmental tasks formerly associated with one stage have been postponed to another or ignored altogether. Multiple tasks have piled up in the same stage, creating tremendous either-or conflicts. Not only the shape but also the *sequence of stages* has been altered. And a plethora of new choices has been opened up by new technologies for pushing the former limitations of biology and longevity.

The most mind-boggling changes of all are in the reproductive revolution. For thirty thousand generations one of the most basic instincts has been to breed as soon as we are able, to reproduce ourselves. In the space of one generation, middle- and upper-middle-class Americans decided to defer childbirth for ten to twenty years. This may be the most radical *voluntary* alteration of the life cycle of all of them.

Now we see on television women in their fifties and sixties proudly announcing they have given birth—to babies whose eggs were donated by younger women. Pregnancy after menopause threatens the ancient concept of the human life cycle. The fact that a woman can now be "fertile indefinitely," even bear her own grandchild, "makes the life course incoherent," according to medical ethicist and lawyer George Annas of Boston University.[20] We must rethink and redesign our own life course. While we're at it, we must give some serious thought to how our cultures should reflect and enhance these new realities.

We also seem to be suspended from our spiritual selves. Václav Havel, the philosopher and former president of the Czech Republic, remarked on the paradox of our times: "Experts can explain anything in the objective world to us, yet we understand our own lives less and less. We live in the post-modern world, where anything is possible and almost nothing is certain."[21] Awareness and acknowledgment of a higher authority have been shunted into the realm of magic and mysticism. The concept of a Creator or an Earth Mother who anchors us in the universe, not for ourselves alone but as an integral part of some higher, self-perpetuating universal order, represents an affront to modern science and technology and gets in the way of arrogant human aspirations. But there must be a reason that we are living so much longer. What are we meant to do with all this leftover life? Surely we are not intended to regress to tribal warfare and cultural genocide. "The only real hope of people today is probably a renewal of our certainty that we are rooted in the Earth and, at the same time, the cosmos," suggests President Havel. "This awareness endows us with the capacity for self-transcendence."

The economic revolution will affect every stage of the life cycle: Young people will have to serve longer apprenticeships and prolong dependence on parents or their surrogates. Baby Boomers in their forties, as they run out of rungs to climb in middle management, will be obliged to find further ways to redefine personal success. Men in their fifties will have to face the fact they have peaked professionally, and rather than gentle, stepped-down transitions to honorable retirement in their mid-sixties, they may be handed a take-it-or-leave-it "package." Women will need to work outside the home for three quarters of their adult lives. We are all casting about for accurate maps and finding the maps woefully outdated.

But foreknowledge is power. Having some grasp of how our own life cycle is changing underneath us should encourage us to take inventory of our personal strengths and skills and to do what survivors have always done: adapt ourselves to accommodate the new age. People at 50 today also stand astride two centuries: With one foot planted firmly in the familiar playing field of the second half of the twentieth century, the other foot is free to dig into the new territory of the next fifty years beyond the millennium. The emergence of a second life to live cries out for new models, myths, heroines, and heroes. Let's hope you will find some in this book who speak to you.

I've learned many things in seven years on this journey, but the one overriding conclusion is this: There is no longer a standard life cycle. People are increasingly able to customize their life cycles.

We are on the brink of discovery. In Willa Cather's *O Pioneers!* it was the open land of the American West that gave drive and purpose to so many lives. At the dawn of a new century it is the adult life cycle itself—stretching it, taming it, bringing it under control, making it yield its riches—that beckons us all, women and men alike. This is the new human frontier.

THE DISCOVERY PROCESS

Research always begins for me with the revelations that come out of real life stories. In 1989 I started collecting life histories of women and men who were living through stages beyond where *Passages* left off. These pacesetters are the primary subjects of my research. They tend to be achievers and risk takers—the natural scouts of any society who are first to spot possibilities in what used to be a terra incognita. This is a book about possibilities. It makes no attempt to give equal treatment to everybody. To describe the new variations in First Adulthood and the provocative possibilities of Second Adulthood is certainly not to suggest that everybody is taking advantage of them. Naturally, economics have a great impact on how free people are to contemplate some of these experiments. But I found that the pacesetters can come from any segment of American society and include those who started from conditions of poverty or racial apartheid.

Some are celebrities, but my interviews with people like Lauren Hutton and Gloria Steinem, Frank Gifford and Hugh Downs were not the glitzy stuff of the "Passages" page in *People* magazine; they were sober self-examinations. In many cases I did follow-up interviews at one-, two-, or three-year intervals, which made it possible to follow a person's passage from onset to resolution.

Most people I interviewed were not famous. To break out of the bicoastal corridor of high-powered personalities in New York and Los Angeles, I made research trips to the Far West, the Midwest, and the South, where very different subcultures suggested different approaches to the life cycle. From a depressed area in Freehold, New Jersey, to a men's health spa high in Seattle's hills to a down-and-dirty discussion with divorced women over 45 in Chicago, I got an earful of the new possibilities and pitfalls being encountered by wayfarers into Second Adulthood. The subject was so fascinating I kept chugging on: Dallas, San Antonio, Santa Monica, San Francisco, Detroit, and back to Baltimore and Boston, down to Louisville and Atlanta, and on to Orlando and Tampa.

Group interviews also turned out to be a powerful experience, particularly with men. On two dozen occasions in different cities, I gathered together from six to twenty men or women in a particular age-group. Having already read their confidential questionnaires, I could raise questions that were close to the bone and let the participants stimulate one another to find universal patterns in the particulars of their experience.

In all, I conducted close to five hundred personal interviews with men and women from age 20 to 70. The people I chose to study range from working-class Americans to those of the educated middle class who have the luxury of choice. These are the pacesetters. First to sense or discover the new passages, they are in a position to plunge in and test out all kinds of possibilities. They usually think themselves unique. It's true that they are on a cutting edge, but they are certainly not alone. Every day more and more people understand that they, too, can join in and be pioneers in this unexplored territory of the new adult life cycle. Reading about them helps us to make sense of our own life by understanding other lives.

The sense of being part of something larger than one's own story may help to explain an unexpected reaction from my interviewees. I had assumed that after sharing their very personal and sometimes painful stories, most people would wish to be anonymous. But after they read their vignettes, the majority of people in the book elected to be identified by name. Even the tough guys from Detroit!

My mentor, Margaret Mead, taught me to appreciate the imprint of the cultures that spawn us. I therefore employ the anthropological method to place an individual's psychological journey in the context of those rules and rituals and often unspoken values of the specific subculture to which a person belongs. Those values color a person's interior emotional life.

I also wanted to look at lives across time and compare the five different generations now simultaneously occupying contemporary history. It would be helpful, I thought, to show where and how the passages have changed with each succeeding generation—beginning with those now in their late teens, twenties, and thirties—and to suggest what they have to look forward to in the most dynamic and unfettered part of the life cycle, beginning in the forties.

The bedrock of my data comes from several years' work with the U.S. Census Bureau. The bureau's data are the broadest cache of sociological comparisons we have in this country. Once each decade the Census Bureau gives us a snapshot of everyone at the same moment in history. When it takes another snapshot ten years later, however, it shows us no continuity. On one of my periodic research trips to the bureau, I asked Phillip Fulton, then deputy director of the Population Division, if there was any way we could sift through its gold mine of cross-sectional data and reduce it down to a richer, detailed comparison of how the stages of adulthood are changing from one generation to the next—purely objective comparisons, nothing psychological.

"If anyone can help you," said Phil, "it's Evelyn Mann." Mann had just retired after forty-two years of serving as New York City's chief demographer. She made it clear from the outset: "We cannot trace Mr. X from 1940 to 1990, but we can trace persons *like* Mr. X from one decade to another and look at the changes in people like him." It was a novel idea for all of us. Census Bureau data had never been used this way before. Mann helped me to create my own tape file, a pseudo-longitudinal data set that would span fifty years, from 1940 to 1990, and would allow us to trace through what happened to a particular cohort—an age-sex group—over its lifetime.

This unique database had a name like a spy movie: the PUMS file. This is a Public Use Microdata Sample. We extracted the same variables from each of the last six U.S. decentennial censuses and cross-tabulated these against age, sex, and marital status. As the big picture unfolded, it documented in hundreds of tables with tens of millions of numbers a clear acceleration of change in the life cycle and all the stages within it.

After several years of interviews and sociological research, I was ready to design the omnibus Life History Survey for men and women in Second Adulthood and to circulate it among a broad population. (See Appendix I for a reprint of the Life History Survey.) It was answered by a total of 7,880 women and men drawn from every region of the United States. A large proportion of the respondents have college educations or some graduate school, they mostly enjoy careers rather than endure jobs, and their incomes are slightly above average. (See Appendix II for more detail.)

For comparison, it was important to find a population of solidly middle-class Middle Americans, to see if they held similar views about the second half of life to those with more education, money, and choices. *Family Circle* magazine generously collaborated with me on this project, making available its selected reader's panel, which is weighted to approximate a representative national sample. (See Appendix III for further detail.) These thousand-plus women and their male partners are mostly not college graduates or professionals but hold white- or blue-collar jobs. Being mostly working class, their views about family and the proper roles for men and women are very traditional. But research has shown that roughly five years after new life patterns and attitudes emerge in the middle and upper-middle class, they are exported to and adopted by working-class young people.[22]

Yankelovich Partners, the social research organization, kindly teamed up with me in reanalyzing its data on attitudinal changes over the last twenty years according to my generational groupings. Harvard Business School invited me to survey and address one of its most famous classes (1949), the Class the Stars Fell On, when they were in their fifties. Ten years later I followed up the same men in their mid-sixties.

Then the real work began: synthesizing the statistical data with the individual life stories I had collected and trying to discern new patterns in the whole crazy quilt. To get through it, I figured I would need at least a third adulthood. From time to time, to keep me from bouncing off the wall, friends helped me to organize expert's groups to discuss phenomena I was picking up in the culture, such as "male menopause." These forums allowed me to try out my findings and ask questions of specialists in the multiple academic disciplines that must now be brought to bear on an understanding of adult development.

There is something about partnerships that is central to navigating through Second Adulthood—not just as a writer and researcher but as a person. Many people have contributed to this book in a myriad of ways (see

Acknowledgments), but I would like to highlight a few of my most precious intellectual partners.

Dr. Ellen McGrath, a friend who is a clinical psychologist with a bicoastal practice in New York City and Laguna Beach, California, and among the most esteemed, cutting-edge mental health experts in the country, is one of the midwives of this book. Dr. Patricia Allen, a friend and gynecologist who is always connecting the tender threads between our corporeal and emotional selves, is another midwife. They offered not only intellectual stimulation but loving sanity points when the work became too solitary. Dr. Ken Goldberg, a visionary urologist in Dallas, partnered with me in exploring "male menopause." (We are both well aware this term is a misnomer, but it is a misnomer that just about everybody recognizes while we attempt to define it more precisely.) Byron Dobell, a friend and editorial colleague from our old *New York* magazine days, also worked with me on the men's studies. And Robert Sind, a brilliant corporate restructuring expert, joined me in researching what men and women can do to offset the human displacement dictated by the economic revolution.

NEW CROSS-CULTURAL EVIDENCE

Is this only an American phenomenon? people ask. Few Britons, for example, think in terms even of inventing themselves, much less *re*inventing themselves. Social class divisions track people from the time they are born and preset their expectations.

When I held a group interview with professional couples in their forties in London, I presented the view that the people who will thrive in Second Adulthood are those who resist the old stereotypes and who plan and prepare for forty more years *after* they hit 40. Plan and prepare! "Nobody in Britain wants to plan anything!" exclaimed Maya di Robilant, a well-known TV news presenter. "Or they don't want to be seen to have planned anything."

The resistance to acknowledging such a disorienting change as a passage from First to Second Adulthood—never mind adjusting to it or planning for it—runs counter to some deep cultural values in Great Britain. A London money manager in his forties expressed amazement. "Do Americans sit down and plan things further into the future than we do? We seem to stumble into things."

His wife added drolly, "It's almost antisocial to be seen as having planned beyond the next dinner party."

The cult of the gifted amateur still exerts a strong appeal on the British. One should not exhibit ambition openly. This tradition dates all the way back to the Renaissance and the English aristocracy. The social analyst Marina Warner elaborated in a conversation with me: "It is a product of the belief that destiny was in command and that those who were smiled upon by fortune (by virtue of their highborn status) did not have to try hard because everything would fall into their laps." This affectation is not only perpetuated by the aristocracy—the higher the status of the duke, the more patches in his tweeds and the rattier the clothes of his son in private school—but it is still aped by many in the middle classes who prefer to look as if they just clomped out of the garden in their mud-spattered Wellies rather than appear to have done a stitch of work.

"England is still a class-ridden society," confirms Professor Robert Worcester, the American director of MORI, Great Britain's leading polling company. But in the very next breath he acknowledges a stunning change. "The last two decades, mainly under Thatcher, have seen the greatest change in the composition of the class structure in a thousand years of English history."

And there is a restless new Liberated Generation in Britain, those under 35, who represent an equivalent to America's Boomers. Many are openly aspirational. Because they will live longer, they are taking longer to prepare for careers and postponing personal commitments and family formation just like young Americans.

"The Boomers in their forties that you write about are redefining middle and old age," says Helen Wilkinson, a project director at the think tank Demos. "The problem in Britain is that we are not yet geared up to giving people second chances."

Are you ready to set off into this big unexplored continent of Second Adulthood? We will meet wayfarers who are stumbling and others who have already leaped over perilous divides. Some of the landmarks will be familiar, but much of the time we will be making up the maps as we go along. And so, before we start, you may want to place yourself in your own generation with your closest traveling companions. People naturally want to know: Where do I fit in? How are the stages of adult life different for me? And how do they remain the same?

Part One

Whatever Happened to the Life Cycle?

1
___

MAPPING LIVES ACROSS TIME

*T*he playing field is quite different for each generation when its young members start the journey into adulthood. The point where you and your friends came in on your culture's history has influenced your choices and attitudes. That distinctive generational coloration affects each stage of life and the passages between them, profoundly influencing which tasks of development you accomplish early, which you postpone, and which you will have to catch up on—or may never complete.

WHICH GENERATION ARE
YOU TRAVELING WITH?

I invite you to join me in mapping your own life across time. Five different generations now occupy contemporary adulthood, spanning birth dates from 1914 to 1980. You will probably find your peer traveling companions among the capsule descriptions of those five generations in this chapter.

To represent each one, I have selected five birth years that make up a definable "cohort group," a sociological term that refers to people who will always share a common location in history. (See Key to Your Cohort chart, page 25.) Not only were members of any cohort born within the same few years, but they have experienced defining events when they were the same age. Economic and social conditions along with technological and medical advances have either sped up or held back their development. Thus people in different cohorts age in different ways.

Drawing on the PUMS file—the unique database created from Census Bureau data that spans fifty years of information on the entire U.S. population—we are able to compare and contrast what is happening at any stage to a particular cohort group over its lifetime, with regard to educational and occupational achievement, labor force status, income level, marriage, childbearing, and divorce patterns.

You can look yourself up in this book and compare yourself to people in your parents' or your children's age-groups. For instance, if you are a woman in your mid-forties, you will find yourself under the Vietnam Generation at every stage you have so far encountered—from *Pulling Up Roots* to the *Tryout Twenties*, *Turbulent Thirties*, and *Flourishing Forties*. Check out the striking increases in your education, professionalism, income, and childlessness compared with women of the previous "Silent" Generation. If you are a man in his sixties from the World War II Generation, you can look yourself up through the *Flaming Fifties* and *Harmonizing Sixties*. Notice, for example, how faithfully married you have remained since your thirties and how unprepared you are to retire at the traditional age of 65.

To highlight the ground conditions when you and your cohort set off on the journey of adult life, each of the five generations described below in capsules are compared during the transition out of adolescence. Pulling Up Roots, as I called it in *Passages*, is the time when we begin detaching from the family and initiating the search for a personal identity. Anything seems possible, but everything is open to question.

The tasks of this Pulling Up Roots passage are to locate ourselves in a peer group role, a sex role, an anticipated occupation, and an ideology or worldview—a tall order.[1] By engaging in these tasks, we gather the impetus to leave home physically and the identity to begin leaving home emotionally. We generally start at this stage by claiming control over at least one aspect of our lives that our parents can't touch. This is a key building block of adulthood. Reduced to its essence, mental health is enhanced by expanding our control over our environment.

This passage used to begin in earnest about age 18 and was usually completed by age 22. Military service, early marriage, or college created a compulsory break away from home. Exposure to a multicultural milieu was much more common when boys had to go to either college or boot camp, where rich and poor, snobs and hicks, North and South, all had to bunk in together. Universal military service ended in the United States in 1973.

Key to Your Cohort

TOTAL BIRTHS IN THE U.S. (Millions)

▮▮▮ — **Birth years of the generational cohorts that are used in this book**

WORLD WAR II GENERATION 1914–29	SILENT GENERATION 1930–45	VIETNAM GENERATION 1946–55	ME GENERATION 1956–65	ENDANGERED GENERATION 1966–80

4

3

2

1

1920   1930   1940   1950   1960   1970   1980   1990

Until 1959, the numbers are live births adjusted for underregistration. After that they are registered live births.

YEARS WHEN COHORTS ARE IN THE DIFFERENT STAGES OF LIFE

	AGED 16–19	TRYOUT TWENTIES	TURBULENT THIRTIES	FLOURISHING FORTIES	FLAMING FIFTIES	SERENE SIXTIES
COHORT OF **WWII** GENERATION	from 1937 to 1944	from 1941 to 1954	from 1951 to 1964	from 1961 to 1974	from 1971 to 1984	from 1981 to 1994
COHORT OF **SILENT** GENERATION	from 1952 to 1959	from 1956 to 1969	from 1966 to 1979	from 1976 to 1989	from 1986 to 1999	from 1996 to 2009
COHORT OF **VIETNAM** GENERATION	from 1962 to 1969	from 1966 to 1979	from 1976 to 1989	from 1986 to 1999	from 1996 to 2009	from 2006 to 2019
COHORT OF **ME** GENERATION	from 1974 to 1984	from 1981 to 1994	from 1991 to 2004	from 2001 to 2014	from 2010 to 2024	from 2020 to 2034
COHORT OF **ENDANGERED** GENERATION	from 1982 to 1989	from 1986 to 1999	from 1996 to 2009	from 2006 to 2019	from 2016 to 2029	from 2026 to 2039

Volunteer military service now attracts only 6.4 percent of 18- to 19-year-old men.[2]

Previous generations of men were desperate to have a paycheck by the age of 21. Supporting themselves was how they demonstrated they had achieved manhood. Young women were expected to be content with an identity confined by traditional sex roles. The message was: You are whom you marry and whom you mother. Thus women were often willing at 19 to make "jailbreak marriages" with inappropriate men just to get away from parental control.

Today, with the economies of the United States and Europe in the midst of a random revolution, men and women of any age feel the control over their lives threatened. To those in the not-yet-ready-for-adulthood age-group, it is particularly disorienting to have the economic ground beneath them shifting even as they make their first test steps. They haven't had a chance yet to develop mature defenses or master any major life crises.

"Youth in crisis." The label is axiomatic for any generation. Do you recognize the generation described in the following commentary from a TV magazine show?

> They feel the rising sense of anxiety and insecurity ... senseless outbreaks of savagery, as race rioting, and they are quick to absorb the new spirit of violence and recklessness.

The accompanying video depicts kids in their early teens smoking dope, buying pornography, and streetwalking to catch tricks. As usual, the finger of guilt for allowing this general decline in the moral health of youth is pointed at the working mother:

> Today U.S. industry is employing hundreds of thousands of women, who before ... were homemakers, devoting their full time to their families ... the latchkey kid, whose working parents leave her to shift for herself at home, is today a familiar ... phenomenon. Everywhere, children of working parents are being left without adequate supervision or restraint.

But this was not Dan Quayle harping on parents of the "X Generation" for failing to instill family values. This was a 1940s *Time* magazine documentary film about "Youth in Crisis," depicting George Bush's World War II Generation. At 19 or 22, its older male members were already away at war, proving themselves as young men in the most traditional way, while their younger brothers and sisters back home were discovering an alternative mode—juvenile delinquency. Herbert Hoover was beside himself about it. Mothers had been "drafted" by society to run the engines of war factories left idle by their soldiering husbands. Society had not foreseen the necessity to provide adequate day care.

So what's new? During the 1970s and 1980s, while total money income levels were declining in constant dollars for men in every age-group except those over 65,[3] wives and mothers were again "drafted" to jump-start the economy. The extra engine driving the economy during the 1980s, so that total income didn't go down more than it did, was working women and wives. The Census Bureau incomes expert Paul Ryscavage corroborated my findings: "Returns on education for women during the 1980s drove earnings for all households in the country."[4] Once again society hasn't caught up with the realities and provided adequate child care for the younger women who need it in order to work longer hours.

Let's look at psychological health in this age-group fifty years ago. One out of every four of the scared young men of the World War II Generation who stripped down for his draft physical was rejected by Selective Service because of a "mental or nervous condition."[5] Of course, the fact that nothing like that number remained psychologically dysfunctional in adulthood suggests that much of the turmoil of this passage is not new. Adolescents have always been susceptible to a "flu of the personality," with brief but severe depressive episodes a fairly common accompaniment to the growing pains of adolescing. Weren't you certain you would never recover from your first broken heart?

And so, while this chapter focuses on disparities in the life cycle from one generation to the next, be aware that important aspects of our inner development remain true to stage.

WORLD WAR II GENERATION

(Born 1914–29)

This generation was young through both the Depression and World War II. The cohort I've selected was aged 20 to 24 in 1945. "I want to fly!" was its motto. The love of adventure that is always the lure of the Pulling Up Roots passage was satisfied for young men by a romance with aviation. They crowded into the armed services, with hundreds of thousands on the waiting list for the U.S. Navy alone. This is the Jack Kennedy, Joe Louis, Jimmy Stewart generation.

The American teenage girl emerged in the 1940s as a consumer with "a mind of her own." Department stores and magazines designed for teenagers began glorifying her, while drugstores hooked her on banana splits and jitterbug clubs introduced her to drinking and dancing. She swooned over a skinny crooner from Hoboken by the name of Sinatra. But her generation, like the current one attempting to pull up roots, was delayed in getting into adult life. Although she was likely to marry between 18 and 19 (about 31 percent in this cohort), she probably had to put her dreams of family on hold while her husband was away at war. If unmarried, she took care of younger siblings while Mom went to work in the war effort. After high school she was content to work as a secretary or in a factory; seldom did her parents consider it worth sending her to college. Without government support and highly involved with marriage and childbearing and raising, this generation's females did not further their higher education. Although about 68 percent of World War II women ultimately finished their high school education, by age 35 to 39 only 6.4 percent had completed college, compared with 14 percent of all males in their generation.[6]

The big difference between youth of World War II and today's "youth in crisis" is that 19-year-olds in the 1940s had confidence in their future. Despite the pessimistic outlook of their Depression-shaken parents, they *knew* their futures would be brighter than those faced by their moms and dads. GIs in our cohort group came home ennobled by having won the last "good" war. They married Rosie the Riveters who had developed skills and learned how to sacrifice. Personal hardships or historical events that demand of us a leap of action before we are ready often have the beneficial effect of boosting us on to the next stage of development in spite of ourselves. And young World War II people in the Pulling Up Roots passage commanded the respect of both older and younger generations.

The dream of nearly every 19-year-old man then was to land a white-collar job in the city. The great majority had no higher education, so only one in thirty of them could achieve that dream.[7] But one who did could rent a room at the YMCA or share an apartment, dress for success, live on weekly earnings of $15 to $25, and still afford to take out a girl two or three nights a week. Meanwhile, almost a quarter of an entire generation was growing up jobless, wondering if they could even earn a living to enable them to marry and establish a home and family.[8] The society greenlighted their efforts to catch up on education and start their families, subsidizing mass college education and suburban subdivisions with the GI Bill. Men in this generation didn't marry until their mid-twenties.[9]

Gender roles were strictly differentiated. Women were defined by their wombs and housewifely skills. The law in some states designated a man's wife and children part of his property, like his horse. Men, mostly veterans, saw life in terms of "missions" and approached the problems of the country with exclusively male thinking patterns. They became organization men, created top-down hierarchies, gave or took orders, built a monumental military-industrial complex, invented and used the first atomic bomb. World War II Generation men became synonymous in the nation's mind with leadership. Indeed, beginning with General Eisenhower and ending with Ronald Reagan and George Bush, they held a lock on the American presidency for almost *forty years.*

SILENT GENERATION

(Born 1930–45)

Although born between wars, this was the "duck and cover" generation, the first to be drilled as grade school kids in how to be prepared for the horrors of thermonuclear war. I've chosen a late cohort group that is closer in spirit to the Boomer generation—those born 1936–40. They were children between ages 5 and 9 when the United States dropped the bomb on Hiroshima, and teenagers during the Eisenhower Fifties.

Born before television, before credit cards, they grew up without tape decks, artificial hearts, word processors, condominiums, or computers. *Software* wasn't even a word then, and no one would think of touching a mouse. Girls wore letter sweaters, saddle shoes, and bobby socks and accepted corsages from boys who wore coats and ties to school dances. These young people had mostly stay-at-home moms, and grandparents in the spare room, since it was before day care or nursing homes. And they were so good: drying dishes for their mothers by hand (before dishwashers), hanging up clothes with pins (before clothes dryers), and washing the family car long before they were allowed to drive it.

As adolescents they drank too much and drag-raced cars as big as tanks with tail fins. The term *rhythm and blues* emerged in 1950, quickly followed by the "doo-wop" sound, and suddenly, springing out of the jazz-based music of the Harlem Hamfats, a musical revolution was launched by a southern white boy named Elvis Presley.[10] Boys grew ducktails to mimic Elvis, but they didn't know about drug raids, only panty raids. In their day, grass was mowed, coke was a cold drink, and pot was something a girl asked for at her bridal shower—preferably in stainless steel. As teens they showed the lowest rates in the twentieth century for almost every social pathology of youth: crime, suicide, illegitimate births, and teen unemployment.

In 1960 our cohort group was 20 to 24, the last gasp of a generation that largely respected authority and believed in American institutions and corporate paternalism. This was the earliest marrying and earliest baby-making generation in American history. One of the main draws was sex, which was not allowable outside marriage for "good girls." Reliable birth control was not available. Many late-adolescent girls stole a brief passion, only to have their lives foreclosed by a "shotgun wedding." A higher percentage of women in this generation had tied the connubial knot at 19 (42 percent) than any generation in this century.[11] By the time they reached the age of 24, over *one half* of Silent Generation males and *70 percent* of the females were married.[12]

Women of this generation also hold the record as among the most fertile of the twentieth century. Three quarters of them had already given birth before they reached their mid-twenties[13] and most stayed home to raise their broods.[14] Ultimately 93 percent of them became mothers. The women in my five-year cohort had an average of 2.85 children by age 40 to 44. (The women at the very beginning of the Silent Generation, born between 1931–35, bore a whopping average of 3.17 children.)[15] And the script for them basically ended there.

The behavior of these men and women, tagged the "Silent Generation" by historian William Manchester, was depicted as a phenomenon of the repressive 1950s. Withdrawn, unimaginative, unadventurous, with no burning causes, they seemed an aberration among youth in America's history. But Manchester followed them only through their high school and college years, which coincided with the height of McCarthyism, when FBI agents were openly conducting campus security checks and Hollywood screenwriters were intimidated into taking loyalty oaths.[16] Whipped up into paranoia about "Reds under the bed," teachers were vigilant about keeping students safe from "Communist propaganda," while the Catholic Church banned books like *Lady Chatterley's Lover.* The American State Department banned travel in Communist countries and fired career diplomats simply because they knew how to speak Chinese.

So it's no surprise that 21-year-old male college graduates lined up passively for interviews with corporate recruiters, prepared for induction into suburban life as the "Man in the Gray Flannel Suit."[17] Their counterparts who didn't finish high school (33 percent)[18] filed through for their induction physicals and went off to Korea to fight in a bloody "police action" that Congress wouldn't admit was a war. Meanwhile, the women who graduated from college by 20 to 24 (5.4 percent, a shockingly small percentage compared with the women in succeeding generations[19]) went comparison shopping in their senior years for the best husband prospects. Very few went on to graduate school themselves. If they had any aspirations for advanced education, it usually was put toward a PHT degree—meaning "putting hubby through." But even at that, only 7 percent of the male Silents in our cohort group had completed four years of college by the time they were 20 to 24.[20]

Nevertheless, career opportunities were plentiful, even for the not-so-bright. Since the Silents were the second-smallest American generation in the twentieth century, job competition was mild. Postwar prosperity was in full swing. It was rare to be a white male and unemployed. But the occupational history of the Silents was the least colorful of all the generations under comparison. One quarter of the white men in their early twenties worked as unskilled operators or fabricators. Another one fifth were clerks or salesmen, and a sixth were laborers or service workers.[21]

By the time the Silents reached their early thirties, however, American society had created masses of white-collar jobs for them, and a shift occurred from unskilled to skilled labor. Business became the most popular vocation, offering the highest return on educational investment. Up to 17 percent of white men became professionals, while almost 23 percent took up skilled crafts, and the ranks of proprietors and middle managers began to swell.[22]

There weren't a lot of expectations that female Silents would turn out to run for Congress or state legislator or mayor or governor. As young women they watched Grace Kelly and Jacqueline Bouvier abandon their careers to marry older princes. One of them later died tragically, but the other survived the myth of Camelot and emerged in midlife with a brilliant career as an editor along with being an attentive parent and grandparent, until her untimely death in 1994.

The lives of this generation were broken up by tremendous discontinuity. The last wave of this generation graduated from college just ahead of "the fiery Boomer class of 1965."[23] The Silents found themselves grown up just as the world went teenage. They missed the Sexual Revolution. "When nobody over 30 was to be trusted, our age was thirty-something."[24] So they had their fling with adolescence in middlescence, creating a surge in divorces and displaced mothers without the skills to support themselves.

Comparing women's lifetime pursuits of education across three generations, I found a remarkable surge in efforts by Silent Generation women to expand their knowledge *after* the age of 40. Only 3.2 percent of their predecessors in the World War II Generation went back to post–high school between the ages of 40 and 54. But fully 11 percent of the Silents went back for some college education in those middle years.[25] In 1991 nearly a million women over 40 were enrolled in college nationwide.[26]

One woman of 50 who was enrolling in law school at New York University met a 42-year-old woman in the registration line. The younger registrant was hestitating: All those years ahead of temping days and studying nights—was it worth the long haul? The older woman spelled out a new consciousness: "I'm going to be sixty anyway. I might as well be sixty with a law degree."

As they turned out, the Silents were not silent at all. Members of this generation were, in fact, the pathbreakers for much of the 1960s-era "raised consciousness"—in music and film, civil rights and women's rights, and multicultural sensitivity—for which Boomers too often claim credit. The Silent Generation produced virtually every major figure in the modern civil rights movement—from Martin Luther King, Jr., to Malcolm X to Cesar Chavez. The so-called Silent women accounted for many of the nation's prominent feminists. In 1964, while 16-year-old Hillary Rodham was playing girls' softball back in suburban Park Ridge, Illinois (no girls' high school athletics teams existed), Fannie Lou Hamer, a founder of the civil rights and feminist movements, was in Atlantic City leading the Mississippi Freedom Democratic party in a protest against the racism of delegate selection for the Democratic National Convention.[27] Four years later Gloria Steinem joined others in bringing anti-Vietnam protest to the 1968 Democratic Convention in Chicago, but was told "no broads." Two years later, Fannie Lou Hamer, Gloria Steinem, and many others formed the National Women's Political Caucus. Never again would women be either "inside" or "outside" the system—they had finally learned the need to be both.

But for the most part, this generation did not come of age angry. Instead, its members developed a highly sensitive social conscience. John F. Kennedy was their icon. A significant number still look upon the Peace Corps as a common bond. They also launched the concept of women helping other women as political partners with slogans like "Sisterhood Is Powerful." That movement found its mature expression in Emily's List, a fund-raising organization that raised the early money that tripled the number of women in the U.S. Congress and made 1993 the Year of the Woman in politics.

As William Strauss and Neil Howe have observed, Silents excel at mediating arguments between others and reaching out to people of all cultures, races, ages, and handicaps.[28] They have a tremendous capacity for asking and listening. It's no accident that among their number are Woodward and Bernstein, Lesley Stahl, Ted Koppel, Phil Donahue, Linda Ellerbee—communicators who set the style for investigative journalism and TV news talk shows. Silents have also produced four decades of top presidential aides: Pierre Salinger (for Kennedy), Bill Moyers (Johnson), John Ehrlichman (Nixon), Stuart Eizenstat (Carter), James Baker (Reagan), John Sununu (Bush), and David Gergen for the first Baby Boom president, Bill Clinton. But they have never produced a president of their own.

VIETNAM GENERATION

(Born 1946–55)

MR. BRADDOCK: What is it, Ben?
BEN: I'm just
MR. BRADDOCK:—worried?
BEN: Well—
MR. BRADDOCK: About what?
BEN: I guess, about my future.
MR. BRADDOCK: What about it?
BEN: I don't know. I want it to be—
MR. BRADDOCK: To be what?
BEN (quietly): Different.

The sullen 20-year-old hero of *The Graduate* gives a quick swipe of a smile to his oversolicitous father before his overdressed mother enters and licks her fingers to smooth down his hair. Benjamin Braddock, class of '67, had just sounded the motto of the Boom generation: *I want to be different.* And at every stage they have been.

Much of the symbolism in this Mike Nichols film is a classic expression of Pulling Up Roots. Benjamin spends half his time underwater, unhearing, unseeing, cut off, expressing the loneliness and isolation of any young person who must reject parental authority before developing any confidence in his own authority. "It's like there are no rules, no one makes them up," he complains. "They make themselves up."

Seduced by the sexy, alcoholic Mrs. Robinson, a woman his mother's age, Benjamin schemes to marry her daughter. The young couple then enacts the coming schism between the generations. At the daughter's wedding, in one of the great adolescent escape fantasy scenes of all time, the young lovers beat off all the stupid adults with a big cross. They break free and escape on a bright yellow bus, like the Beatles' yellow submarine, throwing away everything about maturity that is equated with ridiculousness, perfidy, degeneracy, and emptiness.

Four out of every ten American adults belong to the Baby Boom Generation. Officially these are the seventy-seven million women and men born between 1946 and 1964, although that same postwar generation was born somewhat later in Europe.[29] But as pollsters have repeatedly noted, the formative experiences were radically different for the forward and back ends of the generation. And given the acceleration of the life cycle, a generation is now encapsulated in ten to fifteen years instead of the traditional twenty.

Separating the Boom into at least two subgenerations, the leading edge can be called the Vietnam Generation. Pampered in the childcentric incubator of a prosperous period, with the invisible hand of Dr. Spock sparing the rod, members of the Vietnam Generation grew up believing they could do just about anything. Their World War II Generation parents, determined to insulate them from the hardships they had endured, opened up for their children a world of seemingly unlimited opportunity. The first TV generation, they grew up on *Father Knows Best* and *The Donna Reed Show*, naïve sitcoms reflecting the moral assumptions of their parents, who saw their survival of the Depression and victory in World War II as a demonstration that America was God's chosen nation on earth to civilize and police the world.

Whether blue-collar, new-collar, or white-collar, Boomers have always been highly individualistic and thus irreconcilably divided.[30] They might have been divided at birth, between the Constrained Temperament of highly controlling and cautious types—like Republican Speaker of the House Newt Gingrich, whose anxieties about change cause him to warn in apocalyptic speeches of a "dark and bloody planet" in our future[31]—and the Unconstrained Temperament of more permissive, freebooting types like Bill Clinton and Ollie North. This is also the generation of hellsafire women like Joan Baez, Janis Joplin, Angela Davis, and Oprah Winfrey.

Vietnam Generation babies came to adolescence *expecting* that everything would always get better. And it did, for them. Adolescence had "evolved into a cult, to be prolonged, enjoyed, and commercially catered to as never before," wrote education experts Grace and Fred M. Hechinger.[32] The natural self-indulgence of youth evolved into a philosophy of instant gratification that spread throughout the culture. As teens this cohort's way of claiming some control over their parents' domain was to plug into music that adults suspected as subversive. Their screams were heard 'round the world thirty years ago, when a foursome of cocky young Liverpudlians descended on New York City. With the help of *The Ed Sullivan Show*, the Vietnam Generation launched the Beatles as the most famous rock 'n' roll group of all time. Adolescents had achieved dominion over the music and movie industries for the first time in history. They soon expressed their collective personality: idealistic, narcissistic, antiestablishment, hairy, horny, and preferably high.

The spirit of the Sixties formed their utopian consciousness. They learned to bake bread in rural communes, set up sanctuaries for draft evaders, and had all the fun of sit-ins and love-ins. Hillary Rodham Clinton, who came to political consciousness in the late 1960s, saw those years as "dominated by men with dreams, men in the civil-rights movement and the Peace Corps, the space program."[33] She had written to NASA as a 14-year-old asking what it took to be an astronaut. She was told girls need not apply. "Still," she told me in an interview, "growing up in the Fifties, a lot of us sensed that we could redefine what women do."[34]

And so they did. Women who graduated from college in the late Sixties and early Seventies were living in a time when women *could* assert their independent identities. Hillary Rodham Clinton was only one among the many point women of the Vietnam Generation who marched out of college into the earliest struggles of the women's movement to secure the first places in prestige graduate schools and to infiltrate the old boys' networks and integrate the law firms and corporate boards. Hillary entered Yale Law School the year the undergraduate university first admitted females. And when the blue-chip Rose Law Firm recruited her in 1977, she became one of the first woman partners in a major Arkansas law firm.

But as often is the case in any social change movement, these point women had to hold on to their new status tenaciously, because it was so fragile. Even those on the leading edge had to accept the fact that full equality was not going to come in their political lifetimes. Hillary left the assured professional promise of the East Coast to follow her husband to Arkansas. "I was disappointed when they married," admitted Clinton's own campaign director at the time, Betsey Wright. "She has been absolutely critical to Bill's success, but, then, I had images in my mind that she could be the first woman president."[35]

The group cohort I have chosen is from the earliest-born members: 1946–50. Their motto was: Burn, baby, burn. They came of age at the height of the black power movement when "Black Is Beautiful" was the rallying cry. As the Sixties proceeded, their protest against being drafted into the Vietnam War became symbolic of their resistance to any and all rules and structures set up by an older generation. They were 20 to 24 in 1970, the year the women's liberation movement went public. The Pill was already in widespread use. The number of girls reporting premarital intercourse in surveys more than doubled, as they became knowing consumers of sex.[36]

Women and men of the Vietnam Generation bolted from the tradition of marrying by one's mid-twenties. Almost half the men and 30 percent of the women in this cohort group were still single in their mid-twenties. They launched a strong and healthy trend toward postponed marriage that has continued up to the 1990s. And once these older Boomer women did marry, they balked at spending their twenties barefoot and pregnant. They pitched the birthrate down precipitously from an average of more than 3 children (among women born from 1926 to 1936) to only 2.1 births in a woman's lifetime.[37] In 1973, after years of agitating by feminist organizations, the Supreme Court granted women the right to have abortions. By now the results of all these momentous changes are in: Women born in the 1950s have thus far chosen to have fewer children than any other generation of American women.[38]

The postponing of marriage and the need to defer being drafted allowed these women and men an amazing generational achievement. Forty-three percent of the males had some college or had graduated college by the age of 24, compared to one quarter of Silent men.[39] Females broke even more radically with the past. Almost twice as many Vietnam Generation women had graduated from college by the age of 24 as had women of the same age in the Silent Generation.[40] More impressive, both women and men *stayed* in school (many men to avoid the draft), and many developed a lifelong love of education.

Children of the Sixties were also more inner-directed and spiritually adventurous. They granted themselves a long moratorium on commitments, and a good number left home to live communally, according to their own rules. In search of transcendence from the mean material world, some tried trekking in Tibet or meditating with their personal mantras to reach "bliss consciousness" or jacking themselves up on LSD to reach for a religious vision, often coming down to earth positively *righteous*.

The watershed year was '68: The draft was declared universal, the Tet offensive in Vietnam shook the nation's confidence, and a spasm of violence destroyed young people's heroes—Bobby Kennedy, followed by Martin

Luther King. So strong was the sense of collective responsibility for completing the task of racial integration (after a hundred-year pause) and ending the Vietnam War, the power balance shifted away from society's designated authorities—police, parents, university presidents, elected representatives—and for a moment young people strode like giants through a callous world they were determined to change. They integrated Woolworth's lunch counters, shut down universities, stopped a war, and fired a president. Heady stuff.

But moving into the 1970s, Timothy Leary levitated out of sight and the dour Richard Nixon reinstated the country's natural conservatism. The first American youths to enjoy a prolonged adolescence were shaken out of it in 1980, when John Lennon was shot to death. Our cohort group had already joined the enemy; its members were just over 30. Having spent their passion on their twenties, and remained mostly in a transient state of personal noncommitment, they had a great deal of catching up to do. Overnight it seemed the Vietnam Generation motto switched from Burn, baby, burn! to Earn, baby, earn!

Mickey Kaus, the liberal pundit, had been a college freshman in 1970 who helped organize an antiwar demonstration that wound up setting fire to a professor's office. In a 1988 *Newsweek* confessional, Kaus characterized his cohorts as "an insular generational community, confident of our demographic might, savoring the memories but not bothering to defend them."[41] Notwithstanding, their sense of personal power has remained strong through to middle life. Vietnam Boomers continue to take pride in their uniquely elevated social consciousness, while others often find them judgmental and morally arrogant.

In a 1989 *Fortune* article titled "The Workaholic Generation," they were described as being uncomfortable with leadership roles: "They don't like telling others what to do any more than they like being told." They escape to their work, putting in sixty- to ninety-hour weeks, far longer hours than their fathers ever did.[42]

In 1995 our cohort group is aged 44 to 48, by which age the Silents had mostly come through their midlife passage. But the early Boomers have never done anything the way generations before them did. "They are not parents in the same way their own parents were," points out social analyst Susan Hayward, director at the Yankelovich Partners research and marketing company. "I'm not sure they even recognize midlife crisis yet. That's somewhere off in the future for them."[43]

ME GENERATION

(*Born 1956–65*)

The younger half of the Boomers came of age in the 1970s with a starkly different attitude. It was a period dubbed indelibly by Tom Wolfe as "the Me Decade." If the dream of the Vietnam Generation was to make a difference in society, the new dream was "polishing one's very *self . . .* and observing, studying and doting on it" . . . making a difference in Me!⁴⁴

At Esalen, a famous lodge on a cliff over the Pacific specializing in "lube jobs for the personality," many were initiated into the marathon encounter group vividly described by Wolfe: "Such aggression! such sobs! tears! moans, hysteria, vile recriminations, shocking revelations, such explosions of hostility between husbands and wives, such mud balls of profanity from previously mousy mommies and workadaddies!"

The hippie communes of the Vietnam Generation were taken on a mystical religious streak by the Me Generation, and former radicals enrolled in est, Arica, and Scientology while meditating like mad. The Me's found their political hero in Jerry Brown, the Zen Jebbie, a former Jesuit seminarian and brilliantly perspicacious politician who was among the first to warn of the Age of Limits. Young people who were wary of drugs beyond marijuana, but who still sought the ecstatic spiritualism of hippie life, found it in a revival of fundamentalist evangelical holy-rolling Christianity. This grand religious wave constituted the Fourth Great Awakening in American history.

The Me's missed the idealism of the older Boomers but expanded on their sense of entitlement. They came of age with even more abnormally high expectations. Doing their homework and watching *The Brady Bunch* at the same time, those who went to college often took their own Macintosh computers and spent obscene amounts of money on designer sneakers. In college their heroes were the wonder boys and go-go girls of bare-knuckled Reaganomics.

Prosperity was taken for granted by young people in the early 1980s. Among them were the yuppies wooed out of college by fantastic salaries into investment banking and corporate law and junk bond trading, buoyed by clouds of cocaine and showing off by snapping their red suspenders. One of their heroes was junk bond king Mike Milken, who brazenly ignored the laws and ethics of the securities business and made himself world-famous as the most powerful financier in America, drawing the highest annual paycheck in corporate history—more than half a billion dollars in 1987—while he was still in his thirties!⁴⁵

But the truest symbol of the Me Generation is Madonna. The blatant "Material Girl" thumbed her nose at the self-righteousness of the Vietnam Generation. More than anything else, the Me's identified with her raw, shrewd, incessant striving for narcissistic recognition. As the first youngsters to grow up watching people on TV talk shows, they inhaled vicariously the instant swelled-headedness of public celebrity. Madonna was just a girl from the neighborhood. *So why not me?* Twenty-seven-year-olds were making $250,000 on Wall Street. *So why not me?* Writers were being praised as literary stars in their twenties. Nobody wanted to wait for fame. There was no sense that one had to build through experience. It came to be expected that if you just put on the costume, assumed the role, and practiced your talk show repartee—*why not instant stardom for me?*

To express the Me's I have chosen the last group of Boomers: born between 1960 and 1965. This is the cohort that expected to "have it all." It turned 20 to 24 in 1985, at the height of the excesses of the Eighties— that twelve-year collective denial of reality during which America borrowed from its children and grandchildren to finance one of the great self-indulgent spending sprees of the century. Members of this cohort still saw their parents as a source of supply and showed a decided preference for childhood.

"I'm not married," protests the grown-up Tom Hanks character to his girlfriend in the film *Big*, "I am thirteen." Jay McInerney, the pop-lit figure of this generation who celebrated greed, coke, and decadence in his novel *Bright Lights, Big City*, admits to having enjoyed one of the longest adolescences on record. He describes his early books as having "been about adolescents, almost, who stand at the brink of adulthood and look over the brink and say, 'That doesn't look very promising.' "[46]

When I did a study a decade ago on the pacesetters among men of the Me Generation, their formula for happiness signaled a bold shift of values. In their twenties they didn't want to work hard. They demanded more time for personal growth. Having come of age at the crest of an androgynous consciousness, many were swept up in the new "permissions" given men of their generation. They said that being loving and having children were most important to them, while being ambitious and able to lead effectively were dismissed to the bottom of their priority list. They dreamed of achieving the perfectly balanced life.[47]

Me Generation females have surpassed even the brainy women of the Vietnam Generation. By age 25 to 29 one quarter of the Me's had graduated college, already exceeding the percentage of Vietnam Generation

women who had earned college degrees by their mid-thirties.[48] The proportion of those women pouring out of colleges in the mid-Seventies who
aspired to graduate degrees vaulted over that of men and has remained
higher.[49]

> American women now make up more than half of the degree
> recipients at all levels of higher education except the doctoral.[50]

The hundreds of thousands of women who poured out of universities
and business schools in the mid-seventies were the racehorses of feminism,
spurred on to hit the fast track in formerly male-exclusive careers. In their
asphalt-drab suits and string ties, many set out to prove that marriage was
not essential to happiness and/or survival and that women need not be sub-
servient to men. Having grown up amid spiraling divorce rates, they were
also dubious about the whole marriage proposition. So were men.

There was a distinct surge in women becoming professionals by 25 to 29,
both among married and single females. These women made fools of
demographers who predicted they would fall in line with marriage and
birthing patterns later on. In fact, more of these younger Boomers may
never marry.[51] And a surprisingly large number, perhaps as high as 17 percent, will probably never have children.[52] In a study of single career women
of this vintage now in their thirties, psychologist Florence Kaslow observed,
"They take pride in their accomplishments, and enjoy their autonomy, independence, and freedom. However, mixed in with the pleasure of being in
charge of their own lives is some ambivalence over what they do not have—
a partner with whom to share intimate feelings and thoughts in a committed, durable relationship."[53] And like their single male counterparts, they
feel somewhat conflicted about perhaps never having children. The loneliness they defend against by keeping very busy.

The tables turned on the Me Generation as they began to hit 30. When
the very yuppies who had placed their faith in Ronald Reagan's "morning in
America" woke up in 1992, those aged 25 to 34 found that their median
income had dropped by almost one quarter in constant dollars since
1974.[54] Men in our Me Generation cohort had a median personal income
of $22,600 at age 25 to 29, compared with a $27,600 median income for
men of the same age born from 1941 to 1946.[55] "The Me's were the ones
most shocked by the failure of materialism to make them happy," observes
the research analyst Susan Hayward.[56] But they still wield the power of

demography and youth. In 1994 our cohort group is aged 31 to 36. They represent the largest population bulge in the United States today.

The Me Generation's approach to career, sex and homosexuality, recreational drugs, city life, all of it, is so different from most parents of the Silent Generation, they do not share a culture. The tug-of-war with parents for autonomy now often extends a decade beyond adolescence.

The Catch-30 Passage—a transition I defined in *Passages* as a crisis of contradictions—seems to hold up for those in the Me Generation. They report experiencing it sometime between ages 28 and 32, but the issues they struggle with may be quite different.

It is not uncommon, at the approach to the thirties, to tear up the life structure one put together to support the original dream of the twenties. All the networking a man may have put into advancing himself along a corporate track or building a political base may be chucked overboard, as he feels the urge to strike out on his own or "change parties." Catch-30 often means divorce or at least a serious renegotiation of the emotional "contract" of the marriage. For women who are still single, Catch-30 may suddenly make their career suits feel unbearably confining. They find themselves poring intently over bridal magazines they disdained only a year before. It is the feeling of having double-crossed ourselves that makes it a Catch-30 situation.

This mysterious sense of disruption demands that we alter or deepen our commitments. But for many in the Me Generation it has always seemed easier to live from day to day, with as few serious commitments as possible. Emotional lives can be put on hold. And because gender roles and sexual orientation were so much in flux when the Me's passed through their Tryout Twenties, many delayed declaring a fixed sexual identity by simply avoiding commitment altogether.

"Whether you were male or female, gay or straight, social life in the cities was a marketplace," observes a culturally astute 34-year-old creative vice-president at a hotshot New York ad agency. Dan, we'll call him, was a bona fide yuppie who fled his midwestern roots to join the frantic race for fast fame and easy money in New York during the go-go eighties. "Life was very much about having a really good time in the moment and having a lot of money and buying an apartment. But what was really different for most people in my generation was that you could have sex and just walk away. Nothing was expected of you."

Romance scarcely had a chance in the sexual bartering that engaged the energies and egos of this post–women's liberation generation. Oh, sure, somewhere way down on the brainstem they had a species memory of the "shoulds": *You should have a primary relationship; you should have an emotional life; you should want a family.* But *later* for all that. "Much more exciting was what could happen to you that night," recalls Dan. "Who would you select, or would you be chosen? But the morning after, there was the problem of how to disengage from a total stranger with whom one had struck up a false intimacy. So many bogus promises were made: 'It was wonderful,' or 'You're the best,' or 'I'll definitely call you'—whatever it took for people to backpedal to their 'own space.' "

The technological symbol of the Me's aversion to intimacy is the answering machine. Its greatest utility was to *avoid contact.* It became imperative not to waste time exchanging "Hi, how are yous?" with anybody who wasn't immediately useful or pertinent to one's own life. The first thing one said when calling up a friend was "Are you screening? I know you're really there."

As Dan describes, "We all kept thinking *later.* Later I'll learn to make a primary relationship. Later I'll figure this out. I know this is not the way it's supposed to be, but I'll think about it tomorrow. The other chase—for celebrity and money—was much more enticing."

For those of you now in the middle of your Turbulent Thirties who *are* married and juggling children and careers and probably suffering from sleep deprivation, it must seem as though life will never be anything but breaking your neck just to get from A to B to C. Patience. The thirties always present the maximum role demands.

The romantic getaways and lazy, unchoreographed sex that had been such a joyful part of their twenties is not what Me Generation couples talk about in their thirties. When they do speak about making love, it often sounds more like a fitness regimen—something they have to remind themselves that they shouldn't go too long without.

The number of married mothers working full time who have one or more preschool children at home *tripled* between 1961 and 1991, jumping to 60 percent.[57] And that revolutionary trend will only continue. Projections suggest that new mothers will be lucky to take off *ten or fifteen weeks in total* to stay home with newborn children over the course of their work lives.[58] The more high-powered the job, the more quickly the new mother goes right back to work, fearing that otherwise she will lose her place.[59]

A two-paycheck household is virtually compulsory today. Here is the stark reality:

> Over the past twenty years in America a married couple whose wife was in the paid labor force enjoyed a 14 percent *increase* in real income. But when the wife was not in the labor force, such a family took a 9 percent *decrease* in real income.[60]

This sobering difference goes a long way toward explaining the explosion in the number of wives who work outside the home. And it will only continue to grow. Women of the Me and Vietnam generations, now in their thirties and forties, are expected to spend nearly *three quarters* of their adult lifetimes working outside the home,[61] a current change without precedent in history.

ENDANGERED GENERATION

(Born 1966–80)

This confused Hip-hop Generation has hidden its heart behind a cult of indifference. Its motto is: Whatever. Its members also coined the word *clueless*. They are pragmatic, skeptical, unwilling to be pinned down, and desperately, secretly, longing to belong and to believe in something.

Many social analysts describe them as lackadaisical, underachieving, passive. I would argue that their "whatever" approach is a mask, a defense that announces, "I'm not revealing my expectations (because they'll probably be disappointed). *Whatever.* It just rolls off me." The grunge look—ripped sweaters, baggy tramp pants, clunky work boots with road-kill treads—is worn with a "Fine, fire me, I don't care" look. *Whatever.*

Their views on marriage are somber. Many are haunted by their parents' mistakes and determined not to repeat them. Young women are still dizzied by the eternal problem of how one balances it all—marriage, family, career—without at least one plate crashing. And today many young people do not expect to be married until their late twenties, or thirties, or not at all. Singlehood is growing as never before. Fears are often voiced that they cannot sustain the intimacy expected in a monogamous relationship, and resistance is raised against the stifling of a hard-won sense of personal identity. Living at home longer also puts off the task of learning the give-and-take of intimacy over adolescent self-centeredness.

Having grown up with one broken promise after another, members of this Endangered Generation are reluctant to make any but the most carefully weighed, realistic commitments. But something's missing: fantasy! "I want more romance and mystery in my life—I feel the need for it" was a tremendous yearning registered by members of this age-group in a Yankelovich MONITOR study.[62] They also feel the burden of performing for their successful, achieving Boomer parents.

"Our parents could not bear to see us fail," said one young working woman, "and for them, failing is a lack of financial success." She spoke eloquently for others in the group interview, saying, "We are searching for a conscience. We believe there is more to the life than the warped world we live in. We have seen our parents go through the Me Generation of the Seventies and become the yuppies of the Eighties. We are now fairly apathetic."

While Douglas Coupland's famous novel *Generation X* describes accurately their McJobs and a lot of the waste with which the Baby Boomers left them, the label is widely disdained. One reason that naming this post-Boomer generation has been left up for grabs is that marketers keep expecting them to produce another youthquake. In fact, their numbers are much smaller than those of the Baby Boom youth culture. In 1993 some thirteen million kids who were born between 1968 and 1971 started turning 25. Still, they do form the largest group of 25-year-olds since 1986 in America,[63] and their age-group is ardently wooed by marketers and advertisers.

Why do I call it the Endangered Generation? Because the most important element today's young people are missing in order to accomplish Pulling Up Roots is something previous generations took for granted: safety. If you are in your late teens or early twenties, you will probably be muttering to yourself, "Give me a break. *I'm* not afraid of life," which is the way one should think at this stage. But from my many interviews with people in this age-group my sense is that they are safety-obsessed.

"Our parents grew up in the Fifties with external enemies: communism, the Bomb," said Jennifer Erwin, a student at David Lipscomb University in Nashville, Tennessee. "Our enemies are internal: drugs, guns, the widening gap between poor and elite, and lots more competition for jobs." What is the first thing young people ask about in job interviews today: What are the health benefits? When I asked a savvy focus group of New Yorkers in their mid-twenties, "How safe do you feel—about sex, money, relationships, marriage, street violence, job security?" The response was urgent and unanimous.

"None of the above. Unsafe on all levels. At all times."

And they have good reason. Their universe is not a playground for experimentation but a corridor of epidemics they have to dodge before they even reach the door to adulthood. There is the epidemic in adolescent suicide[64] (quadrupled in the last twenty-five years), the epidemic in teenage pregnancy (the United States has the highest rate of any country in the Western world),[65] and the plague of AIDS that is spreading among adolescents.[66] "People our age were forming their sexual identity with the understanding that we could die for our actions. No other generation has had to deal with this at this stage of our lives," said one participant in a focus group.

Customarily, healthy people in peacetime don't have to confront their own perishability at least until their forties. In the Vietnam Generation war brought death into the living room night after night, and many young men gave up their lives. Dying then in antiwar protests or for the civil rights cause was construed as a noble goal, and it was still shocking when it happened. For members of the Endangered Generation in their early twenties today, the kind of mortality they are grappling with is mostly meaningless. Some of their music reflects it, with its tabloid imagery and desperate energy, its chopped-up chords played at hyperfast tempo. Slayers' lyrics revel in death, chanting, "Kill! Kill!" and asking their audiences, "Do you think you should have a right to choose whether to live or die?"

Although the HIV virus has not spread nearly as much among heterosexuals as it has among gays, heteros tend to be extreme in their reactions to the threat. Some stage their adolescent rebellion by refusing to practice safe sex—in denial of reality—while others are fearful enough to refrain from sex completely. Lisa Peluso, a young actress on the soap opera *Loving,* opted for celibacy at 25. "Sex outside of a marital commitment is only full of fear and anxiety," she told *Mademoiselle* magazine.[67]

Today's young people are forced to think about safety because the world around them has become so much more unpredictable and violent. One in five American high school students carried a weapon to school by 1993. In the same year 37 percent of teen readers of *USA Today* said they *do not feel safe* in their schools. For black teenagers the primary peril is being shot to death; the toys that adults sell to children today load real bullets. White teens are more likely to use cars as a weapon of self-destruction or to collaborate in a suicide.[68] Remember the shock that greeted the demand by students at Brown University that their health service stock suicide pills in case of nuclear war?

Except for TV sitcoms, rap music, the grunge look, and their collective uneasiness about the future, members of the Endangered Generation have not been fused by pivotal events as the Boomers were. Their generational identity is far more diluted and more racially diverse as well—with 14 percent black, 12 percent Hispanics, and 4 percent Asians.[69] Their diversity has the positive effect of making these young people the most naturally accepting of multiculturalism. The great variety of their music reflects a healthy inclusiveness, embracing rap, country, grunge, rave, reggae, heavy metal, hip-hop, and more. Paradoxically, some angry African Americans also show more hostile separatism. While the Vietnam Generation has a true hero in Martin Luther King, Jr., who taught his followers that they could "struggle without hating," African Americans now have their own version of Governor George Wallace, the hate-mongering segregationist of the Sixties. As *The New York Times* columnist Bob Herbert writes, "[Dr. King's] lesson is being turned on its head by the Farrakhans and the Muhammads, who are now teaching young black Americans that they can hate without struggling."[70]

I asked a group of college students of the late 1980s to recall the memorable events they shared as they came of age.

"The *Challenger* blowing up," offered one student, as a searing point of memory comparable to the Kennedy assassination for an earlier generation.

"I was pissed off that it interrupted *All My Children* for hours," droned a young woman. The others all laughed at the irony that is their hallmark.

Others remembered shame when Americans were marched blindfolded by Iranian terrorists across their TV screens. The oldest ones have a collective memory of Watergate, when a president lied, was caught, and all adult institutions came under perpetual suspicion. But the most vivid impression seems to be that they were behind the curve. That idea was summed up in one focus group by Shirley Loh, a graduate of Princeton: "There is nothing left for us to discover. Sex, money, jobs, even drugs—it's all been done. Our big shared event is AIDS."

"I miss that generational identity, too," chimed in a young male graduate of New York University. "It was so great before—and we're not even yuppies."

"*Thank God!*" chorused the group.

Protest has become a gimmick, as they see it. This generation has a high-definition "shit detector." They know they are being hyped all the time. They reject slogans and respond to straight dealing and true value and to humor. Yet their generation hasn't been challenged or inspired collectively by a cause larger than itself. Debating date rape isn't as compelling as bringing a war to an end. Many of the Endangered are determined to fight for a cleaner environment or to monitor human rights abuses or volunteer in their communities, but pragmatic concerns take precedent. Nowhere in Europe are leftist students mounting revolutionary barricades. At Berkeley, famed laboratory for radical causes, the students today wear clean jeans, short hair, ubiquitous Gap T-shirts, and dash from classes to their part-time jobs. It is not a generation that has much time to dream of changing the world. The ever-present worry is that its members are being educated for jobs that may no longer exist.

In the Pulling Up Roots passage, people are too young to recognize an important truth: Setbacks and outright failures are both predictable and useful, and they do not last forever. Change always occurs. Magnifying setbacks can lead to depression. And sadly, the highest-risk population for depression today is late adolescents and young adults.

> More than one third of women in the age range of 18 to 22 are showing significant depression.[71]

For the first time ever, the gap between men and women is narrowing; the risk of depression among young men is rising to almost the same level as among women.[72] This is a worldwide phenomenon. In countries as diverse as Taiwan, Lebanon, New Zealand, and the United States, people under 40 today are three times more likely at some point in life to suffer a major depression than those already over 40—not just sadness but listlessness, dejection, and a sense of hopelessness that keeps them from functioning.

Despite bouts of depression, most young people are functioning with a high degree of responsibility. The Endangered Generation is racking up a record of educational achievement that outpaces any seen throughout the history of the five generations under examination. By 1990 the rate of high school graduation among 19-year-old women was *82 percent*—almost an entire universe—and *four times* the educational level reached by teenage girls of the 1950s Silent Generation.[73] In fact, young women are demonstrating an even greater commitment to higher education than young men today. The numbers going on to college are off the charts:

> By age 20 to 24 fully 58 percent of white women either had some college or have already graduated from college.

Among men, 53 percent have some college or a degree by the same age.[74] The fact that more than half of both young American women and men are gaining higher education is without precedent in any society. Nevertheless, their lives seem to be on hold. When I described the Pulling Up Roots transition in *Passages,* I wrote: "Before 18, the goal is loud and clear: *I have to get away from my parents."* Today, for many reasons, that goal is being drastically delayed.

WELCOME TO PROVISIONAL ADULTHOOD

The bewildering central task of the Tryout Twenties is to choose a life course. The way most people in the World War II and Silent generations dealt with it was to get married and settle into some sort of apprenticeship as a peon at the bottom of an institutional ladder. The Vietnam Generation set a new style for remaining transient through the twenties, resisting any adult commitments and keeping all possibilities open. In the Me Generation the elite were given the chance to be truly grand imposters in their twenties.

But today, in the absence of any clear road map on how to structure their lives and facing an economic squeeze and the terror of unlimited choice, many members of the Endangered Generation have a new goal: *Stay in school as long as you can.* The twenties have stretched out into a long Provisional Adulthood. Most young people don't go through the Pulling Up Roots transition until their mid-twenties and are still in Provisional Adulthood until close to 30, thus moving all the other stages off by up to ten years.

"The statistics bear out your theory," said one of the most thoughtful demographers I know, Arthur Norton, chief of the Population Division at the U.S. Bureau of the Census. "If you hold the prototypical stages of the life cycle constant, and just move off the ages by about ten years, you're not far off. It's even true in the case of behavior that is biologically driven, meaning childbirth."[75] This is part of the uniqueness of the current generation in the twenties.

This age-group has suffered more economically than any other. Earlier generations have managed to keep pace with inflation, while the Endangered Generation has experienced a sharp decline in spending power. The economies of the United States and Europe are not receptive to new graduates. In the early 1990s unemployment among those aged 16 to 24 soared to 23 percent in France, 28 percent in Italy, and 37 percent in Spain, and entry-level jobs are still shrinking. Most young Americans will be unable even to match their parents' single-paycheck middle-class lifestyles.[76]

The average real income—for women as well as men in the Endangered Generation—is 20 percent less than Boomers earned at like age.[77] It is said that the current generation in its twenties is living through a one-generation depression. While that characterization suffers from hyperbole—after all, there are no breadlines, and many new jobs and better-paying jobs in the information industry are opening up—only a tiny proportion of young Americans between 19 and 25 can afford their own apartments today.

In America, as in Europe, more people in their twenties compared to only a decade ago must return home after losing their jobs to live with their parents.[78] The last ten years have seen a 46 percent drop in under-twenty-fives who own housing units and even a 21 percent decline in those who are renting.[79] At best they have to share the rent with roommates or groups. Those who move back home seldom do so because they're lazy or without motivation. They are making an economically sound and usually painful decision for this stage. Society often makes them feel like losers or freeloaders, but it's no fun to share the sink with Dad again or to feel inhibited about bringing home an overnight guest. In fact, this prolonged semidependency on parents runs counter to the dictates of normal development.

The ravishing thirtysomething David Nivenish hero of the British film *Four Weddings and a Funeral* is always a best man, never a bridegroom. As the women in his circle pick off the most marriageable of their lot one by one, he and his footloose pals are left out in the cold. It is the men who are pining to get married; they are completely at the mercy of the women.

What's going on here?

Men are accustomed to being taken care of by women. Now that they can't easily entice girls to marry them and carry their dreams and their offspring while providing for their creature comforts, they are turning back to their mothers. A stunning shift in young male behavior over the past two decades is now demonstrable with statistics:

> Of unmarried American men between 25 and 34, more than *one third* are still living at home.[80]

This is the highest rate ever recorded. Among black men who have never married the figures are even more startling: Two thirds are still living with their families (usually their mothers) up to the age of 30, even though they may have fathered one or more children.[81]

Particularly for divorced mothers over 40, tired of the dating charade, it is tempting to keep a grown son at home as a surrogate husband and general handyman. And many grown sons today don't want to give up the comforts of their more prosperous parents' generation to go out in the world and struggle. Commonly they don't see any reason to pull up roots until they're 30. A good many needs are met for both divorced mother and son. But a woman who settles for that kind of security is shortchanging her own development, while holding back her son's even more. It is a potentially lethal social contract.

Although this new breed of Mama's boy began with the Me Generation, it shows strong signs of continuing as a new norm with unintended consequences. It is soon going to be just as hard for young men to find wives as it has been for older women to find husbands. The PUMS file revealed an important new tilt in women's favor:

> In 1992 there were 121 unmarried men to every 100 single women age 30 to 34.[82]

"Take a guy born in 1967," says Vivian Young, director of strategic services at the Ammirati & Puris/Lintas advertising agency. "By this time [1995] he's almost twenty-eight. If he waits until he's thirty-five to think about getting married, most of the desirable younger women will be gone. [The turnaround in Boomer birthrate began in 1960–61.] The women his age will already have been snapped up by older men, since women are always looking for a man who's successful, and that translates as older." Ms. Young continues: "Who's this guy going to marry? One of the leftovers? He could be single for a long, long time. So young men today are at risk for not finding a suitable mate unless they pluck from the ripe pickings before they're thirty or much beyond."[83]

This means that the mate shortage suffered by those women of the Vietnam Generation who delayed seriously looking for a husband until their thirties is not a big problem for women of the Me Generation. On the contrary, American women who are between the ages of 27 and 35 in 1995 have the advantage, and they will keep it. For these women, there will always be marriageable men.[84]

THE GOOD NEWS

Notwithstanding the early obstacles, things should get better, not worse, for the Endangered Generation. Any cohort group smaller in number than the preceding generation faces lessened competition. By taking longer to educate themselves and test out their aptitudes and interests, this crop of prolonged adolescents will be better able to "package" themselves for fluid careers. Given the necessity to "freelance," they are already far more flexible than the Boomer generations before them. They see an America just beyond the shells of big corporate culture where anyone smart will want to be a free agent. With any talent, why go to work as an insect under the dinosaur foot of a Time Warner or MCA? These kids are making their own movies and pressing their own records. In the sci-fi novel *Snow Crash*, Neal Stephenson's twenties character observes, "Three things our generation is great at are movies, music and microcode."

Today's twentysomethings will also be on the cutting edge of burgeoning fields like brain research and biotechnology. The great race to discover and map human gene sequences will engage young biologists who will start with a known gene and match it to a phenomenon. And they should be the first to hit the ground running when the earthquake of fundamental economic changes in the world settles down and the Digital Revolution finds mass applications. Everything will be different, from the way we do business to the way we shop, farm, entertain ourselves, and take care of our health. The changes will sweep across every sector of our lives.

Once power in the world of cyberspace was wielded only by "propeller heads"—stereotyped as computer geeks who wore beanies with pinwheels. Many of these young men who went to work for the pioneering on-line companies don't read books or dream of writing the great American novel. Their natural skills are not social but numerate. They are the polar opposite of the garrulous, gladhanding traveling salesmen who were the communication system of two post–World War II generations. These people communicate in symbols. But they are the power of the future. They speak the new electronicspeak, and they can write code. From them will come the instructions for how to communicate in this countercultural world that disregards day and night, ignores time zones, penetrates national borders with complete immunity, promulgates visual pornography without regard to community standards, and can crack open almost any information bank they wish.

But the popularity of the Internet has already spread far beyond the asocial propeller heads. Regular kids all over the globe are part of this new social space. Once the electronic superhighway becomes established as the new trade route for buying and selling goods, services, and information, members of the Endangered Generation will be the natural merchants and mechanics. They will own the future.

The fact that the Endangered Generation is marrying later and even more selectively also bodes well for their personal security. The one preventive measure against divorce that holds for every generation is this:

> The older we are when we marry for the first time, the less likely the marriage is to end up on the trash heap.[85]

The Census Bureau tells us where we are now and where we have been, but it also makes projections based on its data. Looking at the cohort I've used to represent the Endangered Generation, officials predict it will have a lower divorce rate than the previous generation. Four out of ten of those who do marry will eventually divorce—down from the famous "one in two" statistic based on the Me's in the 1970s.[86]

The real division between the Boomers and the "Busters" is in their stage of life. Busters are still young. With a slow but steady economic recovery in progress in the Nineties, those in the Endangered Generation may yet end up living better than the Boomers. And they may savor their success all the more because they expect it less.

A dramatic shift—sometimes an astonishing difference in psychological maturity—appears to occur today in most young people toward the end of their twenties. The latest psychological studies confirm the distinctions that I hear in my interviews with people in their mid-twenties compared to those in their late twenties.[87] Kathleen Malley, who has conducted extensive research on maturation in young adults, observes, "The breaking point is somewhere around twenty-nine, thirty. There's something about seeing another zero roll up."

Before the shift men and women feel unable to make clear choices or cope with life's vicissitudes without expecting some help from parents. After the shift they feel confident enough in their own values to make their own choices and competent enough in life skills to set a course—even if that course clashes with a parent's wishes.

Prolonged adolescence ends, finally, when we are not afraid to disappoint our parents.

Today the transition to the Turbulent Thirties marks the initiation to First Adulthood. Everyone *wants to be something more.* It is natural to become preoccupied at this stage with crafting a "false self," a public self that will showcase our skills and talents and, we hope, win us approval and success.

We want validation, and in seeking it, we rely heavily on external measurements: the perks of our job, the size of our office, the feats of our children, the "just right" clothes to wear to the awards dinner. Any of these become showcases for proving our worth. The thirties are a serious dress rehearsal for how we will perform if, and when, we are given the leadership roles.

There is nothing wrong with projecting this false self to the outside world during these early striving years, so long as it isn't too distant or disconnected from who we really are. Later, in the forties and fifties, it becomes imperative to find our way back to the truest things we know and to compose a more authentic self.

Now that you have a rough idea of where you are on the New Map of Adult Life, it's time to get started plotting your course through the Flourishing Forties and the frontier of new passages that beckons beyond.

Part Two

THE FLOURISHING FORTIES

2

THE VIETNAM GENERATION
HITS MIDDLESCENCE

*M*any members of that forever young generation known in America as Baby Boomers find the approach of middle life particularly disorienting. The forward flank of the Boomers, those born between 1946 and 1956 whose early life choices were dominated by the war, the draft, and the turmoil of the late Sixties and early Seventies, represent what I call the Vietnam Generation. They and their counterparts around the world, emerging in the flush of optimism and prosperity that followed World War II, have enjoyed the most prolonged and indulged adolescence of any generation of young adults in history. Now they are running up against the first implacable reality that one cannot change:

They are no longer kids.

Previously, people I studied in their early forties felt older than they actually were. It was as if they had dropped off the edge of a cliff when they turned 40. Suddenly they couldn't find jeans that fit. They looked foolish on the dance floor. They were not part of the youth culture anymore. The cultural messages they were fed about middle life were all about decline and disappearance into the zone of dentures. Not surprisingly, anyone over 40 was hypersensitive to the appearance of the smallest wrinkle or faintest faltering of his or her body's machinery. Believing that time was running out, people had tremors of urgency, or they began the long exhale of resignation. Now, the second half may not begin at 40. It's more like 50. No one can really be certain anymore when he or she hits the midpoint. And more and more people are finding ways to avoid the restrictive identity that used to define middle age. One of the most dramatic changes in contemporary society, as the biggest bulge of the Baby Boom passes the first marker of midlife, is that every year millions of people are turning 40 en masse.

> In the United States an average of twelve thousand people will turn 40 every day during the decade of the Nineties.[1]

What happens when millions of people turn 40 more or less at the same time? The marketplace caters to them and eases the passage. They can take their kids to a Grateful Dead concert or listen to radio stations or go to clubs dedicated to playing Seventies rock 'n' roll, the retro rage in the Nineties. One quarter of the Boomers have already reached or passed age 40, and in many ways the early midlife passage is a unique experience for them. So successfully did these vanguard Boomers delay many adult duties and commitments it's as though they "retired" for their twenties—to play guitar, join the Peace Corps, travel to exotic places, experiment with drugs and communes and unlimited sex, and pledge themselves to ending the draft and winning the civil rights movement. Many got around to real life only in their thirties, whereupon they cut their hair, cut back on the weed, started jogging, and took straight jobs.

Since then legions among this arrested generation have dieted, weight-trained, body-contoured, nipped and tucked, dyed and liposuctioned, until most of them look, and actually believe, they are five to ten years younger than their birth certificates would attest. In many ways they *are* at least a decade younger than 50 ever was. From my interviews and surveys, I find that the image of themselves they carry around in their inner eye usually falls somewhere between ages 28 and 35.

WHO ME, AN ADULT?

It is almost universal to have a hurry-up feeling as we hit 40. The first little fissures appear in our physical shells. Damn, why is the type in the phone book so small? Students start calling you "mister." (Behind your back you know they're probably calling you "that old fart.") Your 14-year-old daughter says, "Mom, how come you're still wearing microskirts?" As the humorist Dave Barry writes, "Teenage boys come to your door saying, 'Hi, Mr. Barry. We're here to have sex with your daughter.'" As a new mother over 40, you have to set down the cell phone from working on an M&A deal to put on your invisible bifocals to breast-feed.

You pull a tendon on the tennis court and ignore it. C'mon, this is the generation that invented triathlons and high-impact aerobics and pounded its calves into bulbs hard as rutabagas, so you keep up your five-mile-a-day jogging routine and wrench your hamstring and have to sit out the next couple of months.

"A man can look at a woman and tell if she's interested in him as a sexual being," says a fortyish Manhattan doctor. "All of a sudden you reach an age where you look at a young woman and—click—you're not even under consideration. That hurts!"

If you manage to avoid mirrors on the wall, you will notice the difference mirrored in your peers. An accountant who has Irish choirboy good looks, a dimpled smile, and a slight build described this startling change: "I've been grouchy as hell the last few months, snapping at people I live and work with, and that's not me. I had a talk with my wife about it. She reminded me I had a fortieth birthday coming up. Oh, wow! I hadn't made that link at all. She was so right. I'm the kind of guy who was always the youngest-looking one in the group. Now I look around me and those peers who used to be younger are older. Somewhere along the line, they switched on me." The reason for all this nervousness and fear of falling apart is predictable:

> You are nearing the end of your First Adulthood, and since you probably have had little experience yet with facing your own mortality, it may seem imminent.

Indeed, an identity struggle often recurs, comparable to that of adolescence. *Who is the real me anyway?* If one is still uncommitted, alone, or childless, the struggle between intimacy and isolation is reengaged but with greater urgency, and the consequences for the rest of one's life will be more deeply felt. Erikson theorized that the central crisis of development presented by each stage must be resolved if the individual is going to proceed to the next stage unburdened by neurosis or constant dread. Of course, the central issues or tasks of one period are never fully completed, tied up, and cast aside. It is when they lose their primacy, and the current life structure has served its purpose, that we are ready to move on to the next period.

But I'm not ready! That is the protest I hear behind the refusal of so many of my interviewees in their forties to acknowledge they are not still 28. *It's not me* is the motto of a generation in collective denial of midlife. Who can embrace the larger meaning of life beyond youth when the most important thing in the world is still *me*?

"At forty you're clearly not a fully mature adult yet," asserted Bob Bookman, a boyishly enthusiastic Hollywood talent agent accustomed to being a *Wunderkind.* When we first spoke in 1992, he was stopping in New York to see one of his clients. I asked Bookman then—he was 44—what he thought he might feel like at 50. The very thought visibly rattled him, but his first response was to reject any notice of the passage of time. "I have no idea how I'll feel at fifty," he said. "I don't feel anything radically changing in my life. And I think like a typical member of my generation."

He was seated like a king on a formal Louis XVI brocade chair in his silky suite at the St. Regis Hotel. The formality of the chair stood in stark contrast with his teenagerish pose, one leg cocked over the other, one ankle constantly twitching. His long gray hair curled over the ears and down to the collar of his grape-striped shirt. Like many of his contemporaries, even though he had children, he had postponed most of the trappings of adulthood. Bookman rejected the very notion of becoming middle-aged.

"I'm almost the fittest I've ever been. Mentally and spiritually I'm still very young. When I watch a Beatles documentary or Bob Dylan's *Don't Look Back,* I cry. And my God, the twentieth anniversary of *Laugh-In*—so nostalgic—that show was *hugely* important to our generation." He then slips into a Sixties stream of consciousness: "Every day, when you got up, you were *engaged* by a new social or political issue. The promise of the Sixties was that the life of the mind was good." He had gone to Yale Law School with Bill Clinton and was in the same class as Hillary Rodham. "I can't compute the fact that a peer of mine is now president."

By defeating a man twenty-seven years older than he, Bill Clinton won the second-greatest (after Kennedy versus Nixon) generational contest for national power in more than a century.[2] But he also shook up members of his own generation. Americans are accustomed to regarding their presidents as father figures. Clinton, by contrast, is the boy king, a *puer aeternus,* an eternal adolescent: charming, bold, full of youthful idealism and energy, but also impulsive, personally reckless, and relatively inexperienced in the larger world. To men of his generation who are clinging to the illusion of youth, his image can be an unwelcome mirror held up to their own aging and a startling clock against which to measure the level of success they have achieved—or not achieved.

"Presidents have always been old guys in suits with ropy necks," spouted radio commentator Garrison Keillor, then 47, speaking for millions of Vietnam Generation men brooding over Clinton's inauguration. "I am 20 years younger than the President," said Keillor, "and now suddenly in January, I'll be one year older than the President." He paused significantly. "Do you know how that feels?"[3]

Bookman, too, admitted to having trouble adjusting to a more mature image since he turned 40. "When they page me at the hotel as Mr. Bookman, I think they're talking to somebody else. I'm not Mr. Bookman. I'm *Bob.*" (He took credit for growing beyond being called Bobby.) "When I look in the mirror, I see this old man with a receding hairline, seriously receding, and it's *not me.*"

What is your inner picture of yourself today? I asked him.

"That's a really interesting question." His ankle wiggled furiously. "I guess in my mind's eye, I'm still twenty-eight."

Why was 28 the greatest year? I asked.

"You still believe all things are possible. *Don't trust anyone over thirty.* We *believed* that, and *now* we think that way about people *under* thirty."

But barely concealed beneath his puppyish warmth and exuberance was something else, a frantic energy, almost a doomy sense of time galloping up behind him. Contradicting everything he had said, Bookman finally acknowledged, "I'm so *conscious of time.*" He rolled his eyes up to the ceiling and blurted out a desperate calculation: "If I've been in business for twenty years already and it feels like I started yesterday, does that mean I wake up tomorrow and I'll have been in business for forty years? *I'd be sixty-five!*" He looked horrified at the thought. (We'll meet an older Bookman in Chapter 3, "Men Redefining Success," where he may surprise you as much as he does himself.)

This dramatic disparity between their actual chronological ages and the inner images of themselves that people in their forties and fifties today carry around in their heads was one of my most consistent findings. For example, in the representative national survey I conducted with *Family Circle,* middle-income men over 45 said they felt eight years younger than their true ages.[4] The professional men I have studied just past 50 are even more bumptious; most still feel like 40-year-olds.[5] The disparity is even greater for women. While the younger women in the *Family Circle* survey feel only about three years younger than their real ages, on average, the women over 45 feel fully *ten years younger!*[6] Commercial marketing surveys find the same age gap.[7] But while many Americans in middle life see themselves as eight to ten years younger, many advertisers are still pitching them as if they were ten years *older*.[8]

Dot Coddington is a good example. An attractive, athletic-looking woman, she stopped to tell me at a book signing that she couldn't find herself in *Passages*. "I'll be forty-four next month," she said, fully anticipating my response: "You look ten years younger." A vice-president for Chase Manhattan Bank, Dot travels light. "I feel like a kid really," she said, "because I don't have any children." She and her husband like to hike. They want to be ready for the first opportunity to move West to pursue their enjoyment of the outdoors. "It's a very now-oriented life. I'm different from the women you wrote about in their forties [who were always sacrificing for someone else]. I've always been a strongly self-oriented person." There is only one area in which she has a hint of time beginning to run out. "It's a little harder to stay optimally fit, which is what you've been used to all your life."

By looking, dressing, and playing as if they were still the kids they feel like inside, many members of the Vietnam Generation can deny that there is any passage at all to be made in middle life. So long as we are buoyed by believing in the collective myth that we are still young and promising, we can steer clear of the dark side, pushing on from one track of vigorous activity to the next. Potency is still high in almost every sphere—stronger bodies through fitness training, better sex through chemistry, bigger accomplishments, higher salaries, later babies—and, oh, how we love to show off our powers at 40! These external proofs defend us well against the need to change—and, too, often against growth.

OUT OF CONTROL

Early in life Boomers got used to having two things: choice and control. A great many members of the current fortysomething generation have been able to maintain the illusion that their choices will continue to be unlimited and that they are in full control of their lives. Since so many of the marker events of adult life have been delayed, the classic early midlife crisis, which used to be concentrated between the ages of 38 and 43, is more likely to be put off today until the mid-forties or later.

But when the storm clouds do begin to gather over their illusions, people in their forties today are likely to feel more out of control than ever. Many men feel they have been hit with economic betrayal, their expectations of continued career progression often frustrated by the sheer size of the "pig in the python." They are arriving at the narrow neck of the career path at a time when the openings for promotion, pay increases, and perks are clamped tighter than ever by downsizing. The system is working less dependably for men at midlife today than at any time since the Great Depression.

Women of the Vietnam Generation are generally more confident than the men. But they too are often conflicted about their earlier choices. As girls they were coded to be traditional women. When they came of age, the new gospel of women's liberation urged them to seize control of their identities, but no one showed them how. There were few role models. Many sacrificed their feminine longings to prove their worthiness in career worlds dominated by men. Others tried to blend the traditional feminine roles of wife and mother with their new appetite for greater independence. Whatever direction they took in their Turbulent Thirties as they tried to put it all together, something was shortchanged. Uneasiness about one's choices naturally resurfaces in the forties. We all become more acutely aware of what has been left out. Is there still time to squeeze it in?

Most men respond to the sudden pinch of time at 40 with a burst of speed in the race for career position: *It's my last chance to pull away from the pack.* A common view was expressed by a New York sales rep, when I asked what 50 meant to him. "Fifty means the end of promise. But forty is getting real close."

You may step up your pace, but the concept of "middle" life hangs over all the frenetic activity. If a violently altered time perspective sets off a midlife crisis, it can take you in one of several directions. Those averse to risk and change will dig in their heels and claim, "It's too late," perhaps finding relief (albeit temporarily) in stoically settling for what is. Others will have a fling or throw over what they have to start again. Still others will not manifest any major changes. It's not uncommon for people in their early forties to be in a mess for a while, stuck in a whirlpool that seems to take them around in circles.

Welcome to middlescence. It's adolescence the second time around. Turning backward, going around in circles, feeling lost in a buzz of confusion and unable to make decisions—all this is predictable and, for many people, a necessary precursor to making the passage into midlife.

"It's the first time in life when you realize you *can't* control it," said Wally Scott, a participant in one of many Midlife Passage group discussions I've attended in recent years. "All of a sudden you have to start listening to the little voices inside: *What do I really want to invest my life in? What do I really care about? How can I construct a life that fits the me of today as opposed to the me of fifteen years ago?"*

Michael Kinsley, the famously liberal political pundit, has been having a slow-mo midlife crisis in public. Accustomed to being an enfant terrible, whose tumult of words in *The New Republic* and hair-trigger cognitions as cohost of TV's *Crossfire* have presumably brought him close to achieving the dream of his Harvard youth—to be recognized as among the most influential voices of his generation—he suddenly found himself an eternal adolescent up against his mid-forties.

"I would say that certainly any male who is 43 and doesn't have a serious relationship is screwed up in some way," he told writer Nancy Collins in *Vanity Fair.*[9] Kinsley is a classic example of the "control freak" who has fallen into the whirlpool of middlescence. A man renowned for the tartness of his logic, he spent a recent year in a stew of indecisiveness, giving yes/no answers to a coveted job offer as editor of *New York* magazine while he wrestled with the idea of giving up his eleven-year post as the author of "TRB," *The New Republic's* watchtower of liberalism.

"The *New York* thing 'started a mild midlife crisis that was resolved by growing a beard,' " he said, sounding impatient and chagrined "that even a rare bird like himself could fall prey to such a predictable passage." He went on to say, "If you think about moving to New York, changing your life completely, then decide not to, you wake up the next day thinking, *So, I'm doing the same thing?* Well, you gotta change something." So this clinically neat man began his middlescent rebellion by growing an unkempt beard.

Among Kinsley's friends who see his angst as the start of a larger transformation is Frank Rich, the *New York Times* writer, who shook himself out of an occupational easy chair as the *Times'* revered drama critic to try a column on the op-ed page. "It's a growth thing," said Rich. "I'm all in favor of encouraging all my friends who are roughly my age to reconsider everything. It's very typical of men our age."[10]

People who do shake themselves out of complacency at this stage are also flourishing. The forties are the gateway to a new beginning, beyond the narrow roles and rules of the first half.

The yearning for community with friends, for a sense of place, for a broader shared purpose, is particularly acute for this generation in its forties. Its members recall well the rallies and protests and sit-ins and love-ins—Woodstock and the Mall in Washington—and all the rest of the body-crushing, mind-blowing experiences of a shared sixth consciousness.

That sense of community is what brought magic into their lives before they peeled off into couples and families and corporate pigeonholes.

When the voice of the Sixties, Paul Simon, turned 50 in 1991, he reassured his flock that "the vision that was planted in my brain still remains, within the sound of silence." Since he and Art Garfunkel went their separate ways in 1970, an entire generation has grown up and gone through college, total strangers to a time that found dark solace and spiritual nourishment in songs like "The Sounds of Silence" and "Bridge over Troubled Waters." On a 1993 world tour Simon was again able to draw together millions from his generation in a communal affirmation, expressing their unquenched yearnings for a world that bridges all differences. The emotional high point was reached when his own estranged partner, Art Garfunkel, briefly joined Simon onstage to perform a replica of their hymn of innocent longing "Bridge over Troubled Waters." For a few moments the oneness of the Sixties lived again.[11]

But these partners have gone different routes in the journey to midlife. Garfunkel refused to grow up. He would have been happy to go on indefinitely singing Simon and Garfunkel songs. At 50 he had the same choirboy aura and the same puff of blond curls under his baseball cap that were his signatures at 17. Meanwhile, Paul Simon had moved on in personal and artistic growth. Using rock 'n' roll, the natural medium of the Vietnam Generation, he forged a musical osmosis with the music of South Africa and South America. The result is a multicultural world music that is understood by young people everywhere.

There is a stunning scene in Susan Lacey's award-winning documentary *American Masters: Paul Simon—Born at the Right Time*, in which the subversive political style of the Vietnam Generation reaches its highest purpose. Simon was performing in China in October 1991. It was the first time since 1945 that the Chinese government had allowed a concert, any concert. As Simon began singing, government leaders turn their shocked and stony faces toward the crowd. Miraculously, after nearly fifty years of Communist mind control, there were thousands of citizens singing the words to the anthem of the Vietnam Generation, "Bridge over Troubled Waters"—in Chinese. By synthesizing his boyish yearnings with his adult powers to effect change, Simon validates the Vietnam Generation's unique approach to this stage of life.

Ann Beattie (born 1949), chronicler of her Sixties generation, has eloquently expressed in her short stories the incompleteness felt by so many of her contemporaries. "A lot of people from my generation got the idea that they were free agents pretty early on . . ." she explained. ". . . [T]he war in Vietnam made people make choices that were either terrible compromises to them or scared them to death, or that embarrassed them . . . the political upheaval made people want to grab on to a life pretty fast. And it didn't often work . . . many of the characters search for, and can't seem to find, a sense of community. They may travel around, often from coast to coast, but they don't seem to know, or care, where they are. . . ." Updating her generation in its forties, she observed, "Today these people are quite security conscious, and they want it on all levels . . . with all the props of the status quo."[12]

The forties are the time to rediscover community on a more realistic plane. Before this decade is out, if you are determined to become authentically yourself, you will find a way to assemble all the parts of your nature into one whole. You will have to stop pretending to be the person you have been and begin to recognize and ultimately accept who, or what, you are becoming.

3

MEN REDEFINING SUCCESS

A generation ago, when people had only one career, men in their forties were secure. If they were trained and on a career path, and if they played company politics reasonably well, they could begin to coast as they got older. Mediocrity was well tolerated by large corporations. And the affirmation men had or had not accrued by age 45 pretty much determined on what rung of the ladder they could expect to play out their lives.*

Just at the point when the forward guard of Boomers reached their forties, however, sweeping structural changes were revolutionizing the American and Western European economies. A Digital Revolution happened under their noses. Worldwide industrial competition grows more fierce with every year. And even as the U.S. and European economies emerge from the ravages of a deep recession, it becomes soberingly clear that serial unemployment and job dislocation will continue to be a problem even in recovery.[1]

Although most members of the Vietnam Generation have long since joined the system, they probably never entirely bought into it. After all, they were the first to discover that certain kinds of work could bring them greater self-fulfillment than leisure. Those who had the education or talent with which to bargain for the better jobs demanded that their work be intrinsically rewarding and socially useful and contribute to their personal development; otherwise they would look for those intangibles elsewhere. Having grown accustomed to downplaying work, they now come upon their forties, and—

*Many of the statements in this chapter could also apply to women in corporate life.

whoops!—the wheel has turned again. The old expectations—that the older a man got, the more leisure he would have and the easier life would get—are insupportable with work forces contracting worldwide.

For many people today, the stepladder of corporate life has been kicked out from under them. Even the wall the ladder was leaning on may be removed. Huge companies shrink to near shells overnight. Mid-size companies start up, merge for a project, then metamorphose into something else to meet market demands. The tenure track is being jumped by "academic migrants" who move from university to university, offering their services by the semester. The pyramid has been flattened. The corporation as parent is dead. Today self-knowledge and communication skills are essential for survival.

Further discomfort from these new realities afflicts men who expected to reach a certain level by dint of their white maleness but who now have to make room for women and minorities as well as their own generational bulge. The old boy network doesn't help them much anymore. The boss may be a woman, or a gay male, or simply a cost-conscious older man who knows he can pay women and minorities less. And fortyish white males are furious when less qualified females or persons of color are chosen over them.

The most stunning change is in the shrinking of men's work that requires more brawn than brains. As information technology takes over, factories, trucking, and construction no longer provide the ready jobs that have traditionally absorbed the largest segment of blue-collar men. Most of the new jobs for people with high school educations or only some college are in "pink-collar" categories classically seen as "women's work": clerical, sales, and personal service (like waitressing and practical nursing). As a result, a shocking number of prime-age men are neither working nor even looking for work.[2]

Their traumatic dislocation was an important factor in the 1994 electoral upheaval in the United States. Angry white working-class men were in the vanguard of the mass migration to conservative Republicanism. Defections from the Democratic party were concentrated among young southern men (18 to 29) with high school degrees or only some college.[3] These are the working-class men who feel betrayed, who are convinced that society and government have turned their backs on them, and who nurse an exaggerated sense of disadvantage compared with women and minorities. Who gets the blame? The people with power in Washington—whoever they are.

Call it the Rise of the Nonworking Class.

RISE OF THE NONWORKING CLASS

Many of the better-educated young Boomer men, on the other hand, see the economic revolution as another benefit of their favored generation. When companies start to sink of their own weight, corporate management seems to prefer toppling whole layers of senior managers, says Robert Sind, a national expert in corporate restructuring. They even have a term for this exercise in human engineering: *delayering.* "Boomers see all these men of fifty and over, above them, falling off the ladder," says Sind. "The Boomers know they're the ones who will pick up the pieces. They're arrogant. They believe their safety net is age. And for many of them, it is."[4]

Even if they are terminated, it will probably be only a temporary dislocation, since trained people in their forties are still in demand and likely to be highly competitive. Smug as they may appear, however, many men of the Vietnam Generation are not gaining the raises and promotions they expected. Their bosses, members of that small but well-trained Organization Man generation, the Silents, are fighting tooth and nail to hang on to the reins of senior management. Those most likely to be in for a shock are usually the least prepared: men who work for gold standard companies in positions that pay best.

> Since 1980 the proportion of the American work force employed by Fortune 500 companies has shrunk by 25 percent.[5]

Many other jobs have been moved overseas. IBM alone virtually cut itself in half—from 408,000 employees to 234,000—in the space of five years. Given the supereducated work force the Vietnam Generation brings to midlife, the pool of qualified managers is constantly multiplying even as companies continue to slash their management ranks. Thus eventually almost everybody is blocked.

People used to think at 45: *How do I prepare myself for the next promotion?* Now they have to think: *How do I prepare myself to make another start if/when I'm pitched over the side?* Companies today treat employees as disposable resources. They hire "contract workers" and call it "outsourcing." Peter F. Drucker, dubbed the godfather of modern management, predicts that "ten years from now a company will outsource all work that does not have a career ladder up to senior management."[6]

Back in their thirties, when Boomer men first faced blockages as they tried to climb through middle management, many of them said, in effect, "Okay, if I'm not going to get my major rewards out of the job, I'm going to flip it around. Instead of being a crazed corporate junkie who sacrifices everything to get to the top, I'm just going to put in my hours from nine-thirty to four-thirty, but I'll make sure that I go to my kid's soccer games, and maybe have a girlfriend on the side, and take my sailboat out every day."

Guess what? They're going to have to hustle again. The very adaptation that these Boomer men made to the hypercompetition within their generation will have to be revised, again, as they approach the year 2000 and their own late forties and fifties.

"I've had to fire one person after another that came from that corporate culture of delegation," says David Birch, president of Cognetics, Inc., an economic research firm in the economically depressed Boston area. "These Boomers have no work ethic, no concept of a twelve-hour day. They go canoeing and kayaking and refuse to give up a tennis lesson, even when there's a report to get out on deadline. I say, 'How about working?' They are not slackers. It's just that they have developed a life for themselves in which work is merely a subset that cannot interfere with other parts of their life. Corporate America has tolerated that, until recently."[7]

THE DOUBLE SQUEEZE

For men, not only does job insecurity threaten their economic future, but it hits them where their egos live: in the center of the concept of themselves as men. A group of white southern men, all of whom work in the health care sector, volunteered to meet with me one March day in Louisville, Kentucky. A freak storm muffled the city in snow that morning. The city's power failed, and the conference center where we were to meet was pitched into darkness. Of course, the men wouldn't come, I thought. But as the first flickers of light reappeared, I made my way to the meeting room. There they were, all six of them: restless, raunchy, unruly as boys in a teacherless classroom, yes, but they were there, and within minutes they had opened up. They were eager to make sense and meaning out of this new territory of middle life. They wanted theory, labels, explanations that would bring some order to the variousness of their experience.

I asked them to start off describing, What was turning 40 like for you? And what does 50 mean to you?

THE PHARMACEUTICALS SALESMAN, AGE 48

"We're dinosaurs."

A pharmaceuticals salesman I'll call Doug was two years away from turning 50. "I really haven't thought a whole lot about it," he said. His only thought was to sock away money for retirement. But when he was asked what he would do with that expanse of after-career life, his screen went blank. He felt threatened by possible job loss or, worse, that his industry wouldn't exist in its present form long enough for him to retire. Doug was the only one of the group who smoked. And being a traveling salesman, he drank a good bit, so it was not surprising that he seemed to be aging faster than the others.

"In the pharmaceuticals business people that are my age—I have twenty-one years with this company—we're dinosaurs. Everybody now is five foot four, weighs one hundred fifteen pounds, has long blond hair, and is a female." Did he feel displaced? "More and more." He had no strategy for changing course before he was run off the side of the road. "I'm facing two kids going to college in the near future. I don't see anybody else willing to pay me the income I'm at now. So I have to play out this string to the end."

Probably the worst thing a middle manager in midlife can do is plan to play out the same string to the end. He can forget about career ladders and pyramids and depending on a company to take care of him. The individual must take more responsibility for designing the right balance of life and work for himself or herself at different stages. Today the smart man will use his early forties as preparation time. What does he need to learn to maximize his ability to respond quickly to a fluid marketplace? Just as the most successful industrial plants are adopting the concept of "agile manufacturing," so the most successful contract workers make themselves agile through developing multiple abilities.

"You have to take responsibility for knowing yourself," advises Peter Drucker, "so you can find the right jobs as you develop and as your family becomes a factor in your values and choices. Simply being well-educated is no longer enough. When you don't communicate, you don't get to do the things you are good at."[8]

A single fixed identity is a liability today. It only makes people more vulnerable to sudden changes in economic or personal conditions. The most successful and healthy among us now develop *multiple identities,* managed simultaneously, to be called upon as conditions change. Recent research also suggests that developing multiple identities is one of the best buffers we can erect against mental and physical illness.[9] When a marriage blows up or the company shuts down or the whole nature of our profession is changed by government reform or technology, we can draw upon other sources of self-esteem while we regroup.

But even if one were able to play out the string to the end of the old natural corporate lifetime, what then? A 20-year-old man in 1900 could scarcely have looked forward to retirement at all; by 1989 a young man could expect to spend at least *one quarter* of his adult lifetime in "retirement" from his original career—at his own discretion.[10] And that was before the Digital Revolution really began to take off. One of the major, slow-acting ruptures to the whole American society is the rise in prime-age men who are retiring much earlier than their sixties or working much less than full time, beginning in their forties.[11] Among healthy, able-bodied American white men with high school degrees, one out of *ten* did not hold a job in 1993.[12]

What's a poor wage slave to do? Should you hold the course, hoping you'll be the hero after all the weaker-kneed fall away? Should you escape to the Golden Triangle with your busty twenty-three-year-old trainer and your old sitar and learn how to grow really dynamite poppy leaves?

There is already evidence of a striking reversal of principle: "I'd be willing to work at a boring job as long as the pay was good."[13] The number of Boomer men just past 40 who agreed with that statement doubled in 1991, compared with their responses five years earlier in the Yankelovich MONITOR surveys. At 40, rather than ask themselves, *How do I become the most perfectly developed person I can be?* this cohort of Vietnam Generation men is more likely to be asking, *How can I hang on to what I have?*

The psychological impact is greatest at midlife. Traditional blue-collar men believe that work and being a provider are the primary activity of their gender. Many are now unable to fulfill the very roles that they use to define themselves as men. When the system fails to reward them sufficiently, they have to depend on their wives, and that leaves them feeling humiliated and resentful.

THE AUTO WORKER, AGE 46

"Forty hurt me bad."

Robert Baker came straight to my men's breakfast meeting in Detroit from working the night shift on the automotive assembly line at the Ford plant. At 46, with a broad middle-European face and his middle-age spread ladled into relaxed-fit jeans, he looked a little green around the gills but eager to get some things off his chest.

"Forty hurt me bad," he blurted. Trying hard to hold on to his youth, his living standard, and his self-respect, he has been essentially repeating his First Adulthood. After being left by his first wife, he married a woman nine years younger. She brought with her two older children, a boy and a girl, but she was desperate to have a child with him. So by now Robert has a 2-year-old daughter. Although he's earning close to $70,000 a year, his chief worry is financial security. As a rear-end man at the Ford plant, he rolls gears all night. He works nocturnally so that he can take over baby-sitting days, while his wife goes out to work; their combined paychecks are needed just to stay even. Robert comes home at 7:00 A.M., just in time to pick up his 2-year-old.

His life is a blur. "I haven't had regular sleep for—I don't know how long," he said. "This marriage here"—his hands boxed the air—"is terrible right now. Strained. Her two older kids don't show enough respect to me. They're set in their ways—everything I say is wrong." His only outlet is talking to the other guys on breaks. They share stepson stories, and they kid about sex. "Oh yeah, I had some sex—last year." On his questionnaire Robert indicated that, in fact, he has sex only once or twice a month, although that is what he most wants from a spouse.

Since he turned 45, he said, he is the same in every respect as he always has been. He presents this rigid stance as a badge of manfulness. He can't think of anything good about being a man over 45.

Although blue-collar men have adopted some of the social values of their less traditional contemporaries, many are still role-bound in ways that interfere with their continuing development. Many of these men have almost no concept that change is good, that change is necessary, that change is the only way to let go and move on to a fuller way of living that can lead them into a Second Adulthood. They adhere to the work ethic that says the most important thing they can do for their children is to make enough money so the kids can live comfortably and go to college. Their workplaces are also much less flexible than professional environments. As a result of these personal and institutional attitudes, many working-class men are missing out on much of the emotional nourishment that nontraditional men are now eagerly absorbing from their children.

A BLACK MAN'S BONUS TIME, AGE 40

The most fortunate of men are those who must redefine success at 40 after having outstripped their early dreams. "As a black cat in America at forty-plus, I'm living on bonus time," says Dennis Watlington, a respected screen-writer. When I first wrote about Dennis, in *Passages*, his future was touch and go. At 16 his world was circumscribed by four blocks of housing projects in East Harlem, where smack dealers and gang leaders were the most readily available role models. He remembers his astonishment when a black person first appeared on a weekly TV series; it was Bill Cosby on *I Spy*. By then, Dennis had already been shooting heroin for two years.

A neighborhood activist rounded up Dennis and his street brothers and harnessed their anger and antic energies in football training. It was 1968. The passage of the Civil Rights Act and the Voting Rights Act by Lyndon Johnson had given vent to a new breeze of opportunity and ripples of black pride. Once Dennis kicked heroin, he was elevated to a symbol of hope by the East Harlem Federation Youth Association. Accepted by the Hotchkiss School on scholarship, he was the first "Afro-American experiment" to be admitted from the ghetto to the tony preserve of Fords and Du Ponts.

From the swarming streets of the projects he was plunged into the win-try isolation of rural Connecticut, where the windows went dark at ten and all the preppies went to bed with dependable destinies under their Black Panther posters. Dennis scared them. He was always big for his age, with dark-chocolate skin. Today he can appreciate the primal fears those attributes awaken in white males. "I look like Willie Horton's sensitive brother," he quips.

But Dennis also cherishes those first six months at Hotchkiss for allow-ing him to break through the crippling stereotypes he and his white class-mates had brought with them. "By that spring, when we came back out into the sun, we either liked or disliked one another based on merit, rather than race ignorance." He can now appreciate the enormous long-term advantage this experience left with him. "One of the reasons I've been able to make my way is that, since I was sixteen, I've never felt uncomfortable in the presence of white people."

But despite his success at Hotchkiss, or, rather, because of it, Dennis's return to East Harlem, where he tried to take up the work of preparing youngsters for prep schools, was a death trap. "At that time you were a traitor when you crossed into the white world," he remembers. He was almost killed in gang wars.

He chose to pursue the dream of becoming a playwright. It was where his talent lay, but the more complex motivation concerned proving himself to the conservative white Long Island family from which he took his second wife. "I didn't want them to feel their daughter got a bum rap by marrying me," he confesses. "I was going to impress them by giving them Mr. First-Nighter seats when my first play opened on Broadway."

He and his wife, Anne, who was racially color-blind, had a son and settled into an empty social corridor. There were long periods when Dennis believed that he would never be fully accepted by either the white or the black worlds. He built his career largely on mentoring relationships with women producers and editors, who, like him, were accustomed to being marginalized and who didn't find him threatening. But, like most people in the theater, he found it impossible to support a family. When commissions didn't come fast enough, he became abusive and drove away his wife and child.

Dennis knows only too well how hard it is to escape the gravitational pull of the ghetto. Fifteen years after he had escaped, following the breakup with his wife, he returned to East Harlem looking for its special brand of solace sold in bags and vials. What he found was a graveyard of the wide-eyed dead. His old street brothers were husks of men, the life sucked out of them by drugs and booze and the doomy certainty that there was no way out. A dealer asked Dennis if he'd like to try something new. Something called crack.

"It's just coke that you smoke," the dealer said. "It's direct." Dennis drew on the pipe and blasted off into the ecstatic edge of consciousness. Within a month the drug owned him. He dropped from 214 pounds to 190 and began living solely to fill his crack pipe.

"Theater had beaten me. I had no idea where I was going." So overwhelming was the addiction to this insidious drug, it destroyed all his friendships and relationships. Except the bond between him and his 4-year-old son, Keelan. Whenever he was able to visit the boy, Keelan would unfailingly say, "Hang in there, Dad."

"It came down to try or die," Dennis recalls. "I chose not to die. It's not often that life comes down to such a clear option." He entered a rehabilitation program, and once he was strong enough, he began attending the first of hundreds of Alcoholics Anonymous and Narcotics Anonymous meetings.

By some telepathic pull, Dennis and I met up again around that time. I urged him to try writing in a form where he could support himself, journalism, starting with his own experiences in surviving crack addiction. Once his story appeared in *Vanity Fair*, Dennis was never out of demand to write magazine stories and later screenplays. He and his wife reconciled and moved to a farm in Massachusetts, a physically healthy atmosphere where

Dennis can remain centered between writing assignments by baling hay and driving a tractor. They had another child. Dennis is buying into the land and plans to build a house on his acreage.

In the middle of high-harvest time in the fall of 1994, success struck Dennis like a thunderbolt. He had just finished seven hours of mowing and baling hay and dragged into the house dripping sweat. Flopping down in his chair, he saw his fax machine spitting out a document: YOU HAVE BEEN NOMINATED FOR AN EMMY AWARD FOR YOUR DOCUMENTARY TELEVISION FILM *THE BLACK WEST.*

This child of the mean streets of Harlem grabbed his wife and ran out into the field waving the paper and the two of them leapt up and down and danced on the crackling golden grass like a couple of kids.

"I am so grateful I had a second chance," he says. His experiences have forged a radical redefinition of success. "When I fell back through the cracks, the black neighborhood had disdain for me," he says. "They had seen me as one of the few survivors, and I had failed them. That straightened me out for good." Today he is seen in the old neighborhood in an entirely different light—as an ambassador to the world of success rather than a traitor. His emotional vitality no less than his body, rock solid from farm labor, are marvels to those of his male friends in their forties who feel weak and hostile and have, in effect, retired from living. Dennis still has dreams. He is committed to writing television and movies that will empower the black middle class by presenting characters that are colorful and complex. On the strength of winning the Emmy, he has formed a company with the director of *The Black West,* Nina Rosenblum, and is working on a documentary about slavery. Once again, Dennis Watlington is held up as a symbol of hope to the children of the ghetto.

How does it feel being in his forties as a solid, successful family man? I asked Dennis.

"I'm *living* the American dream," he began, his musical voice alternating between chords of amusement and awe at the seeming absurdity of it. "It's the dream I never thought was possible. If you took a teenage drug addict from East Harlem in the late Sixties, and told him, 'Twenty-five years from now you will be a successful writer creating your own schedule and living on a farm in New England,' that was unimaginable. My children have grounded me. I know, for the first time in my life, I have people who love me unconditionally. One of my greatest joys is that my children can look up to me as a successful person. That's so difficult to achieve as a black man."

A WUNDERKIND'S HANDICAP, AGE 40

"Today is no time to be a straight white guy."

Men who have been extremely successful, especially those who hit it big when they were young, have the hardest time of all giving up the belief that the riches of life will flow only from reaching and holding on to the pinnacle of their idealized career selves. Some of them become infant gods. This man surrounds himself with subordinates and flatterers who reinforce the fiction: Yes, your word is God. He is not required to be empathetic and supportive with others or remotely in touch with his own feelings. Eventually his emotional register atrophies. He regresses into believing that he *is* a little god who can have anything he wants. And less and less is he capable of loving and being loved because that would demand that he be human. Once he loses the capacity to foster growth and excellence in others because of his own egomania, only sheer ruthlessness can keep this man on top.

"It's *because* of their success that most successful men at midlife have never had to look inside," says Boston University management expert Professor Douglas Hall. "These people are actually developmentally disadvantaged."[14]

Bruce Feirstein was the hot new discovery some ten years ago with publication of his clever book *Real Men Don't Eat Quiche.*[15] "It used to be easy to be a real man," he wrote with tongue in cheek. "All you had to do was steal land from the Indians, abuse women, and find some place to dump the toxic waste. You can't do that anymore." "Today is no time to be a straight white guy," Feirstein told me in an interview, only partially facetiously. "Among newspaper columnists, for example, the pecking order would be a woman first, gay guys second, and very far down the line, yet another balding Jewish New Yorker."

Feirstein left the advertising business, wrote his best-seller, and turned to screenwriting. At 40, he notes, "The equilibrium of life for men has changed so much. I see a lot of friends over forty-five in the entertainment business in serious forms of denial about their age. They're confronting the idea that their careers haven't worked out the way they expected them to." For himself, he is arriving at a decision to stop living on encouragement. "I can't watch another decade disappear. I don't want to be writing *Weekend at Bernie's* at forty-seven." Asked if he foresees a change in what he values most, he says it's already happening. He has begun writing newspaper editorials, a completely anonymous enterprise.

"There's great internal validation. You look at it and say to yourself, 'I did that.' The real change in my thinking is, Okay, I may not be Steven Spielberg. Maybe it's enough to do what you do, and do it well."

Willa Cather, a true American artist whose novels are among the finest of the twentieth century, declared a truth she had learned by the age of 48: "Success is never so interesting as the struggle—not even to the successful."[16]

Put together the unprecedented levels of competition with a shrinking work force, then foist it upon a self-indulgent generation that has reached the stage of life when men and women first glimpse the dark at the end of the tunnel, and what do you have? The makings of an early midlife crisis that can be the springboard out of the trap of premature obsolescence.

THE WUNDERKIND GROWING UP, AGE 47

"You get into the nurturing business."

Remember the Hollywood talent agent we met in the last chapter, the one who, at 44, still saw himself in his mind's eye as 28? Three years later I caught up with Bob Bookman at Creative Artists Agency in Los Angeles. He was now one of the oldest and most successful agents at CAA, where the gene pool is constantly refreshed by tadpoles who come to work in shorts and sneakers and long drifts of crimped blond hair. Looks are obviously at a premium here. Age is about as venerated as cancer.

As Bookman strode across the sunny atrium, I was struck by his conversion. His thinning hair was scoured back over his ears, with only the silver showing. He wore a grown-up dark gray suit and gold-rimmed grandfather glasses, not contacts, grandfather glasses, shamelessly, and instead of twitching he walked with dignity—all of which combined to give him the appearance of an energetic rabbi.

"You look much more comfortable in your own skin than you did the last time I saw you," I remarked.

"Yeah, I can feel it," he said with a smile. The glasses were not some Calvin Klein affectation; he had actually found them in his grandfather's effects. "My grandfather was such an important part of my life it's comforting to me to have that connection." And the hair? "The reason I changed my hairstyle was that I was losing it. I really didn't want to be one of those men who start parting their hair at the back of the neck. That has to be evidence of some deep character flaw." He chuckled. "Anyway, this is what I am."

What seemed to have eased this transition to reality was a new conception of his strengths. Bookman is a walking historical archive of the film industry.

From his movie-crazy days, when he started a film society at Yale Law School and interviewed his hero, director Raoul Walsh, to his current engagement with the baby directors-in-the-making, his knowledge of the industry makes him a most valuable mentor. That is exactly the role he has assumed with the younger agents in his firm. He takes a group of them out to lunch.

"I feel I really have a sense of the past and a connection to the present and maybe to the future more than almost anybody else," he said. "If I can communicate a little of that, I think that's important for them, and it makes me feel good." His smile was relaxed. "You get into the nurturing business." His pleasure in being a professional nurturer has been educated by his personal life. Bookman has a young child from a second marriage, so he can feel the vitality of being a young dad, but he also makes long, regular visits to an older child from an earlier life.

Although Bookman insists that he still isn't using older people as a model, in fact, most of his reference points, both positive and negative, are exactly that. He had just returned from a company retreat. One of the few associates older than he, a man of 60, had shown him the house he had just bought in Montecito, ninety minutes from L.A. in the mountains of Santa Barbara.

"I thought, hmm, that would be a nice way to live when I'm older." He then discovered several other men in their fifties had already escaped the frenzy of L.A. life and were living or commuting part-time from Montecito. It set him thinking.

What was the question for his own life right now?

His foot started twitching for the first time. He folded his arms protectively around his midsection and began a stream-of-consciousness monologue about the possibility of making radical changes. "Are you going to rent your house? Sell it? Store your possessions, or keep your possessions? Do you want to sever your ties to this community? Spend half the time up there and half the time down here? You get bogged down in deciding what it is you really want to do in terms of changing your life." From a boy-man who, at 44, had told me he felt nothing radically changing in his life, Bob Bookman now sounded exactly like a *Wunderkind* in the middle of an early midlife passage.

THE NEW MIDLIFE MAN

Clearly a new perception of middle life is forming among the pacesetters of the Vietnam Generation. Boomers will never define themselves as losers.

Instead they are redefining the parameters of personal success and making a virtue of not being so ambitious.

Being a good father is weighted by Boomers with as much value as being promoted to senior management. It used to be that when older men were fired or induced to take early retirement packages, the acceptable reason to give was "I'm exploring other opportunities." Now Boomer men say, "I want to spend more time with my family." A popular line of folk wisdom in currency is "No one ever cried on his deathbed wishing he'd put in more time at the office."

But there is a paradox here. A man in the Louisville group reflected that paradox as he struggled to redefine success for himself. Listen in:

"I've always looked at fifty as being midlife, because I figure I will live to a hundred." The voice of the 45-year-old mid-level health care executive emanated quiet confidence. "So fifty seems like a nice age of reckoning where maybe I'll understand what the hell's going on." Bruce Bell is his name. A lean whippet of a man with eager eyes and a flaring pink forehead where once there was a full swag of blond hair, he has the viewpoint of a pacesetter on the leading edge of the Boomer generation. I asked Bell how he experienced himself differently now that he had moved into his mid-forties.

"Well, my chest is falling on me, and my waist"—he pinched the marginal excess in the middle of his otherwise slender frame—"since I turned forty-five, I've gotten love handles."

A 52-year-old salesman in the Louisville group with Bell quipped sarcastically, "Don't worry, it gets a lot better."

Once past the annoying physical evidences of aging, however, Bell said he finds much to look forward to about being 50. He looks at life in chapters. Part of his job is to counsel men. "I hear so many older men say, 'If I had it to do over, I would have spent more time with my family.'" Bell isn't going to make that mistake. "My family right now is number one," he said, emphasizing that he gives first priority now to his children "even over the relationship I have with my wife." Having come from a family of ten, Bell learned well how to be a team player. The whole family divides up household responsibilities.

Bell has not escaped downsizing. When his company eliminated a number of positions, he was given more tasks but the same reward. People who work with Bell like him, finding him balanced, positive, and dynamic. He puts in his time, does a good job, but at five-thirty he's out of the office and off picking up one of his kids. Expressing a common value among successful members of the Vietnam Generation, Bell said, "I don't believe in work-ing every week, fifty, sixty hours. I work hard, and I get paid—it's a fair deal—but it's not going to interfere with other parts of my life that I feel are just as important, if not more so."

In earlier chapters of his life he had given his all to his marriage, then to trying to make a difference in society. Then all at once, it seemed, he had children and felt himself shouldering a surprisingly heavy backpack of financial responsibilities. In his mid-thirties Bell took an inventory of his life. "Suddenly I realized that my liberal Sixties giving-to-mankind was hav-ing a negative effect on my family. I didn't feel I could live at thirty thousand dollars a year and raise children." His wife was also restless and resentful. Having put her academic career on hold while their three children were young, she was chafing at 35 to reenter her field and catch up. The values of their twenties, around which they had erected an idealistic life structure, were not holding up against the buffeting of family and role demands in their thirties. Bell made the first of four or five career changes.

He prepared by going back to school for a master's degree in business, which demanded discipline: up every day at 4:30 A.M. to study before going to work at 8:00, then dashing to class in the evenings. He was tired, but exhil-arated, because he felt in control of his future destiny. "I'm really glad that I did it while my kids were young," he told me, "because now all those hours are filled in with their soccer and baseball games and piano recitals."

Bell speaks longingly of the empty nest chapter, that hazy halcyon beach-head when his three children will be gone and most of the financial burdens of putting them through college will be lifted. "Then there will be time for us again, like the period my wife and I had when we were first starting, prior to having children," he tells himself. "I'm figuring, probably sixty, sixty-five, I'll have another career change."

What would he be looking for in a career change at that time?

"Probably something less stressful," he answered. "Idyllically, I'd fade into the sunset at a small campus somewhere, putting forty years of experi-ence into teaching, being able to relay the wisdom of living."

If this carefully calibrated future seems a bit too perfect to be believed, it is because Bell did not disclose in the group the shadow side of his feelings, feelings common for men at this stage. Usually such thoughts engulf him only when he is away from his children at a conference in another city, star-ing up at the ceiling in an anonymous hotel room where the housekeeping staff leaves chocolates on the pillow, as if that would make him feel like a good boy.

Lying there, he looks down a long tunnel at a young man and his buoyant wife: They are in their twenties, child-free, hanging out with friends, listening to their music, turning everything into jokes. The man is laughing. His wife is laughing too. They both laugh until tears squeeze out of their eyes. Who can this man be? He isn't even recognizable. It couldn't possibly be himself. Somehow all that carefree joy has ebbed away over the past five years, replaced by the increasing weight of responsibilities. All at once the missing piece in his life became clear.

"We've forgotten how to laugh."

When I caught up with Bell for a one-on-one interview, he revealed the drizzly backdrop to the sunny self-presentation he had given to the group: "I've been going through kind of a very down, almost depressed period, which I've never really had in my life—a kind of hollow feeling." He had wondered, *Might some disease process be worming its way into my system?* He had visited his internist for a complete physical. Nothing wrong with his body. So what about his head? It had struck him lately how difficult it is to control one's life. "Just when you think you've got things in order and everything's fine, you go around the corner and—smack! You lose your job or some tragedy hits or shit just falls out of the sky."

These are classical statements of the inner discontent common to the early midlife passage. Midlife is the metaphysical point where we recognize the end of unlimited promise and the fact that we *cannot control* many of the *bad things* that happen to us. In a *de*-illusioning period we incorporate those truths, which can weight us down and make us feel prematurely old during the period of transition. But we should also recognize that we do have *increasing control* over the *good things* that happen to us. And that is what makes flourishing possible in the forties.

We know by now what we need and what we like. Ordinarily we have more seniority, more disposable income and discretionary time to invest in a custom-made life structure suitable for this period, plus greater skills of communication to ask for and get the components we need. As for dealing with the bad things, we should have considerable experience in meeting life's passages by now. What have we learned? Which strategies worked for us? Which backfired? The Chinese have a nice image: For a longer, more balanced life, one must wear off the sharp, defensive edges and become more of a ball, well rounded, able to roll with the ups and downs, no matter what happens.

Bell knew what he was looking for, but he wasn't at all confident that he would find it anytime soon. Having enjoyed the prolonged period of noncommitment in his twenties that most Boomers considered their birthright, and having waited for the first child until 30, the past fifteen years had been hard sledding. He had just about forgotten social life, sports, man-to-man friendships, even playing an instrument he used to love, sacrificing them all for the children, who were now only 11, 14, and 16. "It really wears you down—dealing with adolescents continually struggling against limits. I guess I'm tired of giving, giving, giving," he said. "I feel like the emotional bank's empty. But when it comes to trying to pick some things for me or to have fun, nothing seems to interest me. That's where the dullness, the depression come."

In truth, he was tired of being such a good boy.

Most men feel stale, restless, and unappreciated at the precipice of midlife. The "false self" is especially confining for nontraditional men, who, like nontraditional women, suppress cross-sex characteristics in Young Adulthood and leave certain core needs unsatisfied into their forties. Their achievement drive leaves little room for expressing their emotional or spiritual needs. Often angry and defensive, these men look for others to blame for their own (often inexplicable) dissatisfactions. Many pay a high price in poor psychological health in their forties.[17]

Bell's natural need for emotional replenishment as a man in his midforties is now challenged as well by his wife, who brings to this stage her own anger at the lost-opportunity years of her young mothering phase. She complains that her income level will never recover and reach his. They fight. The fights always end like a chapter from Deborah Tannen's book: "God, I just don't understand how you could feel that way."[18] Bell feels his youth escaping but cannot see any respite from the struggle.

"It's not like we're over the hump and in five more years we'll have an empty nest," he said. "We've got ten more years of three children in the whole teenage struggle and then college responsibilities, and that is—that's depressing." By then, God, he'll be 55—old! (Not really old, but that's how 55 looks from the vantage point of 45.)

Many men of the Vietnam Generation have delayed parenthood, and that sets up a whole new timetable for middle life. At ages when their fathers were off fly-fishing and fulfilling themselves, these gray-haired daddies will be making down payments on college tuition. Since the high cost of education and housing may force their adult children to live in their parents' homes even longer in the future, both grown children and the love children of late or second marriages will nibble away at the Boomers' time and money in their middle years.[19] That may slow them down. Look for them to be pushing strollers and corralling sullen teenage children into Club Med family vacations well into their fifties and even sixties.

It adds one more challenge to the passage into midlife for Boomer men. Just as Dad is beginning to freak over his thinning hair and narrowing career track, wondering what he's worth after all, he will have a little beastie slouching around the house in a skull hat, carpenter pants, steel cap shoes, and Malcolm X specs, ready to confirm that Dad is *definitely* over the hill, disconnected from the beat, and hopelessly left behind at the controls of the future by the freewheelers of cyberspace.

Where to turn to make sense of this strange, stalled place in a journey that seemed to be proceeding so well? In the back of Bell's mind are the voices of many men in their fifties who have confided in him during the counseling sessions he used to hold. "You know, I went through two to three years of depression," they often said. "If I had to do it over again, I'd get some help."

Bell is emblematic of the New Midlife Man, both in his curiosity about the possibilities of life from 50 to 100 and in his apprehensions about running the rapids of accelerated change between 45 and 55 without his marriage capsizing. But once a man is older and wiser and, with any luck, more financially secure, the benefits of fatherhood and keeping his family together may far outweigh the protracted burdens.

4

OUT-OF-SIGHT WOMEN

*M*idlife crisis used to be primarily the prerogative of men. For women, if anything, it was a referred crisis: the empty nest syndrome or "what to do after being dumped?" Now that women's expectations include individual achievement and continuing self-development, midlife crisis has become very much a woman's issue.

Women who graduated from college at the end of the 1960s or in the early 1970s were reared under one set of values and expectations, but they were still young enough when the women's movement exploded to adopt an entirely different set of values, which have then shaped the course of their adult years.

The first graduates of the women's movement—point women, I call them—took the greatest fire as they scrambled across the minefield of a society hostile to "uppity" women back in the early 1970s. Many strapped on male values like battle gear. But beneath the jumpsuits and boots their female instincts were suffocated—at least for the duration of their First Adulthood.

Many are still at war with what psychologist and author Dr. Ellen McGrath calls the Traditional Core, meaning a woman's cultural conscience. One cannot overestimate the power of this core of cultural values that "exists deep within every woman and dictates how we must behave and what roles are 'right' and 'wrong' . . . feminine, masculine, appropriate, and inappropriate for us as women."[1]

During the Sixties the dictates of the Traditional Core were shaken by a booming economy. Women were needed to work outside the home. If the Traditional Core is weighted as if written in stone, one can imagine Moses coming down from a renegotiation with the Lord and saying, "Okay, I got Him to take 'obey' out of the marriage vows, but the wife still has to promise to work a double shift."

I talked about this phenomenon with Don Hernandez, chief of the marriage and family statistics lab of the Census Bureau. In researching old Census Bureau data, he found that the long-term historical trend in divorce has been upward since as far back as 1850. And there is good reason for it. Historically people have found three ways to increase their social mobility. First they moved off the farms and into cities, where they could find higher-status occupations and make more money, a continuous trend since at least 1870. The second way was to get more education. Because the World War II Generation was able to finish high school and many went on to college on the GI Bill, they could afford to further their children's education. The third source of social mobility was to have fewer children. A hundred years ago the average child lived in a family with five and a half children. Today the average child has one sibling. With fewer children, parents had more money to spend on health care and education or to buy capital resources or open a shop—or to get a divorce. Thus much that is ascribed to the want-it-all attitudes of selfish Baby Boomers is in fact a long-term, fundamental driving force in the United States, and in all developed countries for that matter.

But as early as the 1940s most people were already taking advantage of these three traditional sources of social mobility. All they could offer a family was a brake against slipping backward economically. That left one other source, untapped since the World War II mobilization: female participation in the work force. Coincidental with this new economic necessity was the publication in 1963 of Betty Friedan's *The Feminine Mystique*, which revealed to millions of women how they had been gulled into serving as handmaidens to their husbands.

By the time the Vietnam Generation women came of age, they were at war with their Traditional Core. They were ready to break the mold. They did it by making dichotomous life choices, either starting out in a strictly traditional direction and doing an abrupt volte-face later, or throwing out the baby with the bathwater in the beginning only to regret and try to rectify it later. Some tried to forge a blend of bourgeois safety and dissident hippiedom. But it's probably safe to say that every fortysomething professional woman with children feels conflicted. No matter what balance she has struck between the traditional and nontraditional, it always feels askew. Somewhere she's *not enough.*

All this produces an identity diffusion that may be unique to this generation of women. It is evident even in the briefest biographical sketches of the graduates of Wells College, an esteemed all-women's school in upstate New York that fostered leadership in women long before it was fashionable. These women, now 45, sent in sketches for their twenty-fifth reunion.

MYRA EGELMAN FEENEY: Bill and I often say we've lived our lives in reverse. We were "retired" for the first eleven years of our marriage, spending our time traveling, boating, bicycling. Then I had an idea that, up until then, I suspected no one else had: "Let's start a family!" And so, now, while continuing to work as a math consultant, mixing dinners with one hand, ironing with the other, I push the vacuum with my foot and enjoy my family life.

While women like Myra returned late to the dictates of the Traditional Core, others like Ginny bought into it in the beginning and later ran into the treacheries of being dependent on the marriage structure:

GINNY FEWSMITH MCBRIDE: June 1968—Out of the cap and gown and into the wedding gown. I spent twenty years living in South Florida. My husband had his midlife crisis, which I refuse to let become my crisis. We were divorced six months ago. He's filed for bankruptcy and stuck me with the debt.

Still others embraced personal anarchy or became hitchhikers along the road of causes and instant gratification. This was one way to be sure of avoiding surrender to the Traditional Core. But the farther one strays into nontraditional territory or alternative lifestyles, the more uncertain and threatened one can expect to feel. And by delaying indefinitely any serious choices or commitments, eventually one is not sure about anything.

The next sketch suggests the effort it takes to integrate a bold career dream (rationalized here as sheer luck) with the need to nurture. The nurturing need wasn't acknowledged until this alumna's mid-thirties.

STEPHANIE WALLACH: I started flying on a lark; it sounded like fun. I had no plans to make aviation a career. I became the tenth woman in the United States to fly for a major air carrier. I'm currently a captain on the

Douglas MD-83. All this, however, pales next to the real love of my life, my 10-year-old son. By the time he came along my career was well established, so I felt ready and able to concentrate on and devote myself to him—and I have.

For many women of this generation the thrill of self-assertion contrasts so sharply with their early encoding in traditional sex roles, it precipitates a full-blown midlife crisis. Religion used to provide many answers. But since it was an article of faith among the Vietnam Generation to challenge all authority, including organized religion, there may be no solid spiritual grounding upon which to construct a mature philosophy. The search for answers is often prompted by the presence of young children, whose metaphysical questions are likely to coincide with—and intensify—the parents' midlife passage: *How do I tell my children what to believe about life and death when I don't know what I believe myself?*

A WOMAN IN EARLY MIDLIFE CRISIS

One afternoon in 1987 I was interviewing a woman in Washington about a research project she was doing on the Vietnam Generation when she lapsed into a most private confession. "I always thought it was men who went through midlife crisis. I identified it with men who ran off with twenty-one-year-olds," she said. "My friends and I used to joke, 'He's just trading down to someone at his IQ level.' But I'd never known a woman to have the same anxieties about starting anew. When I read your book, I didn't identify because I was too young. But now!" This whip-smart well-dressed woman, who exuded executive ability like some new Armani perfume, suddenly leaned across her desk and whispered with some chagrin, "But now, I swear, my generation—all my women friends in our age-group of late thirties to mid-forties—we're all going through a midlife crisis!"

Laurie, I'll call her, helped raise funds to build the Vietnam Veterans Memorial wall, and later set up a foundation to foster renewed idealism within her generation. When I first talked to her, she was 38, and with those successes behind her she felt a firm identity for the first time. Laurie spoke enthusiastically of seeing an emerging activism among her age-group. "It's either a lost spirit they once experienced and want to rekindle or a spirit they felt by osmosis or a contact high during the Sixties they never acted on, and they hunger to express it now," she said. "There's a feeling it's now or never."

As older members of the Vietnam Generation reach the brink of early midlife passage, the echo of early dreams and wishes are expressed oftentimes in a resurgence of the activism and idealism they associated with their youth. Laurie's experience was typical.

She was a college junior at Ohio University during the tumultuous year of 1970, when the Kent State killings of antiwar students shattered the trust between generations. According to the "shoulds" of her generation, she slept around. How many men? "An awful lot, too many. It was just what we were supposed to do in our twenties." She dated a man for almost seven years before daring to commit to marriage. Back then she valued her scholar husband because "he would always be there if I needed him; he was a stabilizing factor for me. This was the man I wanted to grow old with. But I was a different person then."

For some fifteen years between the mid-Seventies and the Eighties, like so many of the point women, Laurie developed at zoom speed. She worked her way up from a receptionist to the executive director of her own organization. She proved that she could be her own corporation. On the question of children, she decided in her early thirties "I'd rather have an identity than a baby." Her learning curve has been pitched very steeply ever since, and her progress through formerly exclusively male hierarchies fantastically accelerated. Laurie's commitment to her career has become increasingly serious. Her cultural and metaphysical interests have expanded. Approaching 40, she viewed her marriage in an entirely new light: She wanted to continue to develop; her husband didn't.

The moment of truth occurred during a two-week driving trip to Newfoundland. Six hours a day in the car, her husband happily occupied with the art of driving, Laurie had nothing to do but read. All the books she had brought were about spiritual growth and inner journeys, a midlife sort of obsession that surprised her. These were not subjects she could discuss with her husband. He was still a linear man.

There was a place along that rugged coast where the tide surges in with almost the force of a tidal wave. She looked forward for the whole trip to witnessing this marvel of nature. They arrived at the spot forty-five minutes before the phenomenon was to occur.

"What a thrill," Laurie said expectantly.

"We can't wait around for something to happen," said her husband. "We have to get to the hotel before dark."

There was no loud argument, simply the sudden unbridgeable gulf between the people they had married and the people they had become. They had come upon the season of divorce.

"I have gone so far beyond my husband, and he just hasn't caught up," Laurie told me. I keep grappling with the same questions: *Why is he so uninteresting now? Should I leave him? Will I then spend the rest of my life being supersuccessful, and alone?* I've been in great turmoil lately. But then I realized, it's not him, it's me. *I'm* the one who has changed. It's not that we married the wrong men. It's because we *had* to change, and they didn't."

Laurie was out on the growing edge again. But there were no trail maps, especially for the point women, and she sometimes felt as if she were hanging off a cliff.

CATCH-40 FOR COUPLES

The striking thing about Laurie's dilemma was that it replicated almost word for word the frustration that used to be expressed by men of 30 about their wives. They used to complain, "I've grown, and you haven't." Twenty years ago in *Passages* I called that phenomenon Catch-30 for Couples.[2]

Both members of the couple felt betrayed. The other was failing to live up to the unspoken contract they had made when they married. No one had warned them that people of goodwill simply change from stage to stage. The result was Americans used to be most likely to break out of wedlock when the man was about 30 and the woman 28.

Today the phenomenon could be called Catch-40 for Couples. The parts are simply reversed. She is now the one becoming bored with a stable, narrowly directed workadaddy, while he is the one envious of her enlarged vision of herself and the exhilaration she feels in her expanded powers. Having faced down so many obstacles to open the doors of opportunity to women, Laurie, like many of her female contemporaries, has become confident and strong and terrifyingly autonomous. Meanwhile, the men of her generation simply developed at a normal pace. They feel overwhelmed by these women and at the same time terrified by their need for women. All around them they see and feel evidences of women's rage, which can be sexually daunting. With all these sociological changes coming to a head at the same time as couples arrive at the edge of middlescence, it is not surprising that the breakup of first marriages for this generation soared in their early forties.

Laurie is emblematic of the flying wedge of Vietnam Generation women. She married a traditional man, and that allowed her to be a maverick. By the time she reached early midlife, she didn't need a man to carry her dream. She had established her own solid identity based on accumulated accomplishments in her work that could not be denied. But there is still the traditional part of her that feels somewhat vulnerable and weak around the issue of her adequacy with men. I asked if she hoped to get remarried.

"The men who really are wonderful, who would appeal to those of us who now have a presence and identity and are doing well, are still married— bless their hearts," she said with muted regret. "And the others, the available ones, are available because they won't change."

Laurie still wishes, vaguely, for a man to validate that traditional part of her. So she's caught in the middle, still battling with the Traditional Core. But she has found a renewed sense of community in her work.

Women born in our 1945–50 cohort group reached a record-high divorce rate of 36 percent between the ages of 40 and 44.[3] Yet Vietnam Generation women are not so frantic about seeking their own identities and establishing their autonomy at 40—they already know who they are—in contrast to women of a previous generation who made personal development secondary to the commitment to husband and children. Boomer women are so much more highly educated and occupationally experienced than women who came before. They outnumber their male contemporaries in higher education by an ever-growing margin, and that gives them the skills and income-producing independence to stretch themselves in all kinds of new directions at midlife.

The income of the men of their generation rose at a very modest rate as they entered midlife. The median income of year-round, full-time employed men who had reached ages 40 to 44 by 1990 had increased only from $32,400 to $34,600 since 1970.[4] In stark contrast, their female peers enjoyed the headiest rise in income, compared to all American women in the last two decades. While the median income for all women working full-time year-round rose 18 percent,[5] the women between 40 and 44 in 1990 posted an increase of 31 percent from $17,400 to $22,800.[6]

Increasingly women who are able to support themselves in a reasonable style are choosing not to remarry after divorce, rather than sacrifice their independence.[7] There is no question that women who remain single or who resist remarriage after divorce—and who work full-time—enjoy the highest economic well-being among all women. The PUMS data revealed that never-married white women racked up a sizable increase in total median money income—up 22 percent—between 1974 and 1992.

> Among white women between the ages of 25 and 65, those who remain single have the highest incomes—compared to women who are married, divorced, or widowed.[8] (See note for full table.)

A recent survey on the confidence level of American women by *McCall's* magazine also depicted a decisive change. Across the board the women felt more independent and sure of themselves than in the recent past. But it was the movers and shakers of the median age 41 who displayed the highest confidence level of all. A synthesis of the results showed "it comes from knowing she can take care of herself. She's learned what really matters in life.... She's well-paid or well-provided for.... She trusts her own judgment. She's not afraid to make mistakes and she doesn't worry what others think of her. What's more, she tends to be outspoken."[9]

BEYOND "ME"—TO ANOTHER
LEVEL OF BEING

When I followed up on Laurie, the idealist who had struggled with a midlife crisis, it was five years after our first interview. I found her divorced, working as the director of development for a continuing-care facility for seniors, and unexpectedly serene. She was now 44. Her blond hair edging toward gray, she was dressed rather primly in a navy blue suit with a white-bow blouse and pearls and looked, from the grooves under her eyes, matured beyond her years, as if she had been to some underworld of the soul and back.

The revelation didn't surface until I asked how her feelings about death compared with the apprehensions about mortality she had expressed before entering the midlife passage.

"I've already had my bout with mortality," she replied. "I had breast cancer." Laurie shifted in her seat for the first time. "Three years ago. On my mammogram. A spot so tiny it wasn't a lump yet." She theorized on how it had happened to her: There was the ending of her marriage, which meant losing her best friend, followed by the loss of a job she loved. It all happened at once and left her with a sense of isolation. "I guess it allowed my immune system to become so suppressed that something would happen," she reflected.

Laurie took it as her challenge to heal. All through her radiation treatments she never missed a day of work. That was part of her healing: to make her job a mission beyond herself. She raises funds for the senior community. To take this dream job to the point where she could fully renew her idealism, she has reduced her lifestyle. In place of a mate or children, she has formed close bonds with the residents whose needs she serves, most of whom also live alone. She has surrendered too to the power of prayer. The day after her lumpectomy she was sitting on the edge of her bed at ten-thirty on a Thursday morning when a powerful tremor shuddered through her body. A surge of warmth and strength came after it, leaving her feeling a calm that was entirely new. She later learned that members of her religious group had concentrated their prayers on her at ten-thirty that morning. There are now a number of studies, some reported in medical journals, that show coronary care patients who are prayed for by community prayer groups have far better recoveries than those who do not.[10]

I reminded Laurie of the passionate consternation she had expressed, at the age of 38, about going through a "midlife crisis." How did it look now that she had come out the other end of that passage?

She chuckled. "Today I would not term it a crisis. Certainly I don't dispute the notion that we hit the first major reckoning around the late thirties or forty, when a whirlwind of change becomes necessary and sometimes we don't know what to do about it. But the term *crisis* has a different meaning for me now. There are ways around it, or under it, but the best way is to move right through it. That's the hardest way, but when you do that, you will come to a new level of being."

As a result of facing her early midlife crisis honestly, Laurie was fortified when she had to confront a truly harrowing challenge. She was describing what I call a life accident, one of those events that we can neither predict nor prevent. A life accident can be very valuable when it coincides with a critical passage in the life cycle since it can force us to confront and resolve the issues of a major transition more effectively.

Laurie never felt as if she were going to die during her bout with mortality. Nothing could upset her, nothing. Her focus became keen. Through meditation she found stillness. Ten years earlier, when a boss blew up at her, she felt sheer panic that she might have done something wrong. Now she doesn't assume that whatever upsets others is her fault, or even if it is, she doesn't have to be perfect. "I'm far enough along to understand that life isn't black and white; it comes in shades of gray. In fact, I am far happier today than at any point in my life," she told me. She has moved a long way inward toward the centeredness that most women are looking for—what we generally call inner harmony. But Laurie has no illusions of immortality.

"Yes, I know I'm going to die. But the flip side of being in a job where death is an ever-present reality is that I've come to realize death is part of life. And that life will continue beyond me. Beyond all of us."

5

THE FANTASY OF
FERTILITY FOREVER

A significant number of women in the Vietnam Generation have chosen not to have children, and not necessarily because they can't. Career concerns often took precedence, or the right partner never came along, or the maternal desire wasn't there—at least not until the eleventh hour. By then it may be too late to prime the reproductive system or, more pointedly, too late to learn how to put someone else first. But before these limits are accepted, there comes the furious scrambling between 40 and 50 to make up for earlier choices.

The myth of perpetual advancement in work success has its counterpart for women of the Vietnam Generation in reproductive success. I call it the fantasy of fertility forever.

A case in point is the dynamic TV news show producer I'll call Olivia. She had never married or had a child, but she didn't appear isolated or alienated or any of the other stereotypes that used to be attached to the single woman over 40. Indeed, I had been with Olivia at a health ranch on her forty-first birthday, and she was full of vinegar. Up until then she had been barreling around the world, putting together award-winning film pieces on deadline, living out of suitcases two hundred nights of the year, and she simply didn't have time for a marriage or family. The one long-term live-in love of her life had left her, and she had spent two years mourning that loss in her late thirties. But she figured she still had time.

Something happened in her forty-second year, however. "I was debating about adopting a child or even having a child. I thought, *Okay, I'm going to see what it would be like. So I'll get a dog.*"

She went out and bought a terrier. "I quickly realized that that was all the responsibility I could muster!" She chuckled. Olivia was an only child. "I don't know if I've lived alone too long, but I know I just couldn't do it by myself."

The upside of this point of passage was a new appreciation of her professional abilities. She was in the edit room one day, furiously trying to make airtime, when she had an epiphany: "There is nothing they can throw at me that I can't do. I have no fears about failing to perform. It just came over me. I *can do* this stuff. My ideas are always going to be interesting." It was an internal recognition. But with the lifting of self-doubts came a new frustration: Her creativity was being thwarted. Did she want to go on forever producing the same boringly perfect show? She began wanting to produce her own TV show, to be her own woman. She stepped up the pace of her already frenetic career. And then, before she knew it, she was standing on the precipice of 45 and the view was altogether different.

Luxuriating in the queen-size bed in her large Manhattan apartment, she would switch off her reading light anticipating a full night's beauty rest. But she began waking up at four, morning after morning. The dog jumps up on her bed. He starts at the bottom and works his way up. She doesn't stop him. Eventually he curls up on the "his" pillow side of the bed. Still, Olivia drifts only into a fitful drowse and then bolts awake with the same panicky thought:

I'm going to be homeless.

When we met for lunch during this period, Olivia was unexpectedly plumpish, hidden inside a loose black sweater. Although she still had the pretty, pixieish face and squiggly long blond hair and cornflower blue eyes that had always made her so attractive, her usual élan was flattened. I asked her if she still had nightmares about being old and homeless.

"Oh, definitely. Because I don't have any brothers or sisters, my mother is eighty-three, and I don't know how much longer she'll live. So I don't have a support system, and I don't have a safety net. TV shows are canceled all the time. I could be forced out on the job market at fifty. What do I do now to prepare myself for that? I'm looking for a way out with some other projects I'm trying to start. The panic comes in because I can't take the risks I could when I was younger, because I'm all alone."

Olivia had followed a life path to this point for which the precedents are rare. She is basically happy with her life choices, but looking at the voyage ahead into the second half of her adult life is like looking into fog. Without any channel markers, she feels stranded. All her success does not defend her from bag lady fears. Indeed, bag lady fears are quite common among successful single women as they get older.

Six months later Olivia called me. She had been going to Weight Watchers and had stripped off the extra pounds; she had also started exercising, and that had lifted the depression. Once she felt more positive, she seriously attacked the proposal for her own TV show: an innovative magazine variety show. "I think it's going to work!" she enthused. The sun has come out in her life again.

LATE BABYMANIA

But for every woman who accepts the consequences of her decision, there are many more women today who seem to believe that the decision to have a baby or not can be put off indefinitely. The new Scarlett O'Hara is the high-achieving woman of 40 who tells herself, "Oh, fiddledeedee, I'll just think about getting pregnant tomorrow." If the marriage doesn't work out, or her career is too exciting and fast-paced even to *think* about making time for a toddler, she can turn off the biological alarm clock and rely on technology to bail her out if and when the desire surfaces. Later she can choose among a sperm bank, a surrogate mother, and that sexy new technology called egg donor baby. Meantime, she'll make do with a dog.

Dianne McMillan was one of the nonchalants. The daughter of first-generation Caribbean-Americans, she was sent to a prestigious all-female prep school in upstate New York. As one of only 18 black or Hispanic students out of 360, she absorbed well the lessons of autonomy and leadership. By her mid-thirties, an import-export entrepreneur, she could boast of being a crackerjack in the business world and show off a portfolio of newspaper clips. As for relationships, sorry, she moved too often. Unattached— no, consciously *detached*, Dianne was breaking faith with centuries-old patterning. Her family urged, "Get a life, get a husband, settle down." Surveying the divorces around her, she sniffed. "Look what it did for them— nothing."

When I first interviewed Dianne, at 36, she was irrefutably certain that she had no alarm clock.[1] "People my age may talk biological clocks; I'm sure they mean something to somebody," she conceded, "but as a human being with intellectual capacities, I think we've been empowered to be in control of our bodily functions." Dianne then firmly believed, "I still have all the options open to me—more in keeping with the way your twentysomethings feel."

Two years later I reminded Dianne of her definitive statement.[2] She giggled. She was married and five months pregnant. "Blissful. I just saw the baby on a sonogram last week. I felt the *quickening*." What had changed her mind? "Seeing what's happening to friends of mine who are ten years older," she said. "They're all obsessed now with getting pregnant. They really enjoyed their younger years and had great success. It didn't occur to them that a child might be important to them on the other side of youth. Now they're very, very nervous about not having any nurturing experiences in their lives. They worry, 'What'll I do when I'm sixty and I have no one around to care about? And who's going to care about me?' "

But like Dianne, they wanted to believe their choices were unlimited by age. "They're forty-three when they start thinking about wanting a baby," she observes. "They're forty-six when they accept it isn't going to happen."

Not all women accept it even then.

The attractive 48-year-old woman perched on the examining table when the big-city doctor walks in is all blushes and titters. "I know it's absolutely silly, and you're going to yell at me, but I have a fabulous new beau, and we've chosen not to use contraception," she says, looking up coyly at her doctor as she wags a tasseled cowboy boot. "We're just going to ride out the consequences."

"That's one way of dealing with passion," the doctor quips, "as long as you're reasonably comfortable that you're not going to get some dreadful disease."

"Yes, but now my period is late," the woman announces with a maiden's blush.

"Well, you're forty-eight; it's not uncommon," says the doctor.

"I want a test for pregnancy," the woman insists.

"I would always recommend that, but it's far more likely that you're just beginning a more serious manifestation of your perimenopause," the doctor responds matter-of-factly. "It's extremely unlikely that you're going to have a spontaneous pregnancy during this part of your life."

The woman will not be dissuaded by facts; she wants too badly to believe. "But I have a friend who's attempting to conceive with in vitro fertilization," she says defensively, "and *she's* forty-seven."

The doctor, muting her disbelief, asks the patient, "Is your friend using her own eggs?"

The woman seems surprised by the question. "Of course"—as if one should expect a woman late in her forties to have great success in producing her own eggs. The doctor thinks, *Why do people need to think that being nearly fifty is the same as being thirty-eight or thirty-nine?* But the gynecologist, who later described this scene to me, is seeing a miniepidemic of these deluded, about to be desperately disappointed women in their mid-forties. She tells them, as she told this patient, politely but firmly, there is no chance she is pregnant. She is starting menopause.

The woman looks as startled as if she'd suddenly seen her own reflection in a fun house mirror, distorted into her grandmother. The image of her inner eye, along with her wish to cement the relationship with her young lover, had fooled her into thinking she really *was* what she wished to be: still a young, fertile woman.

THE GREAT POSTPONERS

Bamboozled all along by these early Boomers, demographers made a big mistake in predicting the life course of Vietnam Generation women. Martin O'Connell, chief of the fertility statistics branch at the Census Bureau, admitted, "In the late 1970s, looking at the low fertility rates among this group of women in their twenties, the bureau was predicting, 'If they haven't had a child by now, they will never have a child.' But Census Bureau surveys on birth *expectations* continuously recorded those same women saying the opposite: 'Yes, I *will* have a child. But later.' Nobody would believe it."[3] Traditionally, if women did not have a child by the age of 30, generally they did not have children at all. The idea of a *deliberate delay* was still relatively new.

In the early Eighties there was evidence in national statistics of a slight increase in childbearing, but it was almost exclusively among women in their early thirties. As that cohort aged throughout the decade, fertility continued to pick up. Clearly it was a phenomenon among the same generation of women that was being recorded as they moved along the life cycle, says O'Connell. In fact, the point women of the Vietnam Generation delayed marriage and childbearing longer than any generation before them. And they are *still* having babies, continuing into their early forties, or at least trying like hell.

Thus an entirely new set of norms has been formed. "I believe that cohort has set the pattern for succeeding generational groups of American women," says O'Connell. In fact, Me Generation women are settling down to reproduce basically the same pattern. And the offspring of Vietnam Generation women—the first of whom will be entering college soon—

promise to continue the trend toward prolonged education and postpone-
ment of family formation. The pattern has not been played out for long
enough to know how it will affect women, their spouses, and in particular
their children as they get older. These Midlife Moms are pioneer women.

One day I met a Midlife Mom who was contorting next to me in a yoga
class. At the end of the class she cracked, "I finished breast feeding just in
time for menopause." Being in your forties with an infant is, well, different. A leader in SDS in 1968, Susan described herself as "your classic Sixties person." Once the war ended, nothing could give her life the meaning
she had found in political radicalism. In her mid-thirties she finished her
Ph.D. and married. After enduring a series of miscarriages, she had finally
produced her first child at the age of 42. She was now 44, and utterly
frazzled.

Up at 5:00 A.M., she feeds and bathes the baby, tries to read the paper,
works all day, and comes home at 5:00 P.M.—to start her second shift.
"This is the part my husband and I miss the most. We used to just wind
down or collapse; we didn't even have to talk to each other. But now the
baby-sitter leaves at five o'clock, and suddenly you're up against a two-year-
old who will swallow anything you don't hide and who wants to play!"

This menopause mom and her mate will give a dinner party, and before
dessert is served, her husband's head will hit the table in a dead sleep. "I feel
deeply middle-aged, at forty-three!" she moaned, only half self-mockingly.
"By the time my husband and I hit fifty, our eight-year-old will be putting
us to bed at nine. Help!"

But for every rare case of the 42-year-old first-time mother, there are
many, many more women who wait until their late thirties or forties and do
not conceive. Their passage into midlife is likely to be a rough one.

Most women assume they have until menopause to get pregnant. They
don't. The cosmic joke today is: *You spend the first half of your adult life trying* not
to get pregnant; then you spend the second half trying to get knocked up.

"The women most aware of their age in relationship to fertility tend to
be those who shouldn't have to worry—the thirty- to thirty-five-year-olds,"
observes Dr. Edward Marut, medical director of the Fertility Center at
Highland Park Hospital outside Chicago.[4] Ironically, it is the women who
flirt with the dangerous edge of fertility who appear to be the most blasé
about age. "The forty-year-old woman doesn't come in and say, 'I'm worried about age,' because her whole mind-set has been to put it off," observes
Dr. Marut. But in the back of her mind is a universal fear: *Will I turn out to
be infertile?* Infertility is generally regarded by women as the most depressing

experience they can imagine. Even younger women don't want to wait to find out. To avoid that possibility, an amazing number of women are seeking "advanced infertility treatment."

Three friends of mine have tried to have in vitro babies. They tell a similar story. When they married in their early thirties, they thought they had all the time in the world to start a family. They started trying to get pregnant naturally. When conception didn't occur, they began to worry. After one or two miscarriages it became an obsession. By the time they got to the fertility clinic, they would sacrifice anything—take out a second mortgage on the house, sell the car, stop taking vacations—all in order to plunk down $8,000 to $12,000 for repeated in vitro treatments or $2,000 a try to get a donor egg from a younger woman.

They are given no guarantees and scant personal consultation. "We are giving women high doses of drugs like Pergonal* to hyperstimulate their ovaries so we can get as many as thirty eggs in one cycle," says one nurse-technologist. High concentrations of estrogen surge through the body (reaching a peak of two to three thousand picograms per milliliter), roughly fifteen times the normal levels of estrogen during natural monthly ovulation. Once multiple eggs mature to a certain size, another drug is administered to prepare the eggs for ovulation. Fearing they might be considered poor candidates, patients dare not show any hesitation by questioning what the drugs they are given could be doing to them.

One of my friends was a corporate lawyer who waited until 38 to try for her second child and eventually turned for help to a New York fertility clinic. Her experience speaks for many: "Every night my husband would stick me in the butt with a needle of Pergonal. Every morning I'd show up before work at the fertility clinic, take a number—like a meat market—and wait with over a hundred other sad, fixated prefortyish women to have a sonogram and my blood drawn. At the precise moment in the month, I'd go in and have multiple eggs 'retrieved.' My husband would be in another room jacking off. Several days later I'd go in to have my eggs 'transferred' back into me, after they had been fertilized with his sperm. My husband never had to touch me through the whole enterprise. Our whole sexual and emotional life—all the tenderness and passion—went right down the test tube. We tried twice and stopped."

---

*Pergonal, purified from the urine of postmenopausal women, is a hormone that stimulates the egg follicles.

It was easier for this couple to "give up" since they already had one child. For the women who start reasonably early and try year after year, doggedly but to no avail, giving up can be one of the most wrenchingly painful events in life. It is easy to understand why some persist as long as there is any shred of hope. But the price in terms of personal development can be very high.

THE PSYCHIC FALLOUT

What are the psychic implications for those who enter the midlife passage with the illusion that technology will allow them to control their ovaries and reproduce themselves, but who fail? Experts report that such women frequently become severely depressed in midlife. In addition to mourning the multiple personal losses—of a baby, a dream, a new love shared with a husband—there is a primal threat to their sense of independent agency over their lives. After all, the typical Vietnam Generation woman seeking help to reproduce in her forties is someone who has been accustomed to exercising birth *control* for many years. She is probably autonomous in every other sphere. She is proud of the social engineering job she has done to establish her identity, marriage, and career before deciding to conceive. She had a life *plan*.

Now infertility rips away the illusion of absolute control. All of a sudden her body is controlling *her*. Her professional and personal lives become hostage to dehumanizing medical procedures like "assisted hatching." Even her emotional life is no longer her own: The powerful hormones used in treatment will buoy up her mood during mid-cycle, when she's also most hopeful of success, then leave her flat at the end of the month, when she's most likely to feel hopeless. Starting over again the next month becomes harder and harder. The woman begins to feel that her body is a factory being readied for experimental production.

She and her partner often put their lives on hold. They don't go back to school or sell the house or make the career change, because they're always waiting. That means they cannot proceed with the normal course of adult development. They're stuck. Repeated failures can be devastating to the woman's sense of self-worth and can lead to denial or desperately futile treatment. The distinguished author Susan Cheever, in her book *A Woman's Life*,[5] distills the feminist analysis of pregnancy adopted by many among the privileged point women of her Vietnam Generation: "Pregnancy is an exercise in surrender." But women who adopt this polemic and postpone indefinitely often find, at a later stage, that pregnancy becomes an exercise in desperation. Essayist Anne Taylor Fleming has written movingly of her own obsession with making up for lost time in her forties, failing to conceive, and feeling betrayed by the feminist message to her generation.[6]

Almost invariably these anxiety-ridden women confess to doctors the same regret: "Why didn't I start trying to get pregnant earlier?" Many bemoan having put career first. They fall into the same guilt cycle common among women who have had therapeutic abortions and later find themselves infertile: *I'm being punished for my past.* Yet typical of their generation, they believe if they just work hard enough they can make anything happen.

WHAT DO YOU MEAN, MY
EGGS ARE TOO OLD?

The women who turn up at infertility centers in Southern California, given that subculture's obsession with nutrition, fitness, and youthful appearance, look like the most enviable specimens of their age-group, virtual Wonder Women. Forty percent of the patients who come to Dr. Richard Marrs, one of the most respected fertility specialists on the West Coast, are women from 40 up to age 50. Their typical profile is high achievers who chose to delay pregnancy for career reasons. They can pay the fees for fancy health clubs or PTs (personal trainers) and go to spas and stay in great shape. They've "made a million," but they don't have a child. And they're desperate.[7]

The following scene is emblematic. A 45-year-old filmmaker is sitting across from Dr. Marrs in his Santa Monica office. Her husband is with her, but he scarcely says a word. She is thin, rich, and reasonably famous. There isn't an unsightly ounce on her tanned body or an unsiliconed line on her face. She is not happy.

"I've done everything," she says. "Tell me what more I need to do to have a baby."

"There's nothing more we can do," the doctor says gently. "You've taken the shots; you've shown up for the tests; you've followed everything we've asked to the letter. That's not the problem." Then the stab to the ego: "Your eggs are not allowing this to happen."

"My ovaries are not working?" The woman is stunned. "How can that be? I feel wonderful. I'm in great shape. Look at me: Don't I *look* thirty-five? I *feel* thirty-five. What do you mean, my eggs are too old?"

"It's true, you don't look anything like forty-five," says Dr. Marrs soothingly. Her husband murmurs his affirmation. "But when I stimulate your ovaries," the doctor says, "there's no question that your biologic clock is demonstrating what it should demonstrate at this age."

"Why can't you make my eggs as good as thirty-five?"

"I'm afraid we can't change the genetics of those eggs."

"Why *can't* you change it?" Anger rising. "You can make eggs, you can freeze embryos, you can insert a sperm into an egg, so why can't you make my eggs the same as a thirty-five-year-old's eggs?"

"It's a good question," says Dr. Marrs. "The answer is that's the way somebody else wanted this process to work."

The patient scoffs at this metaphysical mumbo jumbo. She insists she wants to keep going with high-tech solutions. "Okay, so I respond well to stimulation. I've done three GIFT procedures*; let's do three more. Why stop now? Money's not a problem. Do you want me to stay out here? I'll fly in and stay in a hotel for as long as you want me to. Let's just keep doing this."

"The answer is no," the doctor says. "There is no chance that in vitro will work after age forty-four."

"Okay, then let's use a surrogate," the woman prods, a grace note of panic playing over her commanding voice. "You can just put my embryos into a surrogate because my uterus is too—"

"No." The doctor stops her. "That's not the problem. It's not your uterus."

"Let's try it anyway."

"It costs fifty thousand dollars."

"No problem. Just get me a surrogate."

"No, we're not going to do that." The doctor finally exercises his pre-rogative over the woman's need to prolong the fantasy. "The only other thing we can do is change your eggs."

"You mean use some *other* woman's eggs with my husband's sperm?"

"Yes. An egg donor mother—it's the only possibility left."

"Eeeyou." The woman wrinkles up her nose like a teenager. "I don't want to go through all this for a child who won't even have my genes."

"Then this is where we have to stop treatment."

The husband, who hasn't said a word until now, finally steps in. "Look, he's right. We've got to give this up."

---

*A GIFT procedure is a method of assisted fertilization in which the physician harvests a woman's eggs by laparoscopy, a major operation under general anesthesia. The eggs are then put back into the fallopian tubes along with sperm, and fertilization takes place within the tube.

BUT SUSAN SARANDON DID IT

Doctors tell me in dismay that this is not an isolated phenomenon. More and more Boomer women over 40 are drawn to having a child as a way to delay the aging process. Becoming pregnant in one's forties is an outward sign to everyone around her that a woman is younger than her well-guarded birth certificate says she is.

"In Southern California you can look good for the rest of your life, so why can't you have a baby?" Dr. Marrs spells out the rationale. "The environment perpetuates the illusion. All my forty-three-year-old women are saying, 'Well, Susan Sarandon did it; why can't I do it?' It's competitive."

In certain enclaves of privilege, like Manhattan's Upper East Side, it used to be that well-married women competed for who could remain the thinnest. These living holograms were dubbed indelibly by Tom Wolfe the "social x-rays." Now there is a new form of one-upmanship among women of a certain age: Who has the youngest child? Much more chic than being slim is to be seated at a dinner party with an eighteen-inch clearance for the fetal mound. These Mummy Mommies, as Tom Wolfe might call them, can be heard at dinner parties reveling in nursery school talk and comparing brands of strollers with the hostess's daughter. It's a way of saying to one's peers, "*I'm* still young and fertile, I don't know about *you*." Says one obstetrician who hears this sort of chatter socially: "It's women trying to show up other women, like having a larger diamond ring."

Older women often feel pressure to perform for younger husbands. (Almost invariably you'll notice, older women who want to get pregnant are married to considerably younger men.) Getting pregnant is a tried-and-true way of locking up the deal in a nontraditional marriage. But when these women cannot reproduce the way their younger selves might have done, they worry, *What's wrong with me?* The one thing they always thought they could do was conceive a baby. No one can control her ovaries. No amount of money can buy back the magic. Refusing to give up this false self sets up many such women for an unnecessary sense of failure and makes of the midlife passage a rocky voyage.

But Susan Sarandon did it. . . . They repeat the new mantra.

Susan Sarandon had her first child when she was 38 years old. At 45 she was pregnant with her third child. She is not married. And her lover, actor Tim Robbins, is younger than she is—twelve years younger. The message here is not only that a woman can delay family but that she can find enduring love with a man who was still in kindergarten by the time she got to college.

The charming actress was nonchalant about being pregnant at 45 and said she felt strong and healthy. "I highly recommend waiting," she said at the time. "It's great when it happens late in life, because by the time you get to be forty, you have a better sense of yourself. By that time you've demystified your profession. I wasn't desperate to get anywhere other than where I was." But look where she was: one of the handful of bankable female stars over 40 in all Hollywood.

The TV heroine Murphy Brown is a merciless careerist. When the show centered on Murphy's pregnancy as an unmarried working woman in her forties, those episodes shot to number one. The show's star, Candice Bergen, had to lobby her executive producer to give Murphy more time for the homelife that her character had waited so long to build. Bergen said, "We are sending a message urging single women to have babies. The show has to portray the reality of how difficult it is. It isn't the ideal."

The myth of unlimited choice is perpetuated by novels like Terry McMillan's *Waiting to Exhale*. The heroine, a black woman professional, is blatantly narcissistic:

> I remember the day I turned thirty. I was getting out of the shower and I stood in front of the mirror and stared at myself for a long time. I examined every inch of my body and appreciated the fact that I finally looked like a grown woman. I also assumed that this was how I was going to look for the rest of my life. The way I saw it, I was never going to *age;* I'd just look up one day and be old. And Lord only knows what'd happen to my body if I were to have a baby about now. . . . I can't imagine having a baby at forty. . . . But let me shut up. If I was still able, the right man could probably talk me into having one at fifty.[8]

These movie and TV stars and fictional characters are portraying a new ideal, a customized life cycle, to be sure, but one affordable by very, very few. Ironically, even as the blurring of finite limits on fertility frees women in many ways, it holds up another ideal of flawless and ageless femininity: that a woman should be able to produce a perfect embryo *at any age*. It is as false a myth as the Western anorexic beauty ideal. In fact, it is an unattainable ideal by all but the rich, superhealthy, and very lucky.

A New York psychiatrist, Dr. Graciela Abelin-Sas, says she is beginning to see patients who are dealing with the backlash of being Midlife Moms. She describes a patient who had thoroughly enjoyed being a suburban mother. Her marriage was flagging but solid. At 42, hoping to refresh her life, she had a new baby.

"Now she's forty-seven, looking thirty-five—unbelievable," says the psychiatrist. "But when she drops her son off at kindergarten, all the other mothers are so much younger they assume she's the grandmother." Ashamed, the woman actually began to feel like a grandmother. She finally sought out the psychiatrist because she had started to hate her son. "Ironically, the little boy constantly confronts her with her age," says Dr. Abelin-Sas, "which otherwise would have been assumed to be much younger than she is."

THE FACTS ON INFERTILITY

The descent in fecundity occurs in steps, like aging in general. We go along pretty much the same until suddenly there is a significant change. The body takes time to adjust. Then we plateau until we come to the next step down. Dr. Marrs has identified three different times in reproductive life in which there is a significant change: "From about twenty-five to thirty-seven, a woman's ability to get pregnant is about the same. Then she hits the thirty-seventh, thirty-eighth year, and it drops dramatically. Then it flattens out again until forty—another break point. Somewhere between forty-two and forty-three there's another significant decline, and from then on it stays pretty flat until a woman goes into perimenopause and true menopause."[9]

East coast medical centers are more conservative, in general, about the ages of woman they will accept for treatment with assisted reproductive technology (ART). At New York Hospital–Cornell's Center for Reproductive Medicine and Infertility, directed by Dr. Zev Rosenwaks, 42 is the "quasi-cutoff" age, although it's individualized.[10] "We strongly, strongly discourage women over forty," says Dr. Jamie Grifo. "We tell them, 'Look, this has a low chance of success, so you should consider not trying.'" The center, which can boast of one of the highest success rates for in vitro fertilization in the country, now has over three years' worth of data on a total of 2,668 in vitro fertilization cycles. For women aged 37 to 39, the success rate is slightly better than 30 percent. At age 40 it drops to 22 percent. Beyond age 43 there were only three deliveries out of forty-four attempts. National statistics are even lower.*

*The National Center for Health Statistics found that of women between 35 and 44, *half* had difficulty conceiving or carrying a child to term. The chances of a 44-year-old's being able to get pregnant naturally and have a healthy child are 3 to 4 percent. Of all women in the United States who attempted in vitro fertilization in 1992, 20 percent delivered babies.

"I'm continually amazed at the number of patients you can show these data to," says Dr. Grifo, "and they'll look you straight in the eye and say, 'That's okay, I'm going to be one of the three successes out of your forty-four.'"[11]

I asked Dr. Patricia Allen, the New York gynecologist who has counseled thousands of couples and delivered children to women of all ages, what stage of life she thought was the ideal in which to complete one's child-bearing activities.

"Twenty-eight to thirty-five," she said definitively. "I feel strongly about it. Women seem to be old enough, at the age of twenty-eight, to have separated from their parents. They've had some postgraduate time to look at the options for what to do with their young adulthood. And they've had time to play. I like to see a couple married for a couple of years before having children, so that they get a chance to have fun together. After thirty-five, you may get through the pregnancy and childbirth fine, it's not that, but in families where both the father and mother are too old to play, everyone loses a lot."

Millions of women today are using hormone replacement to bypass menopause. They don't *feel* any different when they stop ovulating. And because of the effect of the hormones, they may still have periods. It's an easy step from there to the fantasy that they will be fertile indefinitely. And now technology fans that fantasy.

Since the first in vitro fertilization seventeen years ago, no genetic break-through has evoked more furor than the spectacle of postmenopausal women giving birth in their fifties and sixties. The media feed us one sensational story after another. One day it's a 59-year-old British woman, married to a 45-year-old man, who produces healthy twins. Next, the world holds a birth watch for a 63-year-old Italian woman, heralded in the summer of '94 as the oldest woman in the world to give birth. These are egg donor births. The eggs are recruited from younger women and fertilized, in vitro, by the respective husbands of the postmenopausal mothers.[12]

In fact, only 250 women in the United States attempted post-menopausal pregnancies in 1994.[13] It may seem an aberration. But the very phenomenon of postmenopausal motherhood has much wider ramifications. The danger is that it sends a message to younger women, who are already struggling just to get from A to B to C, that they can wait until they reach the pinnacles of their careers before they even think about having a baby. But it's rare to reach any sort of pinnacle before 40, whereupon even hard-core careerists are likely to blanch at facing the Barren Woman Syndrome.

SO GLAD I DIDN'T WAIT

Highland Park Hospital's Fertility Clinic sees the failures and rejects from other fertility clinics, many of whom have been told, "You're too old; you're perimenopausal." Although the suburban Chicago clinic will accept women for ART up to age 45, the director, Dr. Edward Marut, has stopped being diplomatic. He tells these women, "Beyond age forty-three, we just don't see pregnancies. It doesn't matter if a woman has had ten children before. If she's been having infertility problems, it's almost impossible after forty-three."

As the window of opportunity closes, these women become increasingly impatient, angry, and frustrated. The failure to conceive becomes an issue of global personal failure. They come to the clinic, pumped up with drugs, having contractions, and lie down to let a nurse check them out with an ultrasound instrument. When she reports, "There's only one follicle this month," the tears break. Frustration erupts. "I've been taking all these drugs, why *aren't* there more eggs?" And there, in the privacy of the examining room, with floods of tears, they let out all the grief they cannot show outside.

Lab technicians who grade the quality of eggs harvested from such patients, before they are selected to be fertilized in a petri dish, say the older egg is often irregularly shaped, dark, and granular. The zona, or outer cell layer, is thickened into a tight mesh that makes it more difficult for sperm to penetrate. A technician at Highland Hospital says: "There's a drastic difference between the egg of a twenty-year-old and the egg of a forty-year-old."

One nurse in a formal interview at her clinic projects the persona of a strong, self-confident, ambitious career woman in the scientific field—until she is asked about her children. She points to the picture of her two children on her desk. Her voice dissolves to something rounded and gentle and full of wonder. For the nurse a "miracle of birth" is not some Old Testament phrase or sappy women's fiction notion, but truly a gift to be considered with awe.

Married at 28, she wanted to enjoy being with her husband for five years. She also wanted to go to medical school. "I could see myself having put off the decision to start a family, going to medical school, and waiting until I was finished to try to conceive," she says. "I had that mentality. Even though I was in the field of ob-gyn, you always think, *It's not going to happen to me. I'm going to be fertile, no problem.*"

As it turned out, she had her first child at 30 and her second at 32. "It was just . . . a moment of passion . . . and irresponsible birth control. I realize now how fortunate that was. I look at these women, and I can see how easily I could have slipped into that. I'm so grateful that I didn't."

Today the nurse is 36 with a pair of children, two and four. Except for her children, *she* would probably be the doctor running the clinic. As a mentor to younger women who are interested in a career in medicine, she urges them to do all their training in their twenties. "If I'd been able to see into the future, I would have gone to medical school right away and waited until a convenient time during the residency to have my children. You can do it as long as you have a support system. That way, after medical school and residency, my family would be started. That pressure would be off, and I would have my practice." The added status of being a doctor would have afforded her more flexibility for parenting than being an on-duty nurse. "You can be a better budgeter of your time."

The nurse has some apprehension that she may never get back to fulfilling her dream of becoming a doctor. She worries that she won't have the confidence to do that piece once she's finished with her major mothering years. But it's much easier to go back to school in one's forties, and produce a graduate degree, than it is to produce a couple of children at that stage.

THE RACE

Pregnancy after menopause threatens the ancient concept of the human life cycle. Until now, when a woman's reproductive life came to an end, she was free to redirect her creativity into a more public sphere or to release it with artistic expression. This allowed her to fulfill the task Erikson posed as central to midlife: generativity, a voluntary obligation to care for and about others in a broader sense. The fixation on prolonging fertility, and the perpetuation of the competitive drive of youth to produce the perfect child, threaten to replace generativity with narcissism.

A new breed of fertility specialists feeds these expectations, and increasingly they do help restore the magic. In fact, an enormous industry is growing up to *franchise fertility*. We have to ask, on a societal level, What is driving this?

There is no denying that the fertility business represents a potential major cash cow to hospitals. The most prestigious hospitals dangle million-dollar offers to the most successful or splashiest fertility doctors around the world to lure them to head their all-star teams, like wooing top baseball team managers. Fertility clinics employ an aggressively hard sell. And the new Fertility Gods—almost uniformly male—are madly competing for market share. Some are financing their own private chains of fertility clinics.

Here are some pertinent facts:

—Infertility is a $2 billion-a-year business.
—There are 250 to 300 fertility clinics in the United States.
—A standard in vitro fertilization procedure costs $8,000.
—In vitro results in four thousand births annually in the United States.
—There is essentially no regulation.

In the latest field of competition, getting postmenopausal women pregnant, an Italian fertility specialist, Dr. Severino Antinori, is the record holder. His patient, 63-year-old Rosanna della Corte, was in 1994 the oldest woman in the world to give birth.[14] He has infuriated his medical school colleagues and divided public opinion in Europe with his controversial techniques. Encouraged by his wife, Dr. Antinori presents himself as a crusader for the rights of the older woman. He told 60 Minutes, "A man can be a father at sixty, seventy, eighty, I know to ninety. For women it's been impossible. Until now women have been thrown away after the menopause. To be able to have children after the menopause is revenge for women."

Revenge? Is that a healthy motive for bringing a child into the world?

Dr. Mark Sauer, an aggressive salesman for pregnancy at any age, holds the current record in the United States. He runs the largest egg donor program in Los Angeles, at the University of Southern California. Dr. Sauer, who will treat a woman of almost any age, talks about "doing the fifty-year-old woman" as if he were doing an eyelid lift. He says it's the logical step after "doing the forty-year-old woman."[15] The sales pitch is seductive. "If Warren Beatty can do it at fifty, why shouldn't a woman?" says Dr. Sauer. But Beatty didn't have a baby. He found a woman a generation younger to have a baby for him. And as Annette Bening herself reminded us about early motherhood, "You're up in the middle of the night, and even if your husband gets up—and Warren does wake up—he can't breast feed her."[16]

Dr. Sauer has what he calls a "stable" of egg producers—young donor mothers who are given massive doses of hormonal therapy to stimulate them to multiple egg production. The eggs are then fertilized by the husband of the procuring postmenopausal mother. Sauer's stable of donors is small and stimulated over and over again, with no regulation and no apparent thought given to the long-term health consequences of these stimula-tory hormones.[17]

The dehumanization of mother and child comes out in the language. Other fertility specialists I've talked to brag, "I got a girl pregnant at 54." Some boast about "getting a seventeen percent take-home baby rate."

I'm not talking now about those rare cases when a couple has lost an only child to a tragic accident or disease. Such an inconsolable loss and the need to make up for it can cause people to find superhuman strength and endurance to be late parents.

But the combination of a growing patient population of desperately childless women and a growing tribe of hustling male fertility doctors has drowned out any meaningful debate on the ethics of reproductive medicine. Eager women argue, "If technology allows it, go for it." Mainstream femi-nists tend to applaud the new developments in reproductive technology as liberating, as a way to extend childbearing options to infertile women, older women, and lesbians.[18] That begs an important question.

This is something we *can* do today. But we must think long and hard: Is this something we *should* be doing? Dr. Marrs has decided for himself: "It's a race that shouldn't be run." He believes that we have to come to grips with this life cycle issue as a nation. "We have to say no. Because we'll be pro-ducing a whole new generation of children set up to be orphans." Dr. Grifo at New York Hospital–Cornell Medical Center sees a cruel irony. "This technology which is supposed to be doing things *for* women may actually be working against them. The message it sends is a very chauvinistic one: The only thing valuable a woman can do is have babies. So prolong the magic at any price. Show your powers. It's very unhealthy."

Accounts of postmenopausal births are convincingly enthusiastic about the new meaning a child has brought the mother and her younger husband. They stress how much time and attention they can afford to devote to par-enting, surely one of the great benefits of older parenthood. "The neat thing," said Don Shearing, a 34-year-old man whose 53-year-old wife gave birth to twins with the help of fertility treatments and donor eggs, "is that Mom can afford to continue to stay home with the girls, and neither of us need worry about the mortgage."[19]

But who speaks even in these accounts about the interests of the child? Children aren't meant to be a tonic to clear up middle-age blues or cement a nontraditional marriage. What will it mean for these children, girls 16 and 17 who will have parents of 68 or 70? How does an adolescent girl identify with and learn her role cues from a woman old enough to be her grand-mother? One of the great banal tragedies traditionally suffered by males is the absence of a loving, playful pal relationship with their fathers. What will be the effect on the little boys in today's late-late second families of having a father *two* generations away from them?

Imagine being 65 when you have a 15-year-old slamming the doors and acting the way adolescents act. Imagine waiting up until two in the morning for your 15-year-old who's out with the family car and the wrong kind of friends. It's not easy to stay up past midnight when you're 50, never mind 65 or 70. The worst case, of course, would be to contract a debilitating or terminal illness before the child has had a chance to pull up roots. Loss of a parent around puberty has proved to be both psychologically and devel-opmentally a devastating experience. It can be mitigated by a close, extended family. But mothers past menopause are likely to have no living parents themselves.

Newspapers report one unimaginable new method after another. Already doctors routinely freeze the extra human embryos that are produced by in vitro fertilization. (Embryos have rights.) Thousands of these little freeze-dried prehuman vegetables sit in lockers around the nation, waiting until cou-ples decide they'd like to drop them into a warm womb and serve them up for a midlife treat. With the creation of the egg donor mother, who contributes her eggs, and the surrogate mother, who rents out her womb, children for the first time in history can have double mothers. Artificial wombs are on the drawing board. Once making babies is seen as a technological rather than a biological process,[20] any connection with a higher power or the realm of the spiritual is severed. It's hard to conceive of a "blessed event" in a petri dish.

Raising children is arguably the most important task we perform as adults. Is it really responsible to take such chances with our children's lives? What duty do we have to a generation that will outlive us? Because of ill-considered social fads like these, a whole generation of women can twist up their lives. Then society is left with a generation of children orphaned by technology and the terror of aging.

All my in vitro friends say the same thing: They didn't *want* to know. And they would risk it all over again. But once they have their babies, they become increasingly anxious and suspicious. With black humor, one woman in an in vitro fertilization program told me, "These babies might grow up to twenty and their heads will fall off, but we want them too badly to ask."

If the need to have a child or to bring another child into one's life becomes overwhelming in the forties or fifties, there are other options. I myself felt my family wasn't complete when I was in my early forties, and saw my adored daughter off to college. I adopted a 12-year-old refugee who had no parents at all. It's been a transformative experience for my husband and me as well as for our second daughter. It's not for everybody, but it is an option. It's what happens to children *after* they're born that matters, not the origin of sperm and egg. Mental health professionals were surprised by a new study of adopted adolescents that showed they enjoyed higher well-being and self-esteem than adolescents nationwide. To families like ours it comes as no surprise to read that both the teenagers in the study and their adoptive parents overwhelmingly rejected the idea that rearing a chosen child differs from rearing a biological child.[21]

There are so many children who are victims of no-parent situations, waiting to be befriended. Becoming a literacy volunteer or a Little League coach is a way to spend time with children and enjoy the good feeling of generativity as well. Publicist Peggy Siegal takes a delightedly active role in the life of her niece, throwing her birthday parties and taking her on vacations. On a grander scale, a childless woman of great talent like Joan Ganz Cooney was able to found the Children's Television Workshop and *Sesame Street* and to know she has a profound impact on millions of little ones. Until these contributions are valued as highly as birthing one's own child, we will continue to see women over 40 flogging themselves for failing to be one of the high-tech fertility success stories.

The truth is, we all have to accept realities at each stage of life. It is very hard to give up the magic of fertility, but when we do, like any sacrifice—if it is consciously made—we have the opportunity of replacing whatever has been sacrificed with something better.

6

PERPETUAL MIDDLESCENCE

*E*ven after hitting an early crisis point in the forties, some people shrink from any suggestion that midlife is upon them. Does this describe you? The more you are made aware of your chronological age, the more oddly estranged you become from it. "Adulthood" seems to describe other people—your parents, your doctor, your boss—but not you.

The alternative for most of those who refuse to enter Second Adulthood is to go in circles, 'round and 'round in a *perpetual middlescence,* a holding pattern that sometimes lasts into their fifties. Middlescence is fine as a transition phase. But a long-deferred midlife passage will rise up later, with a vengeance. You may recognize variations on this phenomenon from several biographical sketches.

HOLDING THE EDGE

"What are you, in your mid-forties?" I take a guess before interviewing the brilliant entrepreneur whom I'll call Charles.

"No, no!" he yelps. "I'm not in my *mid*-forties yet. I'm forty-four. I won't be there for another fifteen days."

A tall, handsome Harvard man, Charles is a late developer, and, like many men of his generation, he is obviously determined to plug up every crack in the Chinese wall that separates him from middle age. Naturally some of the mortar has already crumbled. There is a slight pearishness to his silhouette, but the spidery lines on his forehead and pinstripes of gray in his thick black hair do not show until one gets up close. He sees them, though, and for the first time in his life he feels time pressure. "Big-time," he says.

He confesses that he didn't even begin pulling up roots until his early thirties. "I was on an endless graduate school ride, just lying around having a great time, taking no responsibility." At 30 he settled into a very comfortable job track with a nationwide financial consultancy firm, a groove that would have allowed him to rock along for another twenty-five years, whereupon he could have retired enviably. But the inner impulse to "become my own man" overwhelmed him in his early forties. He quit corporate life, cashed out, and found an ailing consumer research company to buy. Beyond the commercial lure, he believed he could make the firm a major fountain of sociological research.

All swagger and thrust the first few months, Charles swore he would take the company to new peaks of success and national recognition. Indeed, he put that process in motion. Less than two years later, however, as he approached the brink of turning 45, the creative part of shaking up and reorganizing the place had paled into the tasks of everyday management. "I'm tired," he told me. "I spend most of every day just selling the hell out of our services and watching overhead." If he had any illusions of doing meaningful research, they were dashed. As a midlife solution this move did not provide the meaning for which he is looking. Charles has begun to feel more restless than ever. The obsession with prolonging his youthful edge now becomes paramount.

What does 50 look like to you? I ask.

"I'm not going to turn fifty," he replies with a sly smile. "Around fifty, you literally begin slowly to die."

How does he plan to circumvent it?

"I'm going straight to Mexico and get hold of some human growth hormone. Before I ever get to fifty and start losing brain cells."

The fervor over this new antiaging panacea for men was set off in 1990, with a report by Daniel Rudman of the Medical College of Wisconsin on the results of his pioneering experiment of injecting human growth hormone into men over 60. The overall effect on the male physique, reported the investigator, was equal to shedding ten to twenty years.[1] These remarkable results, although not yet replicated, have caused a proliferation of Mexican longevity clinics that offer the drug at a cost of $13,000 for a year's supply. The drug hasn't been approved by the U.S. government because of suspected devastating side effects, not the least of which is the Dorian

Gray—style reversal of magical results unless the drug is taken continuously.[2] Meanwhile, there is no evidence that human growth hormone increases the life span.

"I know all that," Charles says, unblinking. He agrees that there is a male potency crisis in middle life, and he believes it has a sexual component. "But I'm not doing this so I can be a sexpot. Look, when you've grown up all your life knowing that you had something extra in gray matter"—he taps his veiny temple—"I'm doing this because if I lose ten IQ points by turning fifty, I get to be *ordinary.* I can't afford that. The skin is another consideration. The longer I look young, the longer I hold my edge."

Charles is ready to jump right in and deal with middlescence pharmacologically, the way he and his generation have dealt with so much else. He's willing to try an illegal, unproved drug to preserve youth *now,* even if it shortens his life. He will either be the envy of all his friends or go out with style and flourish. "I have it all planned," he says. "At fifty I'm going to take the money and run. Maybe my wife and I will become missionaries."

The next cautionary tale concerns a female version of the male *Wunderkind.* Often such recognized successes, whether men or women, have the hardest time making it through middlescence since they face the problem of following their own act. Addicted as they are to success for the sake of success, the compulsion to prove themselves as top performers prompts them to take higher dares and to need more potent "drugs" to keep up the adrenaline rush. What they really need to do is to listen to other voices in those inner rooms they have kept locked up until midlife. But too often the time pressure at this stage urges them to race even faster in an even narrower track.

A WOMAN ADDICTED TO SUCCESS, AGE 52

Racing against the clock. 'Round and 'round the racetrack, speeding her Ferrari, feeling time blur, faces effaced, the excitement of losing all dimensions, the roar of the engine reverberating in her loins, so thrilling it's almost like anonymous sex—watch out, Mr. Porsche! This is a lady who doesn't like to lose.

Indeed, the lady beneath the racing helmet is accustomed to winning in her world. Jill, I'll call her, is a fashion designer in Dallas who finally became successful enough to have her label on a dress line. But in the world of high-performance racing she is somebody else, a deliberately anonymous, mysterious, and sexy woman who talks cars with men.

"I always wanted to be one of the boys," Jill admitted when I first interviewed her. She was 46 and compelling, her large pale eyes rimmed in black and her body so slim and flexible she could sit on the floor with her legs folded, pretzel-style, like a teenager. "Nondescript" is how she describes herself as a child. But she patterned herself after her brash, extroverted father. When the family moved to West Los Angeles, "we ran into a very Reform, country club Jewish clique. To compete, my father always had the flashiest car. We had the first TV on the block." Her cautious mother, who wanted only that Jill marry rich, tried to intercede with lots of don'ts. Jill ignored them.

Jumping over the ravine was the first dare of her girlhood. Boys did it. Ignoring her terror, she jumped with the boys. But she also made certain all through high school that she had the best boyfriends. "I acquired them," she says. "I wanted those men in my control." At 52 she still relies on her sexuality as the primary source of her power. She acquires men like trophies.

Jill bought the whole male mystique. She developed a wisecracking, confrontational style tempered with seductiveness, an extreme defense against the certain punishment she faced for violating cultural norms as a woman with ambitions. By the time Jill was in her early twenties and working in the fashion business, she felt she was "destined for something great." No specific dream or clear goal formed in her mind, only the need—and total determination—to be a top performer. She married, mainly for her mother's sake. Her husband was agreeable enough, but when he pressed the subject of children, she felt oddly panicky.

"Being a mother translated for me as a loss of sexual power," she later realized. "I did not see anything positive about being a mother—I still don't—which is sad, because I know I'll probably miss not having children or that kind of connection." When she and her first husband dissolved what remained of their union, she realized with a curious numbness, "I just threw away seven years."

In her thirties she was at the top of her game. The chairman of a prestige department store chain spotted her work and offered to double her salary if she would design exclusively for him. She asked for her own in-store boutique and got it, turning it into a gold mine for the company. A few years later she paused in her frenetic work schedule long enough to marry the chairman, at city hall, on a lunch break. "He was fearless. I loved that." Jill was still operating from the mind-set that said the top man is the trophy. "I married him because I was afraid to lose him." She had to acquire him before somebody else did, and in the process she hoped to osmose his power. It worked for a while. They were a formidable power couple.

Jill continued to work nonstop, nurturing her design assistants and lavishing attention on the buyers. This little "home" within the parent company became for her the surrogate for a family. She improved every aspect of the flagship store until it noticeably outperformed the rest of the company. Then the parent company began to slip, and fast. The chairman prevailed upon Jill to take over management of the chain's entire fashion division.

"Our marriage was over the minute I said yes." She can see that in retrospect. "He was very jealous of my happiness and independence. Success was my identity. I *had* to bring up the entire division, both for the company and for myself." The effort pitted her against her husband's authority in one of those competitive power struggles that become all snarled up with sexual politics. *Who's really running this company anyway?*

Their divorce battle was, for Jill, a dare, like jumping over the ravine in her girlhood. Never showing a jot of fear, Jill hung tough and walked away a winner. Once she was out of battle mode, however, the moment of recognition came too late: *I'm doing this all over again—disposing of a life.* By then Jill's pattern was so nearly indelible, she went on to repeat it in a public confrontation with the chairman of the next company where she worked. Given her own label to be marketed nationally, she made an ambitious five-year business plan. But recession cut into her profits badly, and the chairman told her she would have to scale back drastically. She might easily have been adorable and teased him out of it: "Come on, you're a gambler, we'll look at the P and Ls again in a year when you see how much money we're going to make." But she didn't. She saw it as another win-lose confrontation, and if she lost, she would die. So she said the unforgivable:

"I have the balls. I'm up for taking the risk. Why won't you play it out like you promised?"

The chairman wouldn't back down. Virtually overnight Jill was out of business. It was the first professional disappointment she had ever suffered. "I was over it in a week," she told me, shrugging with characteristic bravado. "I've had so much loss in my life I just want to move on."

Failure can be one of the most useful experiences of adult life, but only for those who stop long enough to learn from it. Jill finds it too threatening to dwell on failures. She cuts her losses, cauterizes her emotions, and sprints forward double time to find the next hurdle. Professionally she continued fearlessly taking risks and resisting bureaucratic stagnation. There was no question that she would find another home for her obvious talents. But this defeat had coincided with her long-postponed passage into midlife. The accumulated toll of personal losses and career setbacks was beginning to be apparent when we met for a follow-up interview in the summer of '93.

The woman waiting at a sidewalk café had dropped five pounds. Chic as ever, she was still stunning, but the sides of her face had fallen a bit. She was considering a face-lift. "I'm racing even faster than I was before I was closed down," she said tensely.

Jill had gone back to take up her preadolescent persona—the daredevil girl who was allowed to be one of the boys. Her father had since died and willed her his vintage Ferrari. Jill took it out of storage and reconditioned it. This sleek, souped-up projectile was now the battle machine into which she climbed every weekend, like some dazzling Boadicea in her knife-spoked chariot, to compete on racetracks all across Texas. At the racetrack her identity as a name in the fashion industry is deliberately disguised.

"This sounds so silly, but there is some key in this." She tried to explain. "I've had a great need to be anonymous with men. Dating relationships where my job or my life remains completely unknown. They may not necessarily ever be consummated sexually. I enjoy the 'play' of just having a good time. That's what the car racing is for me."

The symbolism is blatant. Here is a woman who has measured her worth by money and sexual conquest, just like the men who have been her mentors and models in corporate life. But aging undercuts her sexual power. So she has taken on the armor of her dead father. Jill's dream remains unchanged: to be a successful performer. Did she see that she was addicted to success?

"Because of my father? Probably. I was forever trying to catch his eye. I guess I've been addicted to success ever since I was a girl."

She was considering switching to a whole new career, possibly the movie business or performance art, another hurdle on which to prove herself. "It's about accomplishing dreams and being impossibly young always."

At its core Jill's struggle is one we all fight within ourselves, if not at 50, then before: how to accept our own limitations and ultimately our mortality. One hears in her words, and in those of male *Wunderkinder* like her, a more dramatic extreme of a wish many successful people dream of fulfilling: *Once I become the chairman, or the director or the tenured professor, or design the software, or concoct the car, or write the screenplay, or produce the talk show that captures the spirit of the times, everyone will recognize me, admire me, defer to me. I will be a hero, and then I can indulge myself in all the desires I have been denied or denied myself.* Another variation of this gratification fantasy, the Nixonian variation, goes like this: *Once I become rich and powerful, no one can ever make me feel small or second-class again or treat me like a helpless little boy or girl.*

Still driven to be the good-little-girl performer for her father, Jill spells out the fantasy: Each new success is expected to make possible the impossible—"to be young always." Rather than use middlescence to plumb her depths, she will work harder to maintain her youthfulness and sexual power by settling for experiences that are more and more superficial. "If I could just stand still—making pottery, playing pool—maybe I don't have to be a grown-up and have a job," she contemplated aloud. "Maybe, I mean maybe, I could be comfortable living on a plate of hors d'oeuvres."

But what is the price? I asked Jill where she found intimacy. Was there anyone with whom she could share the kinds of fears that wake us up at four in the morning? She was somewhat unnerved by the moment of self-revelation.

"I have such people less and less." She hesitated. "Actually I don't have anyone else to tell my truths to besides my best friend."

Until the next great career leap, she will continue to feed her success addiction with high-performance driving. 'Round and 'round middlescence she goes, testing how fast and how far she can outrace the shadows of the afternoon of life.

"Speed is so exciting. It's the biggest high I've had. You get so high you can't come down from it. It's absolute lift. It's the edge of speed. *It's flight.*"

FROZEN IN TIME

The feminist leader, an archetypal national figure known for her brains and beauty for the last twenty-five years, sat beside me for an intimate chat. She was in her mid-fifties at the time, but no one would have known if she didn't tell. She looked frozen in time. Nothing had changed. With fierce maintenence she was still pencil slim, leggy, flat-tummied, and pillowy-cheeked. Having run through a series of what she calls "little marriages," but never having really settled down, she was still a nomad, dropping in for the weekend with another rich widower. She had always insisted the personal was political and resisted looking inside. But at closer range, a sadness seemed to have settled in her face. She moved without animation, as if afraid to crack the shell that had served her so long, not knowing what, if anything, lay deeper. She was stuck. And she knew it.

"I'd been dealing with aging by defiance," Gloria Steinem told me in that conversation in the summer of '89. "I said, 'Fuck this, I'm going to go right on doing everything I've been doing in the past.'" She would defy aging as she had defied sexism. But imagine the terror, wondering when the morning might come that she would wake up to find the garden of her beauty drained of color overnight and suddenly shriveled, like proud mums after the killing frost. She had countered such images with her earthy sense of humor.

"I was going to become a pioneer dirty old lady, the Ruth Gordon of my generation." She giggled. "A very old lady who dresses very inappropriately." As she sat, immobilized in a deep chintz sofa, still wearing her deliberately unladylike short skirt and long, straight Sixties hair, a recent, painful revelation came out. "It took me a while to realize that although you're defying convention, which is what I've always done, you're not progressing. You're staying where you are."

Eventually the predictable crises of adult life catch up with all of us, even the famously nonconformist Gloria. That was the summer she found herself blocked even in her writing. She was supposed to be writing a book about self-esteem. There was a reason she had chosen that subject, and she had finally stumbled upon it: This was a book she badly needed to read. In direct contradiction to her public image as an articulate, self-assured, utterly original thinker, Gloria acknowledged that she still had not learned to rely on her own authority.

As a child Gloria had reversed roles with her invalid mother, an experience shared by many whose parents were ill, alcoholic, or otherwise unable to function. Taking the part of child-mother had redoubled the culturally female pattern of always being the nurturer, never the nurtured. In order to protect herself from being trapped again in the mothering role, she nurtured others at a distance or collectively.

"I was already in my mid-thirties when feminism came along to rescue me from feeling I had to be a mother," she said. "Even when I got to be fifty and I didn't have children, [I wasn't] saying to myself I should worry about my biological clock. Many of the things that encourage those crises weren't present in my life." As an adult before she ever had a chance to be an adolescent, Gloria had simply reversed many of life's passages or bypassed them.

Never moving from sister to mother, or from lover to wife, or from beautiful young woman to mature woman, Gloria had skirted all those telltale milestones—births, anniversaries, children's graduations, becoming mother of the bride—that of themselves accumulate meaning and leave a proud trail in the wake of rushing years. The meaning of her life was almost entirely externalized: A social movement became her family, along with friends and lovers.

Eventually, however, we reach a point where we can no longer pretend away this passage through middlescence. We have the chance to grow into a full humanity that is beyond the confinements of gender. Even if one waits perilously late to make this transition, it is still possible to pull out of the holding pattern and progress.

"For me it wasn't until I was past fifty that a change occurred," said Gloria, "and that turned out to be a very big change. Exhaustion became my signal."

Like a thunderhead that sits dark and heavy over all the sky one can see, fatigue rose up and overwhelmed her. Worn down, her denied and unlived adolescence began to break surface. Again, Gloria looked to others for what she needed to find within. She attached herself to a rich and powerful man who seemed to require no caretaking at all. And what a wonderful rescue fantasy it was while it lasted—all fun and games, dancing and laughter, cruises and private planes. "Mismatch, desperate, doomed," muttered her good friends. The dramatic contrast between the man's easy wealth and Gloria's daily efforts in the trenches to champion the poor made her feel progressively worse about herself.

After two years she was diagnosed with breast cancer.

She remembers her first thought: "*I've had a wonderful life!* That thought just rose up from deep inside and washed over me." With the stark realization of what she loved about her life, she dealt with the lumpectomy and radiation treatments straight on and recovered quickly. But being a woman in her fifties faced with the life accident of breast cancer represented, finally, a clear marker of age and a warning: That long-postponed midlife passage would no longer wait.

"I tried to say consciously, 'Now, wait a minute, this is important, listen to this, let it tell you that you need to choose what's important and what isn't.' " She recounted the battle with herself. "We always have little cancer cells running around in our systems. The question is, How long can the immune cells keep fighting them off? With an externalized life, and almost no experience at taking good care of myself, my female conditioning had been doing me in—literally."

It was a postfeminist Aha! moment. That understanding, Gloria says, not only allowed her to leave behind an incongruous relationship but also prompted her to rest and take time for the internal voyages that no one else can provide once we are adults. She tried to use this life accident to remind herself of her mortality, an awareness, she acknowledges, that may be harder to come by for those without the visible marker of parenthood.

"For a long time it [aging] felt like a loss," she told me during this period. "Then gradually I began to realize it wasn't a loss; it was another country."

Cutting back on her constant traveling, she took pleasure in creating her first real home out of a chaotic apartment. Gloria Steinem plumping pillows and feeding a cat and giving a damn if the sheets match—yes! It felt very good to mother herself, at last. Ultimately Gloria did look inward, bringing from the depths of her own struggle for self-esteem her best-selling book *Revolution from Within*.[3]

She turned 60 at a surprise party in her favorite soul food hangout, Jezebel's, where the room pulsed with the warmth and love of her many friends. Gloria was already on a new journey, exploring the even freer country beyond 60 in which women, she believes, become themselves at last.

"The victory is not just hanging on to what you already have against all onslaughts," she realized, "but going on to something different, and better."

SINGLE MEN: WHAT ARE YOU DOING FROM FIVE TO NINE?

The age of 50 seems to represent a sort of tollgate, beyond which, having chosen the route and the traveling companions, one expects to be on the same road for a long, long time. Thus people who find themselves approaching 50, unattached—either divorced or never married—are particularly prone to playing out a perpetual middlescence.

Even if they are certain they don't want to be tied down to marriage, there is at least some ambivalence about traveling alone through the unmarked second half of the life journey. This is particularly true of men, I find. Seeking substitute social networks once they drop off the Rolodexes of their married friends, unattached men and women in their forties often develop single-sex circles. I sat in on informal get-togethers of two such circles.

Every Friday night a group of unattached Seattle men between 40 and 50 gets together at a waterfront fish house.* These are businessmen who wolf down *The Wall Street Journal* with jelly doughnuts before sliding into

*The location and identities of the men have been disguised, but all of their substantive comments are verbatim.

their dark, phallic cars, lawyers who accelerate to beat the lights at busy intersections, pols who punch the speakerphone in the car so an intern in the passenger seat is sure to hear them chew out a slack-work aide. By day they endlessly compare and compete over the latest gear they bought for ski-ing or sea kayaking or over the contributions they are making to inner-city school kids. They boast about the vacations they take and about the women they make, or lie about those they don't. But at 5:00 P.M., or 6:00 or 7:00 if they work late, they are painfully reminded of the one thing they don't have, none of them: a real home to go home to.

"Even though one of us sits behind a judge's robe, and another one is powerful enough to take the middle of the day off to fly down to L.A. and date a movie star, we share a secret," said Simon, a 48-year-old magazine publisher. "Each one of us knows that the others are a little fucked up, too." It is beginning to dawn on these men that if they are not in committed rela-tionships by age 50, chances are they won't be able to make the conversion to accept the mores and sexual demands of women in their age-group who have changed so drastically over the past two decades.

The after-work hours are the cruelest. That's the time most of them were accustomed to coming home to the traditional marriage, to wriggling effu-sions from the children, to fussing over by the wife, to the privilege of enthronement in "Daddy's chair" while the man of the house waited for his social life to be arranged for the evening. Those marriages have gone the way of rotary lawn mowers. These divorced men are on their own. Their former wives are catching up on careers; their children are scattered. The weeknight hours between five and nine, emptied of stroking, are now an intimacy void. To nullify the emptiness, these men spend several nights a week at the health club, pulling laps, pumping iron, lolling in the whirlpool, then stretching out on chaises to contemplate the aloof majesty of snow-capped mountains from the club's high floor. Still, that leaves Friday night. . . .

How do I murder time between five and nine?

They seek each other out in this noisy fish-slinging restaurant so they can murder time by trading trivia and telling war stories of middle-aged dating, but mostly so they can stop pretending for a few hours. The necessity to compete is blessedly suspended. As Simon says, "Each one of us knows that the others can say, 'So what if you won the case? We know you're an asshole who can't get a date.'"

Simon arrives first in his hip black loose-sleeved shirt, designer-belted over Polo pants. A red-haired, moderately handsome Jewish man, he sits hunched over at the long trestle table, pursing his lips as if to hold his emotions in check as he tells me his story in monotone.

"Basically what happened, my mother passed away when I was sixteen. My mother was a very sexual being. She was sick with cancer for five years. She would ask me to massage her body. I watched her get thinner." He chokes up. "She died when she was still a young, beautiful woman. I haven't met anybody that can compare with her."

Simon goes on at great length about his phlegmatic aspirations, his conventional twenty-two-year-long marriage: "I was supposed to be the provider; she'd be the housekeeper; we'd bring up children and have a life basically like our parents had." But his wife turned into a radical environmentalist, while Simon hired a gorgeous Filipino girl and tried to turn her into his Woody Allen Asian girltoy. "I was used to always having a young woman work for me, a gofer, like a toy. I was paying this one good money, she was a high school dropout, but I dumped on her too much." He broods. "She left. It destroyed me. I broke down and cried." He was 40 then, with a solid job but no dream, a failed marriage but no insight into why. "I just went on day to day, no crisis. It's only approaching fifty that I feel time is running out."

Consider Simon a man stopped in his emotional development at the point in puberty when his mother took ill. After being quite seductive with her son, she died on him before he was out of adolescence. Mother remains the elusive ideal, a woman who never grew old, a love that was never consummated. Simon continues to look for another mother figure who will devote herself to taking care of him while being dependent upon him. He is still shopping for what he calls "the blueprint Jewish wife."

But it's intimidating out there today. "You're swimming in an ocean you never swam in before." He sighs. "The fish are a little bigger. The competition is with other boyfriends, maybe younger, maybe superrich. All these guys I get together with, at this stage we're looking for companionship. Romance. Flowers. The whole deal. It's the generation. But women today are *personalities*. That's a hard thing to accept."

Before Simon can slip into a Friday night funk, his buddies show up at the fish house. Soon the table looks like a jeans commercial: yuppies sitting around in their Dockers pants, but advanced by thirty years, with their résumés filled out and their jeans elasticized. The waiter takes their orders.

"Give me a Haake-Beck beer."

"I'll pass."

"You have any of that Ariel wine?"

Wimps, the waiter's expression says; these are nonalcoholic drinks. Most of these men have had serious drinking or chemical dependency problems, so they abstain completely.

"I'll take a Jack Daniel's black, straight up," says Bruce, the only one of the group who is married. He's just started on his third wife; she's younger than his daughter.

"Bruce still has neurons to burn," they tease him.

"Yeah, you know why his wife let him out tonight?" The politician retails the latest John Bobbitt joke. "A detachable prick—wives love it. 'Sure, honey, you want to go out with the boys? Just leave your prick on the table. I'll keep it in the fridge.' "

They talk sports trivia, quiz one another on lyrics to old songs and who said which line in vintage movies. Then the talk turns, as always, to the enemy.

"So how'd it go with your movie star?" Simon asks the society dermatologist.

"I blew the date, I was sure of it," he said. "I didn't hear from her for three days. But just before I came out to meet you suckers, she called!" The dignified dermatologist was momentarily reduced to a pimply teenager on cloud nine.

Middle-aged dating is adolescence all over again. The same fears, same roller coaster of emotions—from boldness to acute embarrassment, elation to degradation, passion to despair.

"I met a woman at a party Saturday night that I was interested in," says the suddenly timid judge. "Should I call or not call? Finally I took a chance. Thank God, I just got a message machine."

The biggest risk for these unattached men at this stage in their lives is that a woman will reject them and that the whole aura of success and cocksure confidence might crumble. Their careers no longer pose any real risk. The corporate lawyer could do deals in his sleep; the dermatologist fantasizes about the girls at the health club while he burns the billionth keratosis off a patient; the politician happens to be out of public office. "I'm so depressed and bored," he tells his buddies. "I get up, I know I'm going to have lunch. That gives me something to do. I go home and take a nap and watch TV and wait to have dinner. Even meeting with you bozos, it's better than being home alone with Nancy and the kids gone."

Murdering time. When they were younger, the thrill was in the game, the thrust and parry of competition, the pride and purpose of bringing home the bacon for families. Now there's no one home to cook it. Going out to restaurants, even with a good-looking date, isn't the same thing.

"It's like a lion in the jungle," Simon theorizes. "If you bring the food to him, he's not a lion anymore."

The men study their menus and give their meticulously individualized orders. They talk a little about their relationship to the wider world, where they fit, but soon the conversation drifts back to the same obsession: Is anyone even close to finding a decent woman to marry?

"This woman I met in the pool of my condo complex, you know, the one with the nice body and pretty smile?" Simon picks up his story. "We start talking. Same age, same background, our parents went to the same temple. I'm thinking, *blueprint.*"

"That's a tip-off right there—boring," says the politician.

"No, listen," says Simon. "She brings me right into her home with her children. I'm supposed to sleep with her, with her *mother* there. She says, 'I'm great in bed, and I like wild sex.' But when I got her into bed, I wasn't—and I knew."

"Knew what?" the guys prod.

"I was trying too hard."

"Heavy lifting." One of the men nods.

"Yeah, it was *work.* So I couldn't perform. I slipped out of the covers before she woke up, and I went off to play golf."

"They're all a little goofy, these women today." The politician shrugs. *Goofy* is the group's all-purpose word for the things they can't stand about contemporary women: They're aggressive, they like control, they make their own money, and they're just as likely to be sexual predators as a man.

"Hell, I want to 'go steady' before I graduate from high school." The judge tortures a metaphor. In other words, he longs for romance, security, and, above all, companionship.

"I took out this gorgeous chick the other night," says the businessman. "Something turned me off when it came to the clinch. She's wearing *aftershave.*"

"Who are we kidding?" Simon blurts. "We need them, but they scare the shit out of us. Finding fault with every one of them is just a way to find an excuse not to make a commitment."

The one attached man in the group blots his lips after a big meal. "Well, hell, I'm on my third marriage, and you know what? It's a goddamn relief." This man appears disgustingly happy. The others all look upon him with naked envy.

SINGLE WOMEN: TALES FROM
THE NAKED CITY

I also sat in on groups of formerly married women in their forties. But wait a minute, there was a startling difference here. The old pictures of the weepy, marriage-starved middle-aged woman and the devil-may-care elusive bachelor have switched frames. So confident are successful working women becoming that there is life after youth, many do not waste time clinging to unhappy marriages for economic security in midlife. *Guess what?*

> Among divorced couples between the ages of 45 and 54 it is the *women* who are *choosing* to stay single more than the men.[4]

This is another one of the great revolutions in the adult life cycle over the last twenty years. Divorce is occurring with greatest frequency among people aged 40 to 54. The number of women in that age-group who shed husbands surged from 1.5 million in 1970 to 6.1 million in 1991.[5] As reported by Jane Gross in *The New York Times*, demographers and sociologists agree that increasingly it is women past their childbearing and -rearing years—if they have gained financial and sexual independence—who see a return to wifely status as a bad bargain.

For such women, perpetual middlescence isn't necessarily a drag. It can be a romp for a while, especially if it follows stages of long matrimonial confinement.

The Girlfriends, a half-dozen high-powered Chicago professionals, meet for high tea in the Greenhouse of the Ritz Carlton.* They are the equivalent of the Seattle men in accomplishment: a stockbroker, a couple of lobbyists, a public relations maven, a corporate lawyer, and a former state commissioner. All divorced. All between 40 and 50. All have what Simon would call "personalities." Their teatime is a delicious interlude when they can dish about the last disastrous mismatch before the next blind date.

Three of the women arrive promptly at five, all dressed in the power woman uniform of 1993: black mid-calf skirts each with a slit up to *there* and black stretch ankle boots fitted like a condom. They exude confidence,

---

*The location and identities of the women have been disguised, but all of their substantive comments are verbatim.

playfulness, and sexual energy. All have been up since six and worked out; they give their orders for herb tea and sparkling water, no alcohol. Suddenly Beryl whirls into the restaurant and past the waiter with her felt fedora and fuzzy hair, moving with all the bombast of a Bette Midler. She grabs center stage with her first words.

"I see you're all wearing your FMBs, too." They know she means "fuck me boots."

"You never know." Laura, the former commissioner, imitates eyelash batting. A sexy, animated woman with big dark brown eyes and a generous mouth, Laura jams her long fingernails into her bowlful of curly hair and flips it. She has just come back from a business trip to New York. "Wanna hear?"

"More Tales from the Naked City?" prompts Beryl. "Tell."

"He was at the Plaza, and I was at the Waldorf." Laura builds the drama. "He wanted me to stay afterward, but I felt like waking up alone. So there I was at three in the morning, *breezing* out of the Plaza, I'm feeling great, summer night, the sex had been swell, but the *reeelly* nice part"—she loops a finger through her big hoop earrings and hums deliriously—"I did exactly what I wanted to do. I didn't have to fall in love with somebody just because I want to go to bed with him. I didn't even have to stay till morning."

Always before this, Laura was married. She went from her father's house to her first husband at 20, produced two children, and scarcely paused between divorce and the second traditional marriage. Finding herself single for the first time at—what age? She's reluctant to say . . . "Let's just say, late forties"—she is *loving it.* Laura says she is just coming out of her "Chinese menu phase," meaning the year she has taken to taste the illicit pleasures of sex with an assortment of male lovers, mostly younger: a hot sports star, a baby diplomat. Lately it's a 28-year-old art student. She is discovering the marvelous range of her own sexuality for the first time.

Dot, a divorced attorney from an Irish Catholic blue-collar background, talks about her elaborate evasions of remarriage. "The men I meet take you out for a few weeks and all of a sudden they want to know when they can move in."

"They want a quick answer so they can move on to the next one." Laura giggles.

"They're either very needy or phobic about making another commitment," says Beryl.

"It's part of recognizing they're on the downhill slope," comments Dot. "For myself, I feel *younger* now than before my divorce."

"It's aging to be married to someone you're not happy with," adds Laura. "How's *your* love life, Beryl?" she asks.

"I'm so tired of limp dicks."

Flipping the challis shawl off the shoulders of her business suit, Beryl complains that every single man she's gone out with, no matter how hot the chase and how romantic the dinner and how reckless the disrobing scene, at the last moment *shrivels* and then runs away. She updates the group on the story of the macho CEO who had been chasing her around the office incessantly—"I mean, *panting* after me." She had finally relented and let him take her to dinner. But she laid on the theater tickets, front row center. Afterward she invited him upstairs.

"What happens? He can't get it up. After coming on like Arnold Schwarzenegger, I thought he was going to *die.* So I said, 'It's okay, I'll just give you a massage.' I open the closet where I keep my fifty-seven flavors of scented oils, and he *freaks.* He literally ran out of my house as fast as he could. Later I find out the jerk is married anyway."

Laura offers her critique. "You didn't have to buy the theater tickets. And a whole closet full of oils, the guy must have felt like a bimbo."

"No, no," counters Dot, "he was just hoping Beryl would be his pick-me-up affair."

"I'm not like Beryl," says Laura. "I would *never* pay for a man." Laura is secure enough in her appeal as a woman that even though she's in the habit of advising a governor, in this delicate business of middle-aged dating she lets the man set the pace and style. "I'm open to new experiences."

Her experiences do not necessarily end up wonderfully. Laura updates the story of her "high school romance" with the 28-year-old she met at an intimate club in a summer resort. They danced reggae together, he asked to walk her home, kissed her good night—zowie, the flash! "I told him I was divorced, but I left out two husbands and two children." She chuckles. "He assumed I was much younger." After a steamy month's romance Laura agreed to meet her young man in Mexico.

"It was all over when *his mother called.* She asked me to bring him his allergy medicine. All I could think about was, *Can I get my frequent flier miles back?*" Laura laughs uproariously. But she already has a new love interest in London.

Beryl classifies Laura as one who "always sees the glass half full." She describes herself with deadly accuracy as "one who's always looking for the Prozac around the corner." Single for longer than any of the Girlfriends, Beryl, now 44, lives with her 14-year-old daughter. A rainmaking stockbroker with a nationwide firm, she is always appearing on TV or giving lectures on economics at prestige city clubs.

"This year has been my lowest—the pits," she says. "Externally I've had nothing but fabulous successes. I'm at the top of my game professionally. But internally I keep asking, 'Is this all there is?' " She hasn't had more than a few dates in the past twelve months. At her birthday party the previous Sunday night she did the toast with her usual comic put-down: "I started out this year dancing at the White House and ended up the year on two different antidepressants."

Basically Beryl admits in a small voice, "I feel terribly sad that I'm not in a relationship." She digs her knife into a ripe fig and pries out the succulent pink center.

Despite the many parallels, the Girlfriends' conversation was dramatically different from that of the guys' group. The difference was not in worldly success. The lady commissioner had no better position than the gentleman politician; Beryl, the stockbroker, was no more prominent in her city than Simon, the publisher, was in his. The steam seems to have gone out of the men's ambitions. Once their marriages broke up, their lives dropped away from them. They don't know what to do about it. They are truly alone, treading water. Some will make it out of middlescence, and others likely will not.

For the women it is a thrill to be in the power structure at all and to be able to raise the level of their professional game. Notably the women are not as desperate as the men to get back into marriage. They find it a relief not to have to nurture for once. With the exception of Beryl, perpetual middlescence is turning out to be the time of their lives.

"Adolescence is so much more fun the second time around!" Laura enthuses. "I feel much younger than I did when I was twenty-two and married." Her children tell her, "You never had any time to figure out who *you* were." "Until I was divorced from my second husband, I could *never imagine* living the rest of my life alone," says Laura. "My mother brought me up that you are defined by being married. I find, on the contrary, I *relish* being single. When both my children were launched at the same time as my second separation, it felt like a huge *liberation*."

Laura is prototypical of those formerly married women who, earning enough money by this age to support themselves comfortably enough, are excited about no longer defining themselves through men. When they divorce, their concerns are mostly pragmatic: How much money do they need, if and where to relocate, how to make unfamiliar decisions? "They do well socially because they have friends and bonding skills," points out Frances Goldscheider, a sociology professor at Brown University.[6]

In my observation, these unencumbered professional women—particularly the veterans of traditional marriages—are more playful than their male counterparts, not as uptight, curious about going back to pick up on the experimentation they may have missed by being on the cusp of the sexual and women's revolutions.

"I don't meet many men in their late forties and fifties who are joyful," says Laura. "I used to spend my life juggling everybody else's. Now you want to know my greatest secret pleasure?" She makes an angel face. "On a Friday night to rent two movies and *stay in bed*—what incredible freedom!"

For both men and women a committed marriage to one's best friend is one of the best predictors of high well-being. This truth is validated by study after study, including my own most recent Life History surveys with both sexes and different social classes.[7] But in mediocre or poor marriages, wives are the main losers.

"Marriage is an institution that primarily benefits men," holds University of Washington psychologist Neil Jacobson, whose work on women and depression has won awards.[8] He is among a growing number of experts whose studies have drawn the same conclusion. Men can benefit from marriage even if it's a botched job. Women in good marriages enjoy enhanced well-being, but those in ailing marriages accept the blame and do poorly, as reported in a study of 156 long-term marriages by University of Washington psychologist John Gottman.[9]

"Marriage protects men from depression and makes women vulnerable," says Dr. Jacobson.[10] Ellen McGrath, Ph.D., who chaired the American Psychological Association's task force on women and depression, concluded that "marriage confers a protective advantage on men. As we close the 20th century, we are increasingly seeing women distressed about marriages. They are putting more labor into them and getting back less."[11] No wonder many middle-aged divorcées would rather be dead than wed.

By contrast, men who are unmarried in middle life and later have a very difficult time reaching out for the emotional nourishment necessary to sustain themselves. They often withdraw, become depressed, shut down. Even those with enough money and success to entertain themselves do not fare as well as single women, in general, in terms of overall life satisfaction. Their health suffers. They question their self-worth. "As you grow older," says

Professor Goldscheider, "being part of a social network is more important than occupational success, and men's social lives have always been created by women."[12]

Even Beryl, for all her moaning and groaning about a future alone, would not put up with a replay of the traditional marriage. But the suspended state she is in is nonetheless painful. Those women who have been divorced a long time, becoming workaholics to blunt the loneliness, may well be letting their own immature defenses get in the way.

"What do you really need a man for?" Laura asks Beryl.

"I would like a man to be my best friend and my lover—that's it."

"Maybe that isn't enough for a man."

"I definitely think men want someone more needy," Beryl agrees.

Does she think men might find her intimidating?

"Sure. I have a six-figure salary. I have a lot of clout and company perks. And I have a big personality. But I can't stand to depend on a man for *anything* financially." Beneath the brittle armor of shock humor and all the frizzy hair and stylish clothes and the high-profile persona, there emerges a sad, frightened woman who cannot countenance the near future when her daughter moves out and she faces 50 alone.

Like many divorced women who are well armored against falling back into traditional marriage, Beryl tries to make the relationship with her child the one perfect vehicle for mutual love. The tip-off was last Christmas, when she told her daughter, "I can't stand when you leave me." Inevitably, when one deals with an adolescent, possessiveness is a losing game. Beryl has confused her affiliation needs with her achievement needs. The rewards for one can seldom be applied to the other; they are two separate columns on the balance sheet of life. People don't love us for our work. They may admire us, be attracted to us, envy us, even want to sleep with us to prove something, but the most dazzling work product does not bring people close to us.

But increasingly Beryl's predicament is not the general rule for divorced women of a certain age.

"I'm superbly happy, and I feel so lucky to have gotten to this place in my life," says Laura. "It's not how you're supposed to feel at fifty, is it?"

Yes, today it is. That's what the Revolution of Second Adulthood is all about. Come along for the ride and see.

BOOK TWO

SECOND ADULTHOOD

Prologue

A BRAND-NEW PASSAGE

*J*ohn Guare has been doing exactly what he most loves to do since he was nine years old: writing plays. He soon became good at it, very good, and prolific enough to be one of the rare playwrights actually able to support a family on his productions. The creator of *Six Degrees of Separation* and *The House of Blue Leaves* was described by one of the leading theatrical critics as "the best, most underrated playwright in America."[1] But even a brilliant, boomingly successful playwright like John Guare knows that he cannot rest on his laurels. He was 56 when I mentioned to him that I was exploring our Second Adulthood.

"I was just saying to my wife I've got to reinvent my life right now!" he exploded. "Or we'll be dead. Worse than dead—the walking dead."

Having satisfied the requirements of First Adulthood, now what? Surprise! Look at all the time left. Today there is not only life after youth, but life after empty nest. There is life after layoff and early retirement. There is life after menopause. There is life after widowhood. There is life after coronary. There is likely to be life after cancer. Another life to find a dream for, to plan for, to train for, to invest in, to *anticipate now*. Why?

Because Second Adulthood is not an aberration; it is an evolution. It's almost Darwinian. We have broken the evolutionary code.

The two generations of Baby Boomers—the Vietnam Generation and the Me Generation—are set to become the longest-living humans in American history. Leading experts on aging now predict that if we do things right over the next few decades, at least half the Boomers can expect to live well into their late eighties and nineties, remaining healthy and active.[2] A million of them, it is predicted by the Census Bureau, will live past 100.[3] And their children may live another twenty years beyond their parents.[4] No other change will more profoundly alter the way we live in the twenty-first century.

The first Boomers officially turn 50 in 1996. Approaching that milestone, even the most accomplished and mature members of this generation are loath to be associated with the old labels, burdened as they are with too many negative images. Hillary Rodham Clinton admitted that of all the insulting press criticism she received during the '92 presidential campaign, "the only one that really hurt, and one of the few that was really true, is that I'm middle-aged. . . . I couldn't believe I saw that in print." She was 45.

Although they may not realize it yet, Mrs. Clinton and other women in the Vietnam Generation are on a demographic roll. They stand to gain momentum from the sparks their older sisters in the Silent Generation have already thrown off. Consider this: By the year 2000 of all adult American women, fully 30 percent will be 50 and over! The U.S. Census Bureau predicts that this powerhouse age-group will number nearly forty-two million by then, and it will only swell:

> The fastest-growing age population is women between 45 and 54.[5]

The forward guard of the Boomers, having indulged itself in the longest adolescence in history, betrays a collective terror and disgust of aging. In survey after survey and hundreds of interviews, I find almost no one in his or her forties or early fifties identifies with the unspeakable term *middle age*.

> From this generation's perspective, there is no more middle age.

Here is my prediction, corroborated by analysts in the vanguard advertising agency Ammirati & Puris/Lintas: The women and men who brought us the Youth Revolution that dominated American society for thirty years are in the midst of creating another great quake that will shake up the social and economic landscape.

> Boomers will redefine middle age—as the Adult Revolution.

American society is only in the infancy of this Adult Revolution. Each time Boomers have hit a new stage in the life cycle, they have redefined and changed it. Likewise, they can be expected to find novel ways to express themselves as winners in life during their middle years. And so, in many ways, 50 won't be like what 40 used to be. Boomers will make the fifties their own.

DECLINE OR PROGRESS?

All the early explorers of the life cycle—Buhler, Erikson, Jung, Levinson, Neugarten, Vaillant—observed that the character of adulthood changes markedly between early and middle adulthood. I see Second Adulthood as beginning with a major passage somewhere around the mid-forties. Within the framework of this Second Adulthood, there appear to be two distinct periods. To recap, the middle years between 45 and 65 constitute the apex: the Age of Mastery. The years of late adulthood, from 65 to 85 or beyond, provide the chance for a coalescence of all that has been lived and learned and a period of grace and generosity, what I call the Age of Integrity.

The most neglected portion of this extra adult life is the middle years, the primary subject of the remainder of this book. Research on over-fifties has concentrated on disease, widowhood, retirement, meaninglessness, and impoverishment—that which can go wrong with us. It's high time we look at what goes right with us: the sources of love, purpose, fun, sexual pleasure, spiritual companionship, and sustained well-being that so many people are discovering in Second Adulthood, much to their surprise. At last we humans have the chance to show what feats of mind and spirit our species might be capable of once freed from the humdrum activities of survival, reproduction, family care, and perhaps even from full-time jobs. What a harvest of life!

It is true that women and particularly men lose some of their most cherished strengths in the middle years, but they also stand to gain enormous intensity from being dared to come to terms with the opposing forces of life these new stages present. The real work is nicely described by Carl Jung: "Wholly unprepared, [we] embark upon the second half of life. . . . [W]orse still, we take this step with the false assumption that our truths and ideals will serve us as hitherto. But we cannot live the afternoon of life according to the programme of life's morning: for what was great in the morning will be little at evening, and what in the morning was true will at evening have become a lie."[6]

The first thing we want to know: Is it all downhill from here?

Despite the fact that people understandably resist moving into the middle years, and always have, what really surprised me was the numbers who are now embracing these years for their own possibilities. I became more deeply impressed than ever with clear evidence that people's personalities are still dexterous and open to change—significant and even startling change—well into Second Adulthood.

This new life must be precipitated by a moment of change: the Aha! moment. It forces us to look upon our lives differently. Even a full-out middlescent rebellion can be bracing and healthy, provided we don't get stuck in it or keep going in circles to avoid the risks of moving forward.

Middlescence—my name for the passage leading into Second Adulthood and the Age of Mastery—can be a very active, volatile transition. As we have seen from the stories in an earlier chapter, people in middlescence are in flux and not centered, and they often act as foolishly and capriciously as teenagers. But even while making mistakes, we are in motion. A stimulating middlescence can be a transformative passage, leading us through a second adolescence and into *coalescence*—when all the wisdom we have gathered from fifty years of experience in living begins to come together.

The stage after 45 is exciting more and more women to soar into the unknown. As family obligations fade away, many become motivated to stretch their independence, learn new skills, return to school, plunge into new careers, rediscover the creativity and adventurousness of their youths, and, at last, listen to their own needs. They laugh at themselves for having been so afraid that losing their youthful looks would mean losing their power. On the contrary! Their days become filled with small astonishments.

"At forty-eight I lost forty pounds, looked younger than I did at forty, and took up a long-repressed passion—music," says a typical homemaker. Jeannie enrolled in music school to study electric bass and drums. She now plays in a garage rock band with 18-year-old boys. She already has planned her antidote to "hardening of the attitudes." After 65 she plans to launch a heavy metal band called Guns and Geezers.

Men too feel stirrings in the creative side of their nature. Most hunger for closer intimate attachments. For the first time ever, many men who arrive emotionally bankrupt in middle life are learning how to use not only their rational thinking powers but also "that which is imprinted upon the spirit of man by an inward instinct," as Francis Bacon described intuitiveness. This may open up channels of affinity and love that carry them beyond the peak of achievement.

You may remember the Louisville man Bruce Bell, who has counseled many men over 45 in his work as a mental health hospital administrator. "So often the older men that I've talked with were so busy during their younger years, meeting the financial responsibilities of a family, moving up in their careers, trying to make ends meet. Meanwhile, time races by, and then something tragic happens," he said. "Maybe they lose a job or a spouse, and suddenly the things they've invested all their time in, they question. *Is it really just about going to school, setting up a career, getting married, having two-point-three kids and a dog, and dying?* They start all over, trying to find out what really is the meaning in life."

A powerfully built African American man who joined the older men's group in Seattle confessed, "I grew up in the ghettos in Philadelphia, and quite frankly, I never thought beyond thirty-five because I didn't think I was going to be *alive* past that point."

Having recently hit his fifty-fourth birthday, Chuck Hatten, sober bureaucrat, was suddenly bursting with boyish enthusiasm. Giving vent to his imagination in the past few years, he had come up with an invention for which he had just received a patent. He felt certain he was on the brink of an "astronomical change" in his life. "I have *miles* more perspective on people and how they operate," he said. "I'm a one-on-one psychologist by this time." How surprising it is to recognize the accumulation of our skills and inner strengths: *Hey, I can do this with my eyes closed!*

If we can stop trying so hard to produce, we might awaken to the playfulness parked back in preadolescence. For example, all those harmless things that Alice Lindberg Snyder had enjoyed doing as a young girl—sailing, swimming, whistling, tap dancing—she had set aside for the sake of propriety as a university professor's wife. Once widowed, she wasn't going to spend her second life presiding over faculty teas. Instead she enjoyed a healthy middlescence. "That fun-loving nature of her childhood hadn't died; she just hadn't turned it loose all those years," as described in the book *Gifts of Age*. "She was through neglecting the part of herself that wanted to play."[7]

The task in this transition is not only psychological; it is also spiritual. There is a quickening of reverence in the presence of art and nature, as almost everyone begins to wonder where he or she might fit in the larger scheme of things. We sense that time is growing short and there is no use waiting to settle old scores. It's time to forgive the erring parent, embrace the estranged sibling, let go of disappointments in the prodigal child. Religious faith may be reconsidered or renewed.

This passage allows us to open ourselves to new and more meaningful ways to be alive. Involuntary losses can become the catalyst for voluntary changes in the practice of our lives, altering the efforts we make to connect with others, the values we choose to make congruent with our actions, the habits we change to support better health, the responsibilities we accept for mentoring the next generation and civilizing our communities, country, and planet.

Sherry Lansing, one of the most successful movie executives in Hollywood, confided that she "freaked out" at 45. Still single then, she had intended to be one of those women who just glide through, accepting aging as a natural process. Suddenly she was scared—scared about losing her looks before someone discovered something inside her worth cherishing. As middlescence crept up on her, she began to understand what makes the difference between decline and progress.

"At fifty you have to say, 'What am I missing?'" she reflected. "By that time you can't blame it on circumstance or other people. Whatever is incomplete, it's *you* who has left it out."

FROM SURVIVAL TO MASTERY

The massive shift in the passage to Second Adulthood involves a transition from survival to mastery. In young adulthood we survive by figuring out how best to please or perform for the powerful ones who will protect and reward us: parents, teachers, lovers, mates, bosses, mentors. It is all about proving ourselves. The transformation of middle life is to move into a more stable psychological state of mastery, where we control much of what happens in our life and can often act on the world, rather than habitually react to whatever the world throws at us. Reaching this state of mastery is also one of the best predictors of good mental and psychological functioning in old age.[8]

It is not automatic, however. There is aging, and then there is a successful aging. To cash in on the bonus of Second Adulthood is a career choice. It requires a new focus, energy, discipline, and a whole set of strategies. It must be done consciously. But what is it we are supposed to do?

The first clue is that in order to participate in the potentials and rewards offered by a Second Adulthood, we must construct our own new second adult identity. Sooner is better than later. It means throwing off all the old stereotypes, letting go of outgrown priorities, and developing real clarity about what is most relevant in our lives for the future.

This is not the way the culture trains us to think. People often explain their increasingly sedentary, risk-averse middle years with the cliché "I'm too old for that now." As they see it, they've worked hard, made the money they need, launched their kids, and now it's okay to coast. In one of the early group interviews with men, in Freehold, New Jersey, I heard from a doctor who felt "It's too late." The son of first-generation immigrant parents, he is a short, broad-shouldered man who still affects a street aggressiveness. He knew by the seventh grade he would become a doctor. "And I achieved it," he said huskily. "Did my time in Jersey City pool halls. I was called the hoodlum doctor. I did what I wanted to do." But there was no joy or vitality in his claim; it sounded more like a sworn affidavit testifying to all the effort he had put into proving himself tough and worthy as a young man.

The doctor is now 55, retired, financially set, and mostly miserable. Except for the tinted hair combed over his bald spot, he has clearly not made any effort to reinvent himself for a Second Adulthood. His wife and children had put up a terrible fuss when he decided to retire at 52 and play the stock market. He was adamant. The doctor had had only one full week of vacation in twenty-three years. He was tired and bored. But early retirement did not cure his malaise.

"I feel life is coming to an end," he told the group, "and I haven't done a lot of things I wanted to do, yet I always find excuses not to." He knotted his arms more tightly around his chest, his body language signifying the self-imposed bind of a man still traveling with the old maps. The doctor possessed enough insight to admit, "When I had office hours six days per week, I had a good excuse not to try new things. Now I don't. Meanwhile, my wife is going in the opposite direction."

Men and women are often out of sync in the new middle age.

"Time puts you under the pressure of honesty," says Meredith (a pseudonym), a suburban real estate broker who has followed the conventional age cues for putting together her life. "I just did whatever people in Ohio were doing at the time: I went to college at sixteen, I got married at twenty, I had a child at twenty-one, I've always been right on schedule." And at 38, having launched her children, she started her own successful business, at which point she stopped counting birthdays and, more important, stopped changing. In fact, she has now passed 50, but since there are no instructions or realistic images for how to be a woman of 50 today, Meredith finds herself doing what she's done for the past seventeen years—"I work at home, I work at work, I work in the car"—and every day she feels more weighed down.

The phrase that Meredith runs through her mind is one heard more and more today, rather like a mantra of the Fifties: *This is not a dress rehearsal.*

Look again. Some of the most popular heroes and heroines of the Sixties youth culture already have crossed the great divide at 50—Paul Simon, Barbra Streisand, Aretha Franklin, Mick Jagger, Tina Turner, Joni Mitchell—and they're going stronger than ever. But it is not just celebrities; it's happening within the mainstream of most developed societies today.

What is the meaning of this second act? Is there something special we are meant to do? Without any guide to the *inner changes* in Second Adulthood—which present dilemmas and demands that never had to be part of our calculations in the past—we find ourselves facing a game we don't know how to play. When we don't "fit in" to the old definitions of our age-groups, we are likely to think of our behavior as evidence of our inadequacies, rather than as a valid stage unfolding in a continuing sequence of growth, something we all accept when applied to childhood and adolescence. At this critical point of turning in the life cycle, strange new questions knock at the back of the mind:

- Now that I've done it, what does it all mean?
- What is the purpose of my existence from now on?
- Do I really like the person I turned out to be? Is it too late to change?
- With so many challenges behind me, what makes it worth it to keep trying?
- How will my way of loving change?
- Where do I find a real sense of community?
- How do I build into my life a vehicle for creative expression?
- If I start over again with a second family, will I feel younger or older? Or: Without children, how do I remain connected to the future?
- If I haven't made it in earlier career incarnations, is this the end of promise? Or the converse dilemma, what do I do when I've exceeded all my dreams?
- If I don't subscribe to a formal religion, how do I find spiritual comfort?

- Does middle age bring us to the culmination of life? Or is it simply an anticlimax to be endured?
- Will society recognize us as the wise people or cast us aside as superfluous?

These are some of the deeper, open-ended questions of the second half of the life cycle to which our culture does not provide any convincing answers. We must claim the license to search for those answers and experiment until we find the right answers for ourselves. Life, as we have known it in our young adulthood, is not meant to continue as it was. Second Adulthood has its own joys, tasks, and obstacles and a different scale of relevancy against which to measure what is really important in life. Those who successfully navigate the passage into the Age of Mastery will be much less concerned with proving themselves. Life goes on, but the possibilities and rewards are beyond anything we have anticipated. It is a part of the human experience that we never had before in any significant numbers.

THE "LITTLE DEATH" OF
FIRST ADULTHOOD

Psychologically something has to die before a new self can be born. We must come through something of a mourning phase to emerge and say, "Okay, now I have a new life; there's a new part of me that is allowed to grow." The cycle of death and rebirth has definite phases, although there is considerable variation in the ages at which men and women grapple with each phase of the transition into Second Adulthood. If one has to pick a norm, 45 represents the old age of youth, while 50 initiates the youth of Second Adulthood.

Whether we recognize it consciously or not, women and men in the mid- to late forties are simultaneously undergoing the dying of youth and stumbling into the infancy of Second Adulthood. The striving, competing, proving, and besting of rivals that lent a furious intensity to our young adulthood, forming the basis of our ego identities, now feel more like a dull repetition of duty: *Why do I have to work so hard? What is it all for?* There is also the inevitable anger and frustration at physical changes in the body. A mourning period usually sets in. *Am I ready to accept the ebbing of my physical prowess? Losing the unfair advantage of youthful beauty? Giving up the magic of fertility?* Disillusion and ennui are just as natural to this passage as mood swings are to adolescence. It leads naturally to a pause, an intermission, a "little death" of the perspectives and pretenses and hormonal imperatives of our young adulthood.

Given the phobia about aging in American society and the habitual expectation of decline in every sphere, people often give in to it at first. Their state of mind causes them to give up on sports they've enjoyed or beauty and workout regimens that work for them. They forget about eating and drinking disciplines. They may let their hair go unflatteringly gray or chop it off in some blunt accommodation to "looking my age." Some take on hammocks of flesh, sleep a lot, sink into chronic depression. In the eyes of others they appear to turn "old" overnight. To themselves it feels like entering a winter of the soul.

"To every thing there is a season . . . a time to break down, and a time to build up," as the Bible says.[9] So it is with us. This little death is a necessary winter, to rest, consolidate, nourish, and prepare for the very long growing seasons ahead. Today, in fact, as the end of what seemed the endless spring of our young adulthood comes into sight, there is an opportunity to *reinvent ourselves.* We have probably reached a certain plateau in family and career building. It is no longer necessary to invest all our energies in keeping up that "false self" we concocted as young adults to please or impress or dominate others.

When I described my concept of the little death of First Adulthood to a man who has written about the midlife crisis, the notion made sense to him. "You find out what your strengths are, then you get into that persona, you perfect it and costume it and perform it. It comes to feel like you. But the frustration—if you even recognize it as you come upon that 'little death' you talk about—is the feeling 'That's not the me that I like, or the me that I would like other people to know.' "

The effort expended in creating and defending that persona is exhausting. Once we stop being ruled by the need to prove ourselves to the world and begin to relax our vigilance around maintaining the false self—what a relief—we can start stripping back down to what is real, not false or copied, to uncover our own authenticity.[10]

A study of psychological well-being in different stages of life, conducted by Carol D. Ryff at the University of Wisconsin, Madison, found that the men and women in early middle life (ages 40 to 50) felt the most personal progress. They were also enjoying much greater acceptance of the real selves they lived with every day (as opposed to their ideal selves) than those in young adulthood.

BIRTH OF SECOND ADULTHOOD

Both men and women who emerge psychologically healthiest at 50 are those who, as their expectations and goals change with age, "shape a 'new self,' that calls upon qualities that were dormant earlier."[11] This was the principal finding of longitudinal studies at the University of California, Berkeley. This "new self" then fits into a new life structure appropriate to the second half of adulthood.

Men have always been able to start over, and not once but more than once. What is really new is that now women have the option of starting second lives in their mid-forties or fifties, and increasingly they are doing so. Middlescent rebellion is becoming as common for women today as it has traditionally been for men. Some women admit they became too involved in organizing the details of their children's lives and found it difficult to let go.

"I've let the children fly off into their own lives, but even more important, I've left the nest myself," says Janet Mandaville, a self-employed professional in Portland, Oregon. The break came at 50, when she upped and went off to Australia to take a hard look at her life and stayed for eight months. Her friends carped, "You're just running away from home, it's irresponsible," but for the first time she stopped worrying about what the neighbors will think.

Bushwalking in the outback, carrying her home in a tent on her back, Janet learned the vital difference between being alone and being lonely. "For the first time since I was ten, I had time to sit on a rock and have conversations with myself."

In making the time for that passage, Janet discovered there were many steps in emotional responses that she hadn't walked all the way through. Upon her return she was able to approach divorce not with the indignation or impulsiveness of youth, but with the selective responses that have allowed her to remain friends with her former husband. She also takes the time now to revisit with her adult children the traumatic times of their growing-up years, acknowledging, "I guess I never noticed you were feeling so miserable when . . ." It has brought a refreshing balance to her relationships with them.

Remembering what it was like to be so busy doing the necessary and humdrum, she realizes now there was little room left for magic. "As you get older," she says, "you find more ways to snatch the time to do the *unnecessary and satisfying.*" Now 52, Janet finds that after many years of traditional marriage, living with a lover part-time offers the perfect balance between commitment and protecting her sense of self.

. . .

As we stumble with our first steps into the unknown territory of Second Adulthood, we don't know if we can depend on it. We're not sure what this "new self" might turn out to be, and we tend to doubt it will have as much value as the made-to-please persona that has worked for us up to now. The sooner we accept the idea that life may not turn out as we expected, the easier the transition will be. We have to work our way up to saying, "I'm not going to go backward. I'm not going to try to stay in the same place. That way lies self-torture and foolishness. I am going to have the courage to go forward."

THE MEANING CRISIS

The search for meaning in whatever we do becomes the universal preoccupation of Second Adulthood. It could be called the Meaning Crisis. It is based on a spiritual imperative: the wish to integrate the disparate aspects of ourselves, the hunger for wholeness, the need to know the truth.

Women are more likely to develop their rational thinking functions and enjoy extending their powers into a broader arena, while men are often drawn inward, from thinking to feeling. Many men, however, do not respond positively to this inner impulse toward change; to them, change is equated with loss, giving up, topping off, winding down. They resist mightily the chance to develop the emotions and intuition that were the "unused muscles" of their youthful drive toward success.

The book of the Bible that best describes the crisis of meaninglessness is Ecclesiastes. It is that stage of life when, as we look back, it may seem that we have been "chasing after the wind."[12] It is dangerous to let externals continue to dictate and define who we are. In the first half of adult life self-importance is necessary. We are making a furious effort to develop our egos against the efforts to submerge them that come from everywhere: peer competitors, corporate life, marital partners, parental figures who withhold approval, etc. The start of wisdom is to recognize that things like job titles and outgrown role labels do *not* define us and are ephemeral.

In the passage to the Age of Mastery, unlike earlier transitions, there may be no need for radical rearrangements of our careers and personal commitments. But once caught up in the tempestuous forces that can be released at this time of life, we may be tempted to tear up something important that we have built just to escape the spiritual hollowness we feel. "What needs to happen is inner work, not outer change," urge Jeffrey Burke Satinover and Lenore Thomson Bentz, two contemporary interpreters of Jungian thought. "That inner work increases our capacity for empathy and transforms our experience of what we already have."[13] Healthy development through middle life is a product of how we actually live.

The first hint that Hillary Rodham Clinton was caught up in the crisis of middlescence at 46 came in her stream-of-consciousness speech at the Liz Carpenter Lectureship Series at the University of Texas, delivered just after she had left the bedside of her dying father. "Why is it in a country as wealthy as we are . . . that we lack meaning in our individual lives and meaning collectively, we lack a sense that our lives are part of some greater effort, that we are connected to one another? . . . *We are, I think, in a crisis of meaning.* [italics added]."[14]

One can no longer hope to be "rescued" by the father; approaching 50, we become our own fathers. In the case of the president's wife, the huge task of development that faced her in her first two years as a presidential partner was to reconcile her father's death with accepting full ownership of her own awesome new political powers and the equally awesome level of hostility and suspicions directed at her personally. Mrs. Clinton's vague, vulnerable references to a "politics of meaning" were a sign that she was actively engaged in the transformative work of this passage. In Japan for a G-7 economic summit in the summer of '93, there were signs that the First Spouse was beginning to put a toe in the waters of Second Adulthood. She observed that "one of the big things about being here is to find out how *young* 50 sounds."[15]

Second Adulthood takes us beyond the preoccupation with self. We are compelled to search for greater significance in the engagement of our selves in the world. Another of the men in my older Seattle group made a perceptive comment. "All our lives we create stories and a persona. It's like floating through," said Alan Alhadeff, age 48. "Part of aging is being able to fit into a bigger story."

Do you notice your perspective changing? The way you feel about your way of living will be altered in at least four areas of perception as you make the transition from First to Second Adulthood. Be assured that the following changes are predictable. If you are ready to invest in the future, these shifts in attitude should be welcome. They are the surest signal that it is time to think about composing a "new self."

TIME TO KILL?

In their early forties, as we have seen, people have a hurry-up feeling; time seems to be running out. That is because they are dealing with the notion of limits to the life cycle for the first time. The funny thing is, even the hardest-driving men and women I have studied, once they cross that dreaded line into the fifties, become more certain about the values they stand for and less consumed by competitive drives, though more savvy in strategies for making their professional lives successful. Time seems to pass faster and faster and thus becomes much more precious. The notion of "killing time" goes with youth.

It's as though when we are young, we have seen only the first act of the play. By our forties we have reached the climactic second-act curtain. Only as we approach fifty does the shape and meaning of the whole play become clear. We move into the third act with the intention of a resolution and tremendous curiosity about how it will all come out. We start thinking in broader historical time frames. Time becomes measured more by markers of our parents' longevity and their response to aging, although that can be misleading. We are on a very different clock from our parents.

PUSH TOWARD AUTHENTICITY

The dissonance between the real self and the made-to-order self that the world has endorsed reaches its maximum tension during middlescence. The question that people then need to ask themselves becomes: *Am I going to confine my real self forever in some dark corner?*

"Men don't have much fun in their lives," observed Howell Raines, editor of *The New York Times* editorial page, when we compared notes about the contemporary crisis of middle life. Having studied the subject and written a compelling memoir about his own experience, Raines is acutely aware of the obstacles faced by men when they seek to compose the dividedness of their daylight self and their shadow self—a major task of Second Adulthood.

"Men take on large responsibilities, and in our society they think that they have to work terribly hard, sacrifice their own pleasure, and experience pain," he said. "It's no mistake that football is our national sport—because that's what happens in the game of football. Football is a metaphor for the American corporation. Everybody gets on a team, and they are given a position and a very narrow, rigidly defined set of moves they have to make. They have to confront other men, suffer pain, and get up and keep going— all for the team."

Raines began his voyage out of First Adulthood at 45 and wasn't across the river until 50. It was not one event; it was five years of tossing around in rough waters, trying to answer for himself, *What does it all mean?*

One night Raines sat down to write a story about fly-fishing. For once, he dropped the journalist's objective veneer and visited his own experience. Deep feelings began to surface. He found himself writing his own medita- tions on the soul, spiked with his own quirky southern humor. He let the words run. At one point it struck him that he was actually having fun: *I am enjoying this so much, time goes by and I don't even know it.* The intense pleasure of that night issued into his delightful full-length book, *Fly Fishing Through the Midlife Crisis.*[16]

Navigating the final shoals of his long passage into Second Adulthood, as he wrote in his book, "I came to see that the acceptance of my own mor- tality was the final and indispensable issue for me, that indeed it was hardly worth going to the trouble of having a midlife crisis equal to the name if you were not going to figure out how to be comfortable in the embrace of what Mr. Hemingway called 'that old whore death.'"

This same strong inner push toward authenticity appeared in my interviews with contemporary older women. By the time they reach their fifties, most educated women have acquired the skills and self-knowledge to master complex environments and change the conditions around them. The sense of "being my own person" is profound. They become increasingly the peo- ple they want to be.

Over and over again, with conviction, women who have actually crossed into their fifties tell me, "I would *not* go back to being young again." They remember all too vividly what it was like to wake up not knowing exactly who they were, to be torn between demands of family and commands of career, to be constantly changing hats (and hairstyles) in the attempt to fit many roles, and often losing focus in the blur of it all.

For women the false self is often experienced as the "bad self." Many of us can remember feeling like a bad self in early adulthood, when we were lonely, isolated, and easily made to feel inferior or helpless. When we couldn't make the marriage work, it was the fault of our bad self; or if we purposely didn't get married at all, the suspicion remained that it was because our bad self was too fat, or too weak, or too strident—somehow unlovable. We can remember feeling alternately like a bad mother and a bad career risk, never consistently sure of our own goals and values. Many of us can also remember an Aha! moment when we knew we had to strike out for ourselves, but even that clearer persona was subject to self-censure as a bad self.

The critical work of shaping an authentic identity for a woman (unlike for a man) comes after her biological imperative and most of her obligations to others have subsided. So often women must delay their real dreams. Many of the women over 45 whom I have studied describe goals they didn't achieve earlier but are determined to accomplish now. Commonly, they also say they have *not* discarded the dreams of their forties, such as becoming famous or marrying well.[17]

But with the age of 50 comes a great deal of emotional and social liberation. Since entering this phase of life, most of the women I have studied say they have become more accepting, more outspoken, and less self-conscious.

The majority agree that the struggles that used to claim most of their emotional lives have subsided.

ALIVENESS OR STAGNATION?

We may be accustomed to a background tone of well-being when a sense of stagnation or boredom begins to creep in, signaling the start of a new passage. Whether the world feels foggy or sunny, whether we feel we have a clear direction or are being buffeted by the wind, whether we live in a state of inner assurance or one of quiet desperation, all may depend upon how ready we are to let go of a familiar life structure.

In his play *Broken Glass* Arthur Miller writes about a woman who gave up her career to make a marriage and family for a driven businessman. In her fifties, after years of devoted marriage, she develops a sudden hysterical paralysis in her legs. "It's like I was just born and I . . . didn't want to come out yet," says Sylvia Gellburg. She is at the point of the little death of the false self that served her purposes—and those of others—during her First Adulthood. Now her return to an infantile condition puts her safely beyond any possibility of change. As theater critic John Lahr points out, "She is suddenly excused from . . . the great no man's area that is her life." Sylvia admits, "I guess you just gradually give up and it closes over you like a grave." Her husband, seething with ambition and repressed rage at his long years of sexual impotency, has let himself sink into a well of work. "I kept waiting for myself to change. Or you," he tells his wife in desperation. "And then we got to where it didn't seem to matter anymore. So I left it that way. And I couldn't change anything anymore." Both husband and wife use blame to avoid dealing with the truth of their own inadmissible feelings, and thus they are doomed.[18]

But Second Adulthood is not about giving up or coasting until it doesn't seem to matter anymore. It's about finding a new value in life.

> The secret in the search for meaning is to find your passion and pursue it.

THE TIME FLIES TEST

How do you know where to look for your passion? You can start by seeing if it passes the Time Flies Test. What activity do you do where time goes by without your even knowing it? What did you most love to do when you were 12 years old? Whatever happened to that fiery prepubertal kid who was obstinately passionate about some pursuit or pleasure, back before you began trying to fit into the uniform of your gender? Somewhere in that activity there is a hook to be found that might pull up your dormant self. You may have meant to get back to what you loved to do someday, but most of us become overcivilized as adults or maybe even forget what it is like to have a passion. When Howell Raines gave himself time to sit down and write from a literary rather than a reportorial sensibility, he passed the Time Flies Test.

Adolescents are expected to have rebellions. But what about middlescents? Don't they need to slip the knots of old expectations? Get away to where they can paint or write or dream or try new physical dares? People who have in the past taken the risk of change and made one or more successful life passages are more likely to welcome the chance to renovate their goals in middle life. Having reaped the benefits of purposeful change before, they will feel freer to shape a "new self" that calls upon qualities that were dormant earlier.[19] These are the people who, approaching the edge, are likely to say, "Whoa, there is only one alternative here."

The clue that a new self is forming and the outlines of a new life structure are taking shape is the exhilarating return of a sense of aliveness.

SAFETY OR DANGER?

One more subjective shift in every passage concerns the ratio of safeness and danger we perceive in our lives. As young people we remember being devil-may-care about safety. Of all the people I have studied, the ones who feel most imperiled are not those in their fifties or sixties, but men and women in their forties. Why?

Because the notion of mortality is new to those in the early forties: *Just around the corner I'm going to lose my looks, my knees will go, and then my eyes and my ears and my sex drive, and then I'll just roll over and die.* They are at the beginning of the second half of adult life. Because they have no experience yet in facing the fact of their mortality, it often seems imminent.

By their fifties, paradoxically, some people seem more serene about their mortality. Having almost certainly failed at some major personal or professional challenge along the way and found out they didn't die from it, they are in general more efficient and effective in the way they go about their lives. They may even feel more fit than when they were in their early forties. If so, it is usually because they now give more time and attention to maintaining the body machinery.

Most have at least been brushed by the wing of the raven: confronted with a friend's sudden demise, or the serious illness of a loved one, if not themselves, or a parent who slips away into debilitating age or death. Mortality is no longer just a floating anxiety, as it was during the early passage to midlife. Now it becomes a negotiation: *How long do I want to live? How much am I prepared to invest in my health and mental well-being?* This negotiation calls upon our inner resources and usually prompts a new willingness to devise stratagems for eluding illness and death.

Not everybody can take advantage of a Second Adulthood. Most people don't yet realize the possibilities are there and thus haven't prepared for it. This is a revolution just beginning to happen. It is not possible to give a static sociological profile of all people in their forties, fifties, and sixties, at every class level. Thus the people we shall meet in later chapters will be achievers among the educated middle class. These are the pacesetters in a dynamic, growing movement.

What strengths do we take into the passage to the Age of Mastery? And what do we get out of it? It isn't status or titles. It's deepening friendships, the satisfaction of mentoring, the freedom to explore innate creativity. There are at least two personality characteristics that change for the better as we get older. We usually learn not to depend on the easy but destructive coping methods of scapegoating (always looking for someone to blame when things go wrong), and we rely less on escapism.[20] We can actually reeducate our brains to resist these destructive defense mechanisms.

These Aha! moments may awaken us to a dormant self who was left behind in the rush to make early choices. Too often, however, the need for renewal is not acknowledged until we have a shattering failure: The long-standing marriage simply cannot be repaired, or new technology renders our job obsolete, and suddenly we feel like dinosaurs. Alternatively, we may set back the clock on our wake-up call until we can complete a major responsibility of young adulthood, like paying off a mortgage or seeing the last child off to college. By then the pent-up need to change usually takes a familiarly lurching course: The middlescent "runs away" from home, moving from city to country (or from suburbia back to city), or bails out of a career or a marriage that might have been worth preserving.

How can we make this passage more positively? The many stories in the chapters to follow will show the benefits of intentional inner change.

Part Three

PASSAGE TO THE AGE OF MASTERY

DEFINITION OF A SUCCESSFUL LIFE

To laugh often and much;
to win the respect of intelligent people
and the affection of children;
to earn the appreciation of honest critics
and endure the betrayal of false friends;
to appreciate beauty, to find the best in others;
to leave the world a bit better,
whether by a healthy child,
a garden patch or a redeemed social condition;
to know even one life has breathed easier
because you have lived.

—HARRY EMERSON FOSDICK

7

THE MORTALITY CRISIS

*L*iving on the edge. That is how precarious it often feels when we come to the top of the mountain, or what seems like the top, and are startled to find ourselves looking over the edge. The view is panoramic, breathtaking. But what about the trip down? Ordinarily a sequence of moments shifts the boundaries of our private universe gradually from the concrete concerns of young adulthood to something larger, startling, mysterious. But it often happens that a life accident—one of those events that we cannot predict or prevent—pushes us to the precipice with no preparation. We might suddenly find ourselves face-to-face with the greatest adult mystery of all. And we wonder, we all wonder, How will we behave when we first walk under the hammer of fate?

It could happen to any one of us as arbitrarily as this.

One day you are walking down the street with your life more or less in order, apparently enjoying good health, when a minor physical problem blossoms into one that requires "routine" exploratory surgery.

"Have your wife call me. I'd like to set her mind at rest," the doctor says. He, the patient, does not ask why his wife's mind needs to be set at rest if it is all so routine.

You walk into the hospital off the street, fully active, a man in charge, a busy man with a product to get out and a staff to direct, a man who was probably up late the night before, finishing the work in his briefcase. You are now required to surrender your watch, your wallet, your credit cards, your glasses, your rings. You are asked if you have any dentures, any contact lenses. Within ten minutes from a fully functioning executive you have been stripped down to your essentials. Every possession you own has either been handed over to your wife or put in a Ziploc plastic bag, and you are covered only by a johnny coat too short to come down to your knees, with your buttocks showing in the back, left to lounge on the brittle sheets of a bed not your own while waiting to be called. Waiting on the edge. You have nothing left but the strength, inner and outer, that you have built up to now.

In the next cubicle another man, roughly the same age, is in the same position: lying on his side, staring into space, not reading the newspaper, not making phone calls, not returning phone calls, although he looks like a man who is also accustomed to doing such things. He too has been reduced to a johnny coat striped like a prison garment, too revealing for him to risk walking down the hall to the bathroom, so he shares his fantasy of what it's like to be a man in his fifties awaiting exploratory surgery: "I feel like those men in the French prisons of old. They just lie around until it gets dark. You never know what they're going to do to you until you hear the guards running down to your cell. They throw open the door, drag you out, and that's the first time you know that they're taking you out to chop your head off."

Your wife waits in the flat fluorescent pallor of pinched space allotted to visitors. Sitting on the edge of your life while you are in the operating room, she keeps telling herself that this is just routine, a preventive procedure. Yet she knows that you are lying, pried open like a clamshell, while morsels of your flesh are carried on a tray between floors so the pathologist can rule out the possibility of a cancerous tumor.

People are wheeled out of the recovery room, feetfirst, slabs of meat under white sheets. All that can be seen from the visitors' area at the end of the floor is a hairy arm, or a corona of curls, or a nose with tubes showing over the crest of the sheet. Each time, your wife runs halfway down the hall, hopeful, until she sees the wrong-colored hair on the arm, the wrong corona of hair over the forehead, and she turns away to wait some more.

Night falls. Still no word. The nurse says the doctor is still in surgery, working on another patient—this one a vital young woman who chatted with you from the next gurney while awaiting her turn for an "exploratory."

"You mean she's been in surgery from three in the afternoon until ten at night?" your wife asks the nurse. "Why?"

"We didn't know if the spot on her throat was benign or metastatic. They're doing a total laryngectomy and taking out the bones in the side of her face." Your wife listens to this with a stab of fear, then a prayer, knowing that this could be it; the hammer of fate could nail you just as soon as the next person.

Later your doctor comes down the hall and tells your wife, "I'm sorry. It is prostate cancer. But I—"

She freezes, deafened to the surgeon's next words. He repeats them.

"But I didn't have to remove the prostate. We'll simply radiate. Don't worry. I can assure you, he'll die of old age before prostate cancer ever catches up with him."

Luck of the draw. Living on the edge. Didn't fall off, not this time. When you swim up out of anesthesia, the surgeon assures you this is no big deal. You believe him. You will take the radiation, jog five miles before you go to work every day, and then it will all be behind you. It will not exist in your reality. Your wife gets to stroll out through the sterile labyrinth into the summer night, free to feel the gentle air on her bare arms, able to hail a cab and go home to tell the good news to your children and sip a glass of wine and contemplate a new day tomorrow, while knowing that someone else, a young person, who also went in that morning off the street, will wake up tomorrow missing a throat, a voice, and half a face.

LIVING ON THE EDGE

The man in the story is the husband of one of my good friends; they are the couple I mentioned in the Note from the Author. Peggy is the professor who was planning a trip to France with her good-looking, vibrant husband, Chuck, to celebrate the freedom of an empty nest. This first startling brush with mortality was clearly a turning point that shoved them both to the edge of the mountaintop.

But something like this happens to almost everyone. Whether it happens at the age of 45, 50, or 55, the chances are that an unexpected circumstance will throw us off-balance and threaten the very ground of our being. It need not be an actual mortality crisis. No matter how carefully and successfully we have arranged our lives, disruptions occur. Maybe our occupations are threatened; the power balance of marriage is turned upside down; the sudden slap of lost authority over a no-longer-child can do it, or the somber prospect of taking on the custodianship of a sick parent.

All at once we find ourselves living on the edge. We are plunged into a period of increased vulnerability and heightened potential, and whatever we do will have a crucial and long-lasting effect. But we are not pawns or puppets dancing on a string that is manipulated by invisible hands; we can think and act and plumb the darkness of our motives. We can look at the picture of the lives of others as reference points.

The flame-colored hair was the first thing I noticed about Peggy. As she strode across the San Francisco airport terminal toward me, the freckly white skin and broad swipe of a smile and especially the red-gold hair all struck a chord of recognition much deeper than that of normal social intercourse. She seemed to recognize me instantly too. We were strangers then, meant to meet and drive down the coast to Esalen together. Peggy was one of the hosts of an invitational conference on the New Older Woman.

We discovered so much in common in the first moments. Not just the red hair—we joked that we shared aberrant genes—but a quickness to temper and to laughter, a passion for running and climbing, politics and nature, and both of us were contentedly married to husbands older than we were. Peggy had earned her Ph.D. at the age of 53. She had then taken a postdoctoral year at Berkeley. "Chuck is always incredibly supportive. Any man who could support you through a Ph.D. and menopause at the same time—" Her riotous laugh said the rest. I told her that my husband too was incredibly supportive of my creative life.

Peggy was maybe six or seven years older than I and still raring to go at life full throttle. Such was the rapport between us that scarcely past Monterey she revealed a very personal tribulation. Two years before, her husband had been diagnosed with prostate cancer. But as she told me the story, she emphasized the upbeat prognosis of her husband's surgeon: "He'll die of old age before prostate cancer ever catches up with him." Peggy said it had been a year since the end of Chuck's radiation therapy, and he felt so good he couldn't believe he was coming up on a sixty-fifth birthday. She mentioned that he was due for a checkup while she was away.

The conference was an intimate Sixties-style encounter group, except that for all the personal talkathons we had endured over the years, none of us had ever gathered to talk about being an Older Woman. The participants were savvy and spicy, from 50 to 80, and we bonded quickly. We talked a little about how women in this period of life, free at last of child-rearing responsibilities, often enter a second stage of nurturing when someone in the family gets sick.

On the last day of the conference Peggy left early, saying good-bye to no one. Something told me she must have received bad news. That night, after a cheerful conversation with my own husband, I telephoned Peggy's home.

"I drove up the coast screaming and crying, the only breakdown I've ever had," she told me. "I wanted to drive off the edge because something tells me—" She couldn't finish. The beast was back. Five of Chuck's organs would have to be excavated. All her husband's plumbing would be outside.

The day had brought me delight, Peggy devastation. That is the edge.

So puny I felt, in the face of the spinning recalculations of mortality that had to be taking place inside my friend, that I talked too much. The first thing to remember, I told Peggy, is that people don't automatically die of this disease anymore. Many are cured. Look at all the survivors of breast cancer; they're featured now on the covers of magazines. Even with cancers that medicine can't yet cure, people can live for another ten or fifteen years. Look at Paul Tsongas. Here is a man who left the Senate believing he was doomed by lymphoma. He entered a combat with death, and he won. Four years later he was running for president and winning the New Hampshire primary.

When I finished my little speech, Peggy said, "Uh-huh." Statistics do not penetrate the heart; fear is altogether individual. She felt helpless. So did Chuck. Feeling helpless is the worst medicine for one's immune system. Instead of being passive and "good," they needed to find some ways to take back control. "Do a few things between the two of you," I urged. "Can you go away to someplace magical to prepare for the surgery?"

"Oh, yes, the Sierras, that's our sanctuary," Peggy said.

Learning self-hypnosis can be very helpful, I told her, passing on what I had learned from my friend New York psychologist Stan Fisher and his 1991 book *Discovering the Power of Self-Hypnosis*.[1] The body doesn't know the difference between the benign surgeon's knife and the mugger's assault. A patient can use self-hypnosis to plant the suggestion that the body should be *receptive* to this particular assault, rather than react with tension and stress chemicals. Studies have shown that surgical patients who prepare their tissues in this way heal more quickly. I suggested that Peggy find out if the hospital would allow them to put an audiotape on a Walkman and ask the nurse to plug it into Chuck's ear when he came into the recovery room, to listen to while he was still unconscious. "Tape the meditations now that he'll want to hear: 'You're strong, you're going to heal.' It will give him a feeling of mastery. The main thing is you're not totally their prisoner. You have taken back some control."

Peggy told me she was keeping a journal, but she often had trouble expressing her honest feelings and fears to Chuck since she felt it was her job always to buoy him up. But pretense quickly wears thin in a prolonged emergency. "Try having a dialogue about what you're really feeling. Maybe you could both keep a journal and then read it to each other. It can help you to start working together as a team."

Chuck wasn't comfortable about sharing his fears aloud, Peggy said. But he loved his computer. "Our computers are side by side in the study. I'll suggest we pour our feelings into our own computers and then switch and read the other's thoughts."

This became Peggy and Chuck's armor: dispelling spooks by sharing with gut-wrenching candor what typically goes unsaid. As Camus wrote, "Crushing truths perish from being acknowledged."[2] I kept in touch with Peggy over the course of her ordeal, and from time to time she sent me entries from their lives in progress. She and Chuck ultimately self-published *Dialogue of Hope: Talking Our Way Through Cancer* as a little gem of a book.[3] From excerpts, and my talks with Peggy, we can follow one couple's revealing experience with living on the edge.

LITTLE VICTORIES

PEGGY: We worked as a team, playing off each other: touching, imaging, preparing Chuck for the surgeon's scalpel.

CHUCK: The medics weren't going to get a number, a case history, a medical anomaly. They were getting *me:* a person, a husband, a father, a grandfather; feelings, sensitivities, needs. No way were they going to forget who I was. I was going to prepare my body for them. I lay on the hot Sierra granite, turning myself into butter so the knife would meet no resistance. I willed myself part of the surgical team.

When I talked with Peggy before the daunting surgery, she said Chuck was strangely ebullient. They had gone to each consultation prepared with intelligent questions to ask. She asked the questions he was afraid to ask, and vice versa. Chuck did learn self-hypnosis so that wherever he was, if anxiety threatened to overtake, he could slip into an inner room for a few seconds and calm himself. "But ultimately there is so much that we can't control," Peggy said.

And paradoxically too much willful, planful preparation can stand in the way of a deeper, even transformative passage of the soul. "But it sounds like you two are operating as one pair of eyes and ears and feelings, interchangeably"—I encouraged her—"and that is probably what is making Chuck feel so confident."

Extreme stress like this forces us to awareness of the presence of the spirit. The spirit finds an opening in the brokenness, where smooth functioning has broken down, and comes up through the cracks to create a breeze beneath our wings. It releases love and desire. When Peggy talked about the weeks of constant uncertainty they had just been through, it produced a giggle. She and her husband had been together in all the doctors' offices and together driving to and from tests, holding hands and making eyes and blowing kisses and making love wherever the spirit moved them, and it moved them often, prying open those latches behind which we all guard our love, letting it tumble out like sheets knotted together and stretching for miles in an unbroken lifeline through all the random events life was throwing at them.

Real devotion is an unbroken receptivity. And the ultimate cure, I am reminded by reading the ancient philosophers, comes not from logic but from love.

PEGGY: We invited our friends to our home to celebrate Chuck's going into the hospital to win back his health. We filled our patio with every bright thing we owned... Santa Fe pottery, buckets of impatiens, sparkling music. All were asked to bring pictures of themselves snapped at joyful moments in their lives. I would make a collage of the images and hang it on Chuck's hospital wall directly in front of him—the first thing he'd see out of surgery. I was determined to bring into the hospital all the "uppers" we had collected in our eighteen years together—children, friends, special places.

On the morning after his ten-hour operation, Chuck awoke to a web of tubes. Ominous whispers could be heard outside his room. Then the medieval procession known as grand rounds began, and seven sober residents and interns entered single file and circled his bed, holding clipboards against their chests like dueling shields. Peggy felt violated for her husband—he seemed so vulnerable and exposed—but his first words let her know he was still fighting for control.

CHUCK: "You have to understand... anyone who works on me has to touch me." I reached out to the Chief, who took my hand and held it. With my other hand, I reached for an intern: "That means everybody." Like awkward schoolchildren, they looked to their Chief for permission.
[An intern stepped forward, introduced himself, and touched Chuck.]
CHUCK: "Good, that may be the best medicine you'll ever dispense."

Every night while Chuck was in the hospital, his room was filled with laughter, as he regaled his children with tales of growing up in Baltimore in the 1930s. Peggy was relieved to hear him sounding so happy and full of life, but somehow there was too much energy in that room. When everyone else left, she still had to be up.

CHUCK: I needed Peggy, I needed her so I could feel safe again, so I could fall asleep, confident that I would wake up. "Christ," I thought to myself, "if I don't wake up, I won't even know it."

Drained, Peggy dragged herself down the highway night after night to the same depressingly familiar motel. When I couldn't reach her by phone, there was a good reason. "I realize we've left something out of our carefully crafted scenario: a support system for me," she finally admitted. "I was feeling sorry for myself, and I was ashamed of feeling that way. I just holed up in the motel—you know, all incoming telephone calls cut off, the TV turned on for company. But every night I became more isolated, and I felt more abandoned."

We talked about how indispensable it is that the caretaker take care of herself. It was September, most people were in a busy back-to-school mode, but Peggy had lightened her teaching load at the college where she taught political science and had suspended work on her first book. She had nothing in her life except battling with the beast, secondhand. She needed full-service friends on call to meet her for lunch or a movie, comedy tapes for the car; she needed to be able to tell someone just how shitty she felt. From now on, sex with Chuck would be only a memory. She wondered if it would be that way with everything. Would they ever see the French countryside again, for instance? Peggy needed some sustaining hope to hold on to, one thing that wouldn't be taken away.

"Maybe I'll suggest to Chuck that we try to make a trip to Provence next May, to smell the lavender."

Chuck's miraculous recovery allowed him to leave the hospital three days ahead of schedule. The doctors—while touching him—told him he had broken all records. In that tiny sterile room he and Peggy had invaded an impersonal machine, made their own rules, created warmth and love. It was a small victory.

Homecoming, for Chuck, the balm of sea air, the mentholated freshness of Monterey pines filling the lungs, the sight of his own house were overwhelming. He took Peggy's hand. "It's going to be all right."

Two months later Peggy was running as fast as she could but always falling behind. She was back to commuting four hours a day to teach at Santa Clara University. "Guilt follows me everywhere," she told me. "In my office I feel I should be with Chuck. At home I worry my students are getting short shrift." Was she doing anything nice for herself? I asked. "I did plan a celebration for our anniversary—dinner at an elegant restaurant. Ten minutes into our salad, his bladder bag gave way."

But it was Chuck's rage and humiliation that most worried her. When she kissed him good night at home that night, he had exploded. "I'll never leave this property again!" he said.

Leave it alone for a while, I suggested. Later she might start leaving around some enticing travel articles. By now I needed to believe as much as Peggy did that Chuck could resurrect himself. I was eerily identified with her struggle.

Two months after the surgery Chuck was back on a nearly normal work schedule and flying around the country on business trips. He began to notice the stack of travel articles Peggy had left around to remind him there was a world beyond Monterey. Leafing through them, Chuck remembered French villages, the smell of freshly baked bread, the sound of boules being played on the square, the hot sun warming the stones of a ruined castle. "Why not?"

"I came home carrying midterms, dog-tired," Peggy later recounted. "As I headed for the study, I stopped short. There was Chuck in his paisley shorts. He was speaking slowly in his old, fractured French. 'Oui, monsieur, une chambre pour deux avec une vue.' I caught a whiff of lavender. With any luck we'll be in Provence by May."

I didn't get in touch with Peggy for a while. *The Silent Passage* was published that May; I was swept up in the publicity tour, and I assumed—no, I wanted to believe—that luck had taken Peggy and Chuck off to their beloved French countryside. It was June before I called to find out if they had made it to smell the lavender in Provence in May.

"We like to say we took a raincheck," she said carefully. The reality was, Chuck had been back in the hospital for several more surgeries or massive infections. They were living day to day, learning when to pull back and husband their energies and when to "grab the day." Still, they had plans. They were going to hike the gentle rain forests of the Olympic Peninsula. Peggy had found an apartment in San Francisco that felt very Parisian; with the right music and posters, she would create a French experience in their own backyard.

That night I had a gruesome nightmare. The next morning I awoke at four, shaken, crept out of bed not to wake my husband and went out to sit in the garden and let it seep into my soul in all its Juneness. The lawn carpet was so thick the robins had to waddle to get through it. It was that time in the country when one can no longer conjure up the drab gray stillness of winter, when the splurging urgency of June makes one aware of every moment to be caught, like a butterfly, or it's gone.

I realized why I hadn't called Peggy. This was what I must have feared, that the beast she was wrestling with would invade my own security and like some feral creature contaminate me or mine. This must be why most of us retreat so cruelly from those with cancer—business associates stop calling, friends often arm themselves with indifference, even relatives sometimes withdraw and wait for the victim to die, in effect, burying the victim alive—when what we should do is turn to face the beast. That was what Chuck was doing.

In other cultures death is often accepted and colorfully ritualized as a natural part of the cycle of life. Not so in America's youth culture, where death is viewed as a failure, as something private and almost shameful that should be hushed up. Our general attitude toward death is to deny it. Everyone lives as if no one "knew."[4] So when a button is pushed, as it was for me by Peggy and Chuck's experience, the sudden fear of death seems to edge everything else with heightened menace. Yet somehow we have to incorporate the reality of our own death and move beyond it.

A month later, when I worked up the nerve to call Peggy again, there was a new reality. A new tumor had been found. But the alchemy of their love had created in Chuck the most precious form of courage. He and Peggy had talked it over. Chuck made a decision which he believed affirmed life and offered him dignity and an opportunity to enjoy some peak moments with Peggy and his family and closest friends, while he was still symptom-free. He had stopped all forms of aggressive medical treatment, except for pain medication.

Peggy sounded relieved, almost buoyant. "Each day we have together counts for a little bit more. We're already looking at the chance to sniff lavender in Provence next spring."

It is only too obvious that not everyone has the chance to engage or enjoy fully a Second Adulthood. Even if we do everything right, there is no guarantee that we will avoid being assaulted by some dread disease. Nor can we be sanguine that we will have a compatible spouse to keep us company all the way to God's waiting room. Peggy walked through the mortality crisis. Chuck went as far as he could. But Chuck's was not a story of defeat. Even though he had picked a bad card, he refused to be reduced to a medical problem. The memorable thing about this man is that he went all the way to the end fighting to preserve the fullness of his humanity. This is a victory in itself. Chuck showed us how to go out with a shout.

If we deal with the mortality crisis at this stage, and do it honestly and well, we earn the license to travel over to Second Adulthood. Otherwise, when the seas unpredictably become rough, the wave may break over us and we'll begin losing ground. In order to continue to enjoy life and be productive, it is particularly important at this stage to feel anchored in something. We need to know what is absolutely relevant about our lives. If we don't know already, this is the time to work at finding out. It will provide a sense of direction and an anchor.

COMPOSING YOUR OWN
PROGRESS NARRATIVE

Each of us tells our own personal life story to ourselves, every day. The "mind chatter" that rushes through our brains at two hundred words per minute when we're not concentrating on something else *becomes* the story we are living. *I should have done this,* or *I'll never get over that.*

The mind is formed to an astonishing degree by the act of inventing and censoring ourselves. We create our own plot line. And that plot line soon turns into a self-fulfilling prophecy. Psychologists have found that the ways people tell their stories become so habitual that they finally become recipes for structuring experience itself, for laying down routes into memory, and finally, for guiding their lives.[5]

As Søren Kierkegaard wrote, "Philosophy is perfectly right in saying that life must be understood backward. But then one forgets the other clause— that it must be lived forward."[6] Charlotte Buhler, a pioneering theorist in adult development, proposed back in 1933 that most people's lives seem to have an inner coherence or unifying principle; she called it "intentionality."[7] This principle, she wrote, becomes particularly apparent in interviews with individuals over 50 or 55. "When asked to tell the story of their lives, they usually end up with a summarizing statement: 'All in all it was a good life,' or 'It all came to nothing.' "

Most of the time we live day to day. You might be surprised, if you take time at the midpoint, stop, and look back over the first half of your life, to see that it does have direction, to register just how far you have come. One of the arresting results of my survey of Professional Men was the deep satisfaction they take in looking back. In doing so, they write, the majority feel "aware of progress in important parts of my life."

A generation ago the same men almost surely would have felt on a decline. Today they can appreciate the progress they have made *and are still making*. Many of them say they are not as angry, driven, or selfish as they were when they were younger. And even if they do wrestle with such demons, they are better able to manage them. These results, along with the surveys, historical research, and many life stories I have collected, form the basis of my concept that many people at 50 today—probably for the first time in history—see their lives as a progress narrative, as opposed to the decline narrative that used to be standard to describe middle life. Once we become aware that we are on a progress track, it can give us the courage to go on, confident there is still more progress to be made.

Literature is undergoing the same revolution in storytelling. In novels the familiar decline narrative of the middle years is being replaced. We now have a midlife-progress narrative for very nearly the first time in Western literature. In her book *Safe at Last in the Middle Years* Margaret Morganroth Gullette shows how early novels by authors such as John Updike, Saul Bellow, Anne Tyler, and Margaret Drabble depicted young adulthood as a threatening and overwhelming time.[8] But as the writers themselves moved beyond that dangerous age, they and their characters discovered the benefits that can follow lost youth. Macon Leary, protagonist of Anne Tyler's novel *The Accidental Tourist*, looks back over his earlier years from the perspective of his early forties and proclaims, "I'm more myself than I've been my whole life long."[9]

Updike was almost 50 when he wrote *Rabbit Is Rich*. The selfish, angry, violent Harry Angstrom, who had been tracked by his creator through his tempestuous twenties and thirties, now, at 46, emerged "hearty" and "huge" and "serene in his middle years." Having moved on into another state of being, "He sees his life as just beginning, on clear ground at last."[10]

Playwright Wendy Wasserstein complained that "nobody in Hollywood says, 'Oh, boy—let's do a play about a fifty-four-year-old woman who falls in love, who still has possibilities.'" But Wasserstein showed them by doing just that in *The Sisters Rosensweig*, her comedy about three accomplished, still-lusty sisters, which went from a small production to a hit run on Broadway.[11]

When people experience their "awakening" into the Age of Mastery, they often revise their personal narratives. B. Cohler observed that this need occurs in both women and men at adolescence and again in middle age.[12] There is a need at this time to reorganize our perceptions in order to give coherence to our continuing life story.

Some people appear to go through calm, uneventful midlife transitions. But by the time they are in their fifties, when some life accident inevitably brings home the mortality issue, it throws them into a deeper, darker crisis. Something in the psyche has been repressed longer and comes up with a greater wallop. A very successful woman in television told me that even when she had cancer, at 45, it never crossed her mind that she wasn't immortal.

"I just wanted to prove how well I was, so I plastered a smile on my face and went right back to working."

What knocked her flat—and she has to laugh when she admits it—was the death of her dog. "Barney and I had been through separation, divorce, cancer, courtship, and remarriage together, and we kept moving, always moving. Suddenly I said to myself, if Barney can die, anyone can die. I've never been the same again."

Rationally, of course, the death of a dog and cancer are not comparable in danger. This relatively small triggering event mushroomed into a major life turning point because by then the women was 55. She could no longer drown out her anxieties in her high-powered career, and she no longer wanted to do so; workaholism had exhausted her enthusiasm for life. She wanted to detach from the career that had for so long been her primary source of identity. But then what would she be?

Her inner thoughts articulate the inchoate fears of many: "If you realize that you can die and begin to accept it, then what do you want to do with the life you have left? It's an incredible passage. Some people never quite pull out of the depression; they come out the other end thoroughly defeated. Others just keep on playing poker and never look up at the window. We're all going to be executed at dawn. The ones who never look up are the people making millions on Wall Street: If they can do one more deal, if they can kill one more competitor, they think they can keep on playing poker forever. But there are many of us who play our hand and watch the window all the time. And when we start seeing a little light in that window, it's a tremendous crisis."

This woman had also chosen to be childless. That choice can render the passage to the Age of Mastery a more difficult one. For the childless woman or man, the future represents primarily time subtracted from *me*.

The inevitable narcissistic wounds of aging are not ameliorated by a sense of continuity of generations and the connectedness to the future that one naturally feels through grown children and *their* progress. It is a one-generation progress story. For a person with children, the future also represents gains, such as watching one's children grow and flourish and become, eventually, more caring of you, together with the ultimate joy and stimulation of grandchildren. How often do we hear men or women in public life say, "I'm doing this to try to leave the world a little better place for my grandchildren." The progress narrative continues.

Let me put a question to you: Will your personal life story in Second Adulthood be conceived as a progress story or a decline story? To a large degree, *you* have the power of the mind to make that choice. Yes, you will encounter losses in Second Adulthood, some of them irrevocable. But you will also have the accrued experience and judgment to adapt to them along with the confidence of a firmer identity and far greater self-knowledge than you ever had in First Adulthood. You also have a greater capacity to love and to be loved, in ways far deeper and less selfish than when you were younger. The opportunity is to get on with the real work of your Second Adulthood—the feeding and crafting of the soul.

As you begin to put your own adult life into words, you will probably find that the story can be told in many different ways, depending on the kind of future to which you think it is leading. This should start you thinking about the possible relationships between your past self and your future self. In his book *A Search for God in Time and Memory*, John S. Dunne suggests that we think about our life as a whole, all the elements of drama in it, which will provide a sense of how our lifetime fits into the larger historical and generational saga of our times.[13] "Composing a personal creed . . . the object of the search would be to find your God . . . to know what you personally believe in and act upon."

Some see it as an act of selfishness, or at the very best self-indulgence, to sit around and think about where one has been. Yet one does not discover the passage to be made without taking the time to glance backward over one's life. By reflecting on that series of apparently unrelated actions that constitute our own story, we should become conscious of a pattern. By 50 the formlessness has taken form. The pattern of our lives is as clear and repetitive as the narrative of a novel or the theme and recapitulation of theme in the symphony. And if we *choose* whether to find the joy or pain in our pattern, we make of fate a human matter.

Oedipus, blind and bedeviled on all sides by vengeful gods, has one of the most triumphant Aha! moments in all literature: "Despite so many ordeals, my advanced age and the nobility of my soul makes me conclude that all is well." He recognizes that he would not have discovered his full humanity without his mistakes and suffering. The mortal then assumes ownership of his fate and proclaims it progress.[14]

PEGGY'S PROGRESS

The friend whose ordeal I described earlier in this chapter definitely felt her life was in decline as she watched her husband die organ by organ. But a year after Chuck's death Peggy Downes told me of her own progress. "I still can't talk about loneliness. I miss Chuck terribly," she said. "But it's ironic. When nothing bigger can happen to you in a negative sense, you feel invulnerable. Since he's gone, I'm more *me* than I ever was. I dare more. My first question now is always, Well, why not? I've done, for me, some pretty strange and unpredictable things." She laughed. "I call it my wild hair. When I don't have my wild hair, I'm sad. But when I have it, there's a certain elation."

Peggy had just come back from three weeks in the Canadian Gulf Islands, diving into the sea at dawn. "It made me feel like I can be a spicy woman again." She was back on track professionally, teaching a full load, designing a pilot course on the politics of aging, and coauthoring a book.

Like Sisyphus at the foot of the mountain, about to roll his rock uphill one more time, we will always pick up our burdens again. But even Sisyphus, in his descent, like the blinded Oedipus, concludes that all is well. Who knows? This man, described by Homer as the wisest of mortals, may have had the best of both the mortal world and the underworld. Having tricked the gods into allowing him to come back from the underworld to punish his wife, he stays on with her, delightedly, facing the sparkling sea and ignoring the gods' many recalls and living out the fullest of Second Adulthoods. Furious, the gods designed for him a task meant to be the ultimate in futility. But instead of going back to the darkness of the underworld and death, he was given a challenge that would keep him active, in the light of the world, forever. "The struggle itself toward the heights is enough to fill a man's heart," asserts Camus. "One must imagine Sisyphus happy."[15]

GUIDES AND TEACHINGS

You may find guidance for composing your own personal narrative in science or religion, philosophy, psychiatry, or poetry. I find that each of these systems of thought offers valuable illumination along the journey.

Science tells us that mastery of stress is one of the basic sources of self-esteem and self-confidence. Mastering a major life transition or rising above a life accident not only helps us avoid psychic scars; it can also enable us to make a *brain passage*. The brain is like a collection of computers of different kinds, but they don't work together as a unified system! As the brain receives information and raw impressions from the outside world, through a variety of sensory receptors, a series of logical operations is performed on that input. Associations are made with the perceptions of our inner world and perhaps with our accrued knowledge. This enriched information is converted into coherent images that we call thoughts and feelings. The brain is then capable of initiating action on the basis of these images.

But the brain is different from, and vastly superior to, an electronic computer. It is remarkably plastic. When one observes the gifted neuroscientist Eric Kandel at his pioneering work on brain research at Columbia Presbyterian Medical Center, it becomes clear that the brain is able to change its images and therefore its performance and even its coping strategies *as a result of new experience.* This holds true whether that new experience is unintended or consciously introduced. Therefore we can actually produce new passageways in our brains by learning how to *think* ourselves into another state of physical as well as emotional well-being. In that state of arousal we are capable of making leaps of competence, modifying our self-image, identifying self-defeating behaviors, and learning new coping skills. We are also in the best state of mind to spot an imaginative solution to a major life passage.[16]

But what to do about the anxiety if you are feeling overwhelmed by a life accident as you try to make the passage to the Age of Mastery? A memorable image was described by a psychiatrist I interviewed, Dr. Patrizia Levi, who often works with people facing mortality crises. Imagine yourself in the ocean. Sometimes the current of life is fairly calm, and you can move along with it. Even if it's choppy, you can take the waves, perhaps readjust your course, and push forward. But at other times, when a storm blows up, the waves swell so high they threaten to overwhelm you. At that point you don't fight the waves; you go with them. And you try to retain a sense about yourself that you will eventually find your sea legs in spite of the storm. The chances are that if you remain calm and alert, you will land safely.

A former Duke University economics professor, Thomas Naylor, his psychiatrist wife, Magdalena Naylor, and Duke's dean of the chapel, William Willimon, developed a seven-step process for addressing the most important quest of the second half: *The Search for Meaning*, as they call their useful book.[17] "By facing the abyss, the end, by going to Hades and back, we face the meaninglessness," Professor Naylor tells participants in his workshops. "The confrontation with the abyss, with meaninglessness makes us *wise*. We can come back with incredible skills of honesty and self-awareness, with patience and lovingness."

Traditional religions, of course, are predicated on the Resurrection story, and a majority of Americans believe in life after death. Dean Willimon told me he sees "passage" as a secular way of describing what is termed in Christian religion a conversion experience.

In the ancient teachings of Tibetan Buddhism there is also a concept very similar to that of passages, the intermediate states or transitions known as bardos. Occurring continuously throughout both life and death, bardos are "junctures when the possibility of liberation, or enlightenment, is heightened." Just like passages, whatever one does at these highly charged moments has a lasting effect. Sogyal Rinpoche, who brings the teaching of the *Tibetan Book of the Dead* into the realm of living, thinks of a bardo as being "like a moment when you step toward the edge of a precipice."[18] Living on the edge—we're back to our original theme—and once again it is depicted as a positive preparation for liberation.

The greatest and most charged of these points of passage or bardos, or opportunities for conversion, is the moment of death. But we don't have to wait for the shock of terminal illness, or for the rageful sorrow at watching helplessly while someone very dear to us dies prematurely, to force us into confronting the meaning crisis. We can begin, here and now, to find meaning in our lives. The Tibetan masters say the true attitude toward change should be "as if we were the sky looking at the clouds passing by." That is, let go, let it happen, accept the impermanence of the previous stage while preparing to relish the new life to come, *without grasping*. William Blake elevated that attitude in poetry:

> He who binds to himself a joy,
> Does the winged life destroy;
> But he who kisses the joy as it flies
> Lives in eternity's sunrise.[19]

Part Four

FLAMING FIFTIES: WOMEN

8

WOMEN: PITS TO PEAK

Fifty-two. Standing up here right on top of the middle of it has to be the happiest time.
I mean, it's the only time you get a three-hundred-and-sixty-degree view—
see in all directions. Wow! What a view![1]

—EDWARD ALBEE, *THREE TALL WOMEN*

An attractive woman friend confided that when she turned 50, she felt like one of those park statues that turn green, weather-streaked, and crumbly, the kind that no one, not even the people on the benches right in front of it, notices anymore.

The first clues we have to our own aging are the ways other people see us—or stop seeing us. By her mid- to late forties a woman knows that she is walking the edge of losing her looks. That advantage, taken for granted in youth, no longer counts for free points. "All of a sudden I feel invisible" is the ubiquitous lament. Oh, if your hair has just been tinted and done in a particularly breezy style, and you're in a thin phase, and your skirt is short and bouncy, and you have on dark glasses, it's as though you had been reborn for the day. "Hey, Mama, you is beyoodeeful," shouts the New York trucker. Buoyed up for an instant by the wind in your vanity, you may catch yourself succumbing to the sort of sexual evaluation you haughtily scorned when you were still young and pretty enough to be an object of male lust whether you liked it or not.

From the number of women who describe such moments I can only say they are as common—and as politically incorrect—as rape fantasies. Our concern with how we look as we age may be superficial, but it's natural. We shouldn't be ashamed of obsessing about it from time to time. After all, this is one aspect of the passage to the Age of Mastery that all of us face, men as well as women. But for women the worry about losing their looks is only one symptom of a much larger phenomenon.

Women I have interviewed often describe a "pit" or "low" during their mid- to late forties, complicated in many cases by the confusing symptoms of perimenopause. Even those women who emerge from the surveys most satisfied with their lot have not magically avoided patches of despond and problems. In fact, fully half of them have suffered from at least one serious depression. Looking back, however, they feel grateful for what life has given them.

Around 50 they begin to take off. Straight through their fifties the women studied showed gains in inner harmony, mastery, and life status as they register—with considerable surprise—that they are more fulfilled and enjoy greater well-being than at any other stage of their lives. Of the total of seven thousand women who answered the national surveys, those with the poorest sense of well-being were, on average, 47 years old—the pits—while those enjoying the highest sense of well-being were 53—the peak. What accounts for this slump? And how do women come out of it?

FIRST, THE TERROR

Lauren Hutton is no ordinary woman, but she is emblematic. The supermodel strutted nonchalantly just out in front of the lives of a whole generation. She carefully worked out the pose, the look, the gestures and facial expressions to suit each stage of a woman's life. When I visited Hutton in her Soho loft, she spread out the photographs from her thirty-year career, a stunning visual record of the culture's refusal to equate female beauty with real life, passion, blood in the veins, or current in the brains.

In the Sixties, when Hutton was in her twenties, women tried to copy her blank baby-doll stare, the blond falls and miniskirts. In the seventies, when Hutton was in her thirties, she became the Revlon "girl," and women loved looking at her dozy sexuality in wet bikinis and clinging T-shirts. As she grew older, Hutton struck younger and younger poses. By the age of 40 there was no aliveness left in her face. She let stylists trowel on three hours' worth of makeup, hack off her long locks, load her up with hair spray and lip gloss. The Greek chorus in studios that used to purr, "Oh, darling, you're beyond deevine," now treated her as if she were lucky to be photographed. Hutton internalized their image of her: *I know I'm over the hill. . . . Whatever beauty I have left, take it.*

All anybody had paid and praised her for all through her First Adulthood was her outer appearance—her false self. "I'd been striking stances, and imitations of stances, all my professional life," she says. "They were getting further and further away from the truth of how I felt." She tried to shift into movies, but according to Hutton "they were mostly cheesy movies. Nobody can make a cheesy movie look good. I started acting late, so I didn't have enough of a craft to make something good out of the movies." By age 44 she was certain she was "bottoming out." By then "I had lost my real self," she says. Then she pulls out Exhibit A, the last modeling picture taken of her before she dropped out of sight.

"This was the pits for me."

The bony woman in a strapless bodice with a cinched waist, frizzed-out frosted hair, magenta lips, sunken cheeks, and eye sockets that look bruised because they're loaded up with purple shadow and heavy black eyeliner, looks, well, let Lauren Hutton suggest the caption: "She's gaunt. She's frightened. She's desperate. She looks like a bad sixty-five."

Hutton was actually 44. She had just started perimenopause. "And I was so frightened by then, I felt so out of it, and so out of control of myself, I wouldn't stop them. I felt they must know how to make me look good."

But photographers knew only how to make her look like a girl. (It was a long time before she understood that society did not have pictures of *women;* it had only pictures of girls *pretending* to be women.) That photo shoot when she was 44 was the occasion of Lauren Hutton's "little death." She felt she had become a complete fraud. Menopause heightened her sense of loss. "I didn't have a family, I didn't have an art, and I hadn't made peace with myself."

As she descended into the pits, Hutton began to have horrifying dreams. "I was the figure on top of a one-hundred-foot-tall Venetian chandelier wedding cake. In a giant hoopskirt. Everybody was stuck in it—the whole crew. My job was to fly this giant apparition through rooms and find ways to get out into the open, to fly it through the town streets. People were chasing us, and I had to do something. I wasn't keeping it up in the air anymore."

She spent lots of time alone in her early to mid-forties. Seeking out haunts in Noho where no one she knew could see her, she sat reading newspapers. Then it was home to the loft to go to bed with a book and a pot of okra. The terror of facing the decay of her false self in the lens of a camera or the eyes of her friends was unbearable. The only escape she knew was to slip inexorably into a Garboesque self-exile.

Hutton was pushing 45 when the photographer Steven Meisel thought of featuring her in a now-famous Barneys New York ad. She rejected the job again and again. "I hadn't looked at a fashion magazine for five years because it was too painful," she says. "Everybody in them was twenty-five years younger. There was no one from my generation. I kept feeling further and further away from beauty. Old. Worn-out. Faded." Once again Hutton mirrored what many women of her generation were feeling.

Finally she agreed to see Meisel. "I can't pose," she told him. "I don't know what modeling is anymore." She was dressed in overalls and desert boots and wore an ironic smile that said, "Okay, now I get the joke."

"Guess what?" the photographer said. "*That's* what we want."

Weeks after the shoot Hutton was hiding in her Sunday morning hangout to read *The New York Times.* The paper fell open to a full-page picture of a woman—not a girl—who was absolutely beautiful. "It took my breath away," says Hutton. "I didn't recognize her." The "her" was Lauren Hutton.

From that Aha! moment, realizing how separated she had become from herself, Hutton has undertaken to transform herself personally. The Barneys ad turned her into the Poster Woman for over-50 glamour. "Women began to come up to me in the street and say, 'You make me feel so *good.*' I felt useful for the first time in my life. It was thrilling." She now has a cause: to help change a phony system that promotes the lie that beauty is only youth. More important, by projecting a blend of clarity, curiosity, spirituality, and the glow of good sex, all wrapped up in the positive message that accompanies her Revlon ads—"This is our prime time—let's make the most of it"— Lauren Hutton has become the icon for millions of women coming out of the pits and looking forward to the peak.

THE VANITY CRISIS

Lauren Hutton's story is, of course, a highly exaggerated version of the vanity crisis. It is particularly hard on those accustomed to being appreciated for their looks or those paid for looking pretty, such as actresses and models (and Hutton makes no pretense that looking as good as she does in her fifties is not possible without the strict discipline of a professional model). But many other jobs, from hotel reservations manager to retail salesclerk, are biased toward the hiring of pretty young things. What to do? Become consumed by the struggle to hang on to the few remaining strongholds, dangerously dieting and running to colorists and skin specialists and cosmetic surgeons—the Helen Gurley Brown model? Or should one give up and let oneself go into instant grandmotherhood—the Barbara Bush model? Isn't there a middle ground between panic and relinquishing your sense of yourself as a woman and sexual being?

The truth is, it is virtually impossible to uphold the cultural stereotype of the taut-skinned, pouty-lipped child-woman with her thin, leggy, high-breasted, tight-bottomed young body. Those who put all their efforts into trying to maintain their youthful physical plant do so at the expense of cultivating the mature psychological strengths and the intellectuality and achievements that are the natural prerogatives of middle life.

Second Adulthood is not about repeating ourselves; it's about finding a new version of attractiveness. It's making the most of whatever external beauty we have, but also activating sources of internal value and defying the "beauty myth" that constrained us in First Adulthood. Once we begin to accept and enjoy the roundedness and normal weight gain, the wrinkles and sags that come naturally with maturity, we become grounded. And being grounded, we can build on the two pillars that make the New Older Woman such good value: her complexity and her uniqueness.

Some of America's favorite singers have found a second wind in their fifties—but not without first assuming that it was all over. Even those who once relied on their seductiveness are now composing a more fit, streamlined, and self-assured sexuality appropriate to their Flaming Fifties.

Tina Turner, fearful at 53 that "you can't be a rock 'n' roll old woman," tested the waters on tour in the summer of '93 and proved exactly the opposite. Seeing Tina Turner live in concert made vivid the contrast between the charms of young beauty and mature beauty. Despite all the years of dancing that have toned her, Turner's body has matured from the feline sex kitten to a shapely roundedness, with the slightly thicker waist and fuller hips that are natural to maturity. She still looks provocative in her minidresses, but she is able to project even greater physicality—without trying too hard. The superthin postadolescent twin backup dancers who jump around beside her, while they're adorable sex objects, exude no personal power. They are essentially meatless and weightless; all their beauty comes from the outside. With Turner, it's gathered into a core that has gravity—pain converted into personal power.

Having escaped sixteen years of beatings by Ike Turner, Tina published her midlife autobiography to put an end to that chapter of her life. Both the best-seller *I, Tina* and *What's Love Got to Do with It?*, the hit film based on the book, are progress narratives that emphasize survival and resilience. "I stood up for my life," she has said.[2] But she didn't have the courage to stand up until she was older.

When you are young, you can rely on so little. If your skin is smooth and your eyes sparkle and your body looks smashing in a miniskirt, people respond to you automatically before you open your mouth. You don't need much help. But all the attention to your physical charms can easily distract a woman from developing deeper core attributes.

Trading on physical charms becomes more and more difficult to pull off with age, because a woman's beauty is simply not as enchanting as it was in her twenties or thirties—just as a man no longer possesses the physical strength and speed on which he prided himself as a young lion. Therefore, if there is no core value, you cannot go very far. You are threatened by everything. Even illness becomes a threat to your beauty. And if you have counted on another person as the mirror defining what is relevant about you—by playing the pretty accessory wife, for instance—that becomes another trap.

"The only way through our narcissism is to feel the mortal wound," writes Thomas Moore in *Care of the Soul.* "Narcissism is not going to be cured by literal fulfillment of the grandiose expectations for ourselves we may have entertained in fantasy. That false ideal has to be let go, so that an 'other' can appear."[3]

But fantasy itself can work magic.

"I'm much more attractive to men now than I was as a young woman," says Pat Pickens, a button-eyed businesslike woman who works as a guidance counselor in a Queens, New York, elementary school. "It doesn't have to do with prettiness," she insists. "It's all about keeping your chemistry alive." This is a woman of color who, two weeks away from turning 50, had no intention of giving up on herself as sexually desirable or desirous. Her secret appeal? "I'm always looking at men to pick out my candidates"—that is, candidates for an imagined idyll on a desert island. A dimple winks wickedly in her smile. "You have to decide what it is in men that attracts you and then actively use the fantasy anywhere. When you go through an airport, instead of looking down and being shy and demure, you look around and say, 'Oh, my God, now *he's* a candidate,'" she suggests. "Then you let the chemistry happen. Just the sensation, the fantasy. It's wonderful."

Her husband, William Pickens III, a sweet man and an extrovert, joins in the game. "He doesn't mind my fantasies because I'll tell him whenever there's 'a girl from Ipanema' coming down the street, and he'd better look at her," says Pat. "I have to keep my home fires burning too."

As the years go by, your warmth and curiosity, your ease in relating to people, your intelligence and imagination, your wit and sense of irony all become far more important than looks to the package of attributes that people appreciate about you. If you cultivate more of those qualities and begin to rely on an internal mirror, you will not be so preoccupied and self-conscious with how people are going to see you as you enter a room. If you enter with curiosity and a twinkle of good humor, *expecting* to meet some-body who will be interested in what you have to say and *be interesting back*, if you perhaps drop an unexpectedly ironic remark, clearly something is going to happen in that room. People will be drawn to your easy self-assurance and your curiosity about *them*. If not, it wasn't the right room! There will be another room.

THE NEW FEMALE PACESETTERS

The female in her fifties today had a lot of catching up to do. She broke out of Fifties conformity into Sixties revolution, Seventies feminism, and Eighties ambition. With everything she had learned, she roared into the 1990s, having already detonated the expectations others had for her—and those she had for herself.

The passage to the fifties and the Age of Mastery has been radically altered. Many women now at this stage in life find themselves blazing with energy and accomplishment as never before in history. Call it the Flaming Fifties.

In 1993 alone it seemed that every time one picked up a newspaper another woman in her fifties was assuming a command position: U.S. Ambassador Madeleine Albright (at 56), shaping world policy at the United Nations; Janet Reno (at 55), balancing the scales of justice as America's first female attorney general; Cabinet Secretary Donna Shalala (at 52), helping foment a health care reformation. Ruth Bader Ginsburg (at 60), once the backseat wife encouraging her husband to go to law school, stepped up to the Supreme Court bench. Kay Bailey Hutchison (at 50) became the first woman from Texas to be elected to the U.S. Senate. The unimaginable happened in California in 1993. Not one but two members of the "wrong" sex, both Jewish and from the same part of the state—Dianne Feinstein and Barbara Boxer—beat their male primary opponents and sailed on to the U.S. Senate.[4] And a whole new class of congresswomen, most of them in their fifties, won seats as freshwomen legislators in the nation's Capitol.

Clearly, contemporary women now moving into their fifties are transforming the whole concept of middle life. And those moving up in public life are turning the old stereotype upside down—from decline to rule.

It may be a revival of women's ancient roles as priestesses and healers, a shift necessary to revive sick patriarchies and address a health-care and environmental crisis in the waning days of the twentieth century. To explore this phenomenon across social classes, beyond the anecdotal evidence from individual stories, I conducted three different national surveys. (For a complete description of each survey sample, see Appendixes II, III, and IV.)

Of the 687 business and professional women who responded, more than two thirds are 45 or older (average age, 50). The majority followed a traditional path through First Adulthood, marrying on the average at age 22 and having the first of two or three children at 25. Half divorced, usually in their mid-thirties. By now more than three quarters have college degrees—an extraordinarily high percentage who have reeducated and reissued themselves as polished career women, most of whom feel fortunate to be paid for doing work they enjoy.[5] One in three is a business manager; others are in teaching, counseling, or nursing; and 14 percent are professionals with advanced degrees. They believe their work is useful and gives them an opportunity to use their talents while contributing to society. Their average personal income is $41,000.*

There is a dramatic shift in what these women most value. In their twenties it was independence and romance. At 50, although they still rank family commitment above all else, they are more interested in power and their potential for creating social change. For younger women, power is a loaded word, often connoting aggressiveness, stepping on people, being unfeminine. This survey revealed that as women grow older and place less emphasis on their own personal problems, they see power as a tool for pursuing their more socially connected goals. Indeed, seven out of ten of these busy professionals are devoted to causes larger than themselves.

These women are among the pacesetters. They are on the cutting edge of the new definition of Second Adulthood for women.

---

*Only 7 percent of the 687 business and professional women earn a personal income of more than $100,000 a year.

WORKING-CLASS WOMEN: FINDING
FAITH IN YOURSELF

Many women approaching 50, however, still suffer from internalized images of themselves as tired, shapeless, sexless, and superfluous. They don't have anything like the fame or money or God-given attributes of a Lauren Hutton or Tina Turner. Some continue with behaviors that contribute to accelerated deterioration, such as smoking, drinking (more than two ounces of liquor or two glasses of wine a day), and eating fatty diets, any one of which can exaggerate the symptoms of menopause and increase vulnerability to heart disease and cancer. Indeed, a shocking leap in the number of overweight Americans took place during the 1980s, according to recent national weight surveys.[6] The age-groups showing the greatest increase in obesity were women between the ages of 45 and 54 (40 percent are overweight) and women between 55 and 64, almost *half* of whom are carrying much more weight than is healthy for them.

This pit is one that people usually dig for themselves, becoming increasingly sedentary even as their metabolism is burning up calories less efficiently. An adult over 45 who watches TV four or five hours a day, rides in cars or public transportation instead of walking, and takes in the usual excessive thirty-seven-hundred-calorie daily American diet, is a living recipe for obesity. Blue-collar working women and wives, in particular, may look and feel a decade older than professional women, especially if they overeat or drink to compensate for low self-esteem or because they see their middle-class status being threatened by global economic realignment.

For a solidly middle-class sample to compare with the Professionals, I turned to *Family Circle*, the popular magazine, which has a mass readership of 26 million. The magazine distributed 2,000 of my Life History surveys, asking each woman to give a copy to a "significant other." (For a complete version of the survey that was sent to *Family Circle* readers, see Appendix I.) A total of 1,024 people responded, including 385 matched pairs of husbands and wives.

This group of women is radically different from the Professional Women. The majority of *Family Circle* respondents have *not* graduated from college, and half have family incomes of less than $40,000 a year. (Nationwide, half of Americans earn less than $30,000.) Almost all these women are mothers, and few have ever been divorced. Most still adhere to the Traditional Core sex roles. These women do all the housework and twice as much of the child care, although almost two thirds also work outside the home either full- or part-time. The jobs they hold are traditionally white- or pink-collar female positions—clerks/secretaries or teachers, social workers, nurses, or managers/administrators—for which they earn less than $25,000 a year. Their contribution to the family budget is usually seen as supplemental, so there is little concept of career development.

There appears to be an economic threshold below which women do not have the economic or physical security to allow for flourishing in Second Adulthood. That magic threshold in my surveys is a family income of at least $30,000.[7] Women whose family incomes fall below that level find taking any kind of risk, much less making a major life change, far more remote and terrifying than it would be for an educated business- or Professional Woman who has escaped from many of the restrictions of traditional roles and attitudes.

Given these material and cultural differences, it is striking how many of my broad theories about women and men in Second Adulthood are confirmed in the *Family Circle* sample, a reliable indication that they are probably true for a wide spectrum of people and not limited to those more privileged.

Ann Stunden, for example, came out of a working-class background and put herself through graduate school before getting married and having three children. She tried to stay home and fulfill the traditional role of good wife and mother, but eventually she found she needed the stimulation of outside work. She was divorced at 38. By her forties she held down a responsible job in hospital administration. But at a deeper level, Ann didn't feel she deserved this status. And she resented having deprived herself of so much natural joy in life to reach it.

She began to live a double life: "I was a workaholic and single mother during the long week, and a weekend drunk," when she was able to escape to a party or travel for business. Her self-regard flagged all through her forties.

"When I was forty-seven, forty-eight, those years were horrible," she admitted in a group interview with Rochester women. "I was working in a job where I wasn't appreciated, they could fire me at any time. I put on forty or fifty pounds. I wasn't comfortable in my own body, and the white male system certainly didn't appreciate a fat, irreverent woman. Physically I wasn't well because I was drinking too much."

Ann comes from a family of alcoholics, and her standard defense was simply "I just need to drink a little less." But late at night, alone, after cleaning out the freezer of ice cream and emptying the bourbon bottle, another thought would snake through the haze: "In my fifties I am going to be dead."

Just as she was bottoming out, a friend who happened to be a psychotherapist, Beth Streuver, took her off to a women's workshop. On that dark February day in her forty-ninth year, Ann realized whom the speaker was describing. "Oh, my God, she's talking about *me*. I'm an alcoholic. Now I know what it is, and I can do something about it."

To her utter amazement, "my fifties have turned out to be glorious." Her fiftieth birthday was the first she celebrated in sobriety in many years. With that scaffolding of self-respect beneath her, Ann was able to reach out and land a rewarding job directing a computer center at a major midwestern university. "I feel loss about having left Rochester," she says honestly, "but my job is wonderful, my home is beautiful, my kids have followed me, and I've had two younger men fall in love with me in the last couple of years!" (We'll meet Ann again, in Chapter 15, "Men and Women: The New Geometry of the Sexual Diamond.")

Economics greatly influences the possibilities of pulling out of the pits. Women who are poor cannot easily change their lives or find meaning in their work. Education is a key factor.

> Most of the women in all my surveys who measured near the top on a scale of well-being have completed college or earned graduate degrees.*

Ann Stunden, for example, had scrambled before she married to get the college and specialized education she would need later in life, and which, once she was sober, allowed her to relocate and find a job in which she commanded greater respect and rewards. This advanced schooling gives women a number of advantages associated with high well-being:

- Better jobs where they exercise authority
- Ability to be self-employed
- Broad expertise or skill base
- Fluidity in their careers

Most of the high-well-being women have made dramatic life changes: returning to school, beginning new careers, generating new dreams, or

---

*Embedded in the Life History Survey is a complex instrument for measuring well-being.

escaping marriages in which they couldn't grow—or all of the above. And having taken risks in almost every part of their lives, they feel the thrill of powers they didn't know they had. Many have rekindled dormant careers and are getting a tremendous kick out of their work. This is an area where they can control the outcome and make things happen much more easily than in a marriage. Indeed, work often becomes the surrogate marriage partner. Having empowered themselves at home, at work, and in the community, they feel more competent in managing life's complexities.

Women who cannot seem to pull out of the pits share a very different profile. The great majority of the unhappiest women over 45 wish they could make a career change but feel they can't. Many designate their career as homemaker. Others have low-paying, dead-end jobs. They feel trapped by financial instability or preoccupied by family problems.

Tellingly, these women of low well-being do not feel they have the "permission" to make a midlife passage. They have great reluctance to do anything for themselves. Generally their husbands and children do not see them as having careers, but rather as holding down jobs to supplement man-as-breadwinner. No one encourages them to take time to extend their educations or to start at lower levels on different career paths that might ultimately become more rewarding and lucrative. They are supposed to keep punching the clock and bringing home the extra salary and getting dinner on the table. These women often mentioned in interviews that their husbands resent and envy any efforts they do make to improve themselves, complaining, "Hey, you're making me look bad."

As a result, at a stage where they see their children leaving and their husbands becoming more rigid and resigned, instead of soaring, some working-class women feel tied to a treadmill. Half feel lonely. Most feel fat. When they hit rough spots, they usually pretend there is no problem or overeat or drink. They are plagued by an average of *seven* physical or psychological problems, from tiring easily and insomnia to frequent headaches and constant anxiety.[8]

By contrast, most of the high-well-being women don't even feel fat! In fact, the vast majority of the Professional Women surveyed follow exercise regimens to maintain their health and extend their endurance. More than a third also color their hair, have regular massages, or practice yoga. In all these ways they demonstrate their optimism, by making a greater investment in their health and longevity. For the most part they have stopped trying to reproduce their younger selves. Only a fraction of the most satisfied Professionals have had cosmetic surgery.

SURPRISE! YOU'RE NOT GETTING OLDER,
YOU'RE GETTING HAPPIER!

The results of all the surveys strongly suggest that by Second Adulthood the dominant influence on a woman's well-being is not income level or social class or marital status. The most decisive factor is age. Older is happier.

> Among the Professional Women in the Flaming Fifties, almost all—90 percent—say that 50 feels like "an optimistic, can-do stage of life."

The finding about the benefits of being older holds true for most of the working-class women. More than half of those over 50 in the *Family Circle* survey say that they are delighted with their lives at this stage. They are more satisfied with their work and finances and their own personal growth and development, and even more content with their body and physical attractiveness than the younger women (most of whom are self-conscious and certain they are too fat). To find this positive attitude among such a broad spectrum of older women all over a country as large as America represents a major social change.

Today's women are truly the pioneers in the new country of Second Adulthood. They are on a different timetable from men.

> College-educated working women over 45 believe they won't hit middle age until 60. And women in their fifties and sixties today do not expect to feel "old" until they are about 70.

This evidence of dramatically changing age norms coincides with the startling new recognition that one has a huge unmapped territory to fill in with another life. It is a perspective that doesn't really become clear in terms of time organization, however, until women pass 50. But a new wrinkle emerges. Since most women are married to men older than they, a woman's feeling "This is my time to fly!" may be dampened by a husband's sense of the foreshortening of time. A woman entrepreneur in upstate New York admitted her fears: "My husband is fifty-three and considering an early retirement. *That* is scary. Guess I'll have to be working indefinitely." She has seen the future.

Having started their income-producing work so much later than men, most women of the Silent Generation cannot afford to stop working. Indeed, while more and more of their male contemporaries are taking early retirement, women in their mid- to late fifties are more likely to be out working full-time than ever before.[9]

Here is an astounding figure: Three quarters of employed women aged 60 to 64 who are divorced, widowed, or not living with spouses are still drawing full-time paychecks![10] This trend will only mushroom.

> Women age 45 to 54 will show a 300 percent increase in job holding by the year 2000.[11]

WOMEN'S HISTORICAL PROGRESS ACROSS TIME

It used to be that the people at greatest risk for depression were middle-aged women. The pits for women had a label: "involutional melancholia." In 1980, a decade after the women's movement took off in America, that disorder was expunged from the psychiatric handbook.[12] Today we discover a totally different reality:

> Psychic prowess actually builds in women as they age.[13]

Clinical disorders, including depression, continue to drop off in older women. (The peak age for depression now has descended into the mid-thirties.) "There is a psychological maturing among women that continues well into their *sixties and seventies,*" confirmed Dr. Frederick Goodwin, director of the Center on Neuroscience, Behavior and Society at George Washington University.[14]

Even fresher and more exciting is to note the *cumulative progress,* from one generation to the next, in women's flourishing in the second half of their lives. This pits-to-peak phenomenon is not sui generis to the Silent Generation. Women have actually been breaking through in middle life for some time, going back at least to educated women of the World War II Generation.

The first suggestion of this generational progress spilled out of a 1974 follow-up to the 1954 Midtown Manhattan Study.[15] The late Dr. Leo Srole was surprised to find that as women move beyond the age of 40, they enjoy marked progress in mental health. Two different generational groups of older women, twenty years apart, were tested with the same mental health measures. On further observation Dr. Srole and his colleagues came up with an even more startling conclusion: *The improvement in mental health and well-being among older women was accumulating generationally.*

When the first of these results were published, a tremendous wall of resistance went up in the social science community.[16] The existing precept was that as women get older, they get depressed, and there were vested interests in perpetuating that erroneous assumption.

I asked one of Dr. Srole's last coworkers, Joel Millman, Ph.D., if we could go back into the data and probe more deeply for gender differences. The questions that form my well-being scale are similar to those used in a follow-up to the Srole study that explored how happy people were at particular ages and stages. These happiness questions have been asked of tens of thousands of people in the United States and of hundreds of thousands around the world.

"The men didn't vary much in their happiness by age," Dr. Millman reported back upon his reanalysis of the data, "whereas the women show very interesting patterns." Among women, again, we found a *very* strong correlation between happiness and age. The women who were aged 40 to 59 in 1974 were much happier with themselves and their lives, and showed far fewer mental health problems, than women of an earlier generation who had been those ages in 1954. When both sexes and every age-group in the study were compared, the happiest people of all were the women aged 45 to 49 (in 1974), followed by the women aged 50 to 55 who were "pretty happy." The most likely people to say they were *un*happy were men aged 50 to 59.

Since the late 1960s, when the great transformation of women's lives began in this country, new scholarship has poured forth offering fresh theories on the complex nature of female growth and development. Psychologists Norma Haan and Ravenna Helson at the University of California at Berkeley; Jean Baker Miller (1976); Nancy Chodorow (1978); Judith Bardwick (1980); Carol Gilligan (1982); Ellen McGrath (1992); Kathleen Day Hulbert and Diane Tickton Schuster (1993) and others, have studied women's lives across time and turned our thinking around.[17]

In her work on the psychologically healthiest women and men at age 50 drawn from the Berkeley studies, Florine Livson, Ph.D., fleshed out some fascinating detail that again verifies the pits-to-peak thesis historically.[18] Livson divided the women into traditionals and nontraditionals. The latter were the liveliest, most intellectual "doers" as adolescents; they had dreams of achievement and seemed to be progressing toward a firm identity.

By age 40 these nontraditional women appeared to have regressed. As the caregiver role disappeared, they became angry, thin-skinned, and bothered by demands, and they no longer used their intellectuality well. They complicated simple situations. The originality they had shown as girls was consumed now in fantasy and daydreams. Each one appeared to face a shattering identity crisis, as she confronted the empty shell of her other side—that girl who had a drive to achieve.

But by 50 these nontraditional women enjoyed a stunning rebound. They opened up intellectually and flowered emotionally. Their verbal fluency was again high. They had become more spontaneous, humorous, and expressive than the traditional women. But the traditional women, too, had reached a higher level of psychological health by age 50.

Educated women, in particular, generally undergo greater personality change in Second Adulthood than men do. Ravenna Helson, Ph.D., director of the Institute of Personality Assessment and Research at Berkeley, is the principal investigator of a respected study of 101 women graduates of Mills College.[19] Followed across twenty-five years—from age 22 to 52—even these moneyed and educated women were more dependent, insecure, and self-critical in young adulthood than their husbands or male partners.[20]

But once over 50, it is the women, and not their husbands, who exhibit more self-confidence. The men are becoming somewhat more dependent and less certain about their future goals. The Mills women reconsidered themselves totally in middle life. Their renaissance is not tied to giving up the parental role, which had been the prevailing theory offered by David Gutmann.[21] In this study of more contemporary women, their competence and self-confidence increased *regardless of whether they had children.* Those who held career positions of high status increased in forcefulness and independence, but most of the women enjoyed a burst of self-assurance and independence regardless of their job status.

In my own earlier work, a study of well-being among sixty thousand Americans conducted in 1979–80 and reported in *Pathfinders,* life satisfaction was also found to dip among women in their late forties but to come back strong in the early fifties.[22] This observation was emphatically confirmed after the publication of *The Silent Passage* in 1992, when I had an opportunity to travel the country and talk to thousands of women in their fifties who are enjoying "postmenopausal zest."

Thus in one study after another we find the pits-to-peak phenomenon. It is also apparent that consciously looking back to affirm the movement from survival to mastery in one's own life is a key strategy in accomplishing the passage to Second Adulthood.

In search of other working-class women who had found their way up from the pits to the peak, I made a trip to the Oregon coast. There I came to know a dozen feisty women in their fifties for whom vanity and status were the least of concerns. I will never forget the story of Justine Heavilon, the daughter of a cleaning lady. She had the wit and courage to find her passion in her fifties, outside conventional life, in a way rarely dreamed of by her mother's generation.

A SURVIVOR WHO FOUND PASSION AT 50

"Passion is about allowing yourself to get lost in something."

Picture Justine at 19: cabbage-pale face dented by a battering husband, body bagged out from four births. A high school dropout, she spent her nights standing the swing shift in a dark, cold, sulfurous-smelling factory, candling eggs, speechless against the din of machinery. She had no models beyond other uneducated women with bad teeth and beaten-up wombs, women who were old at 25. But she felt things, powerful things. She knew she had creativity inside her. (Almost all the women I've interviewed recall a wilder, creative spirit from their preadolescence.)

In her twenty-eighth year her third husband left her with no job, no car, five children, and a ninth-grade education. She was crushed. But Justine spent the next twelve years squirreling away enough money from child support, school loans, food stamps, teaching fellowships, and "garbaging" in Dumpsters to put herself through high school and college.

At 34 Justine was already a grandmother. By 40 she had earned a Ph.D. in psychology. By 44 she had sent her last child to college and started her own psychotherapy practice. But for all her accomplishments, after thirty years of silence during which her gender role crowded out any time or space for creativity, Justine still had not found her voice. She felt empty. Her mother had always talked, worshipfully, about "moving from the hot South to Oregon, to the ocean." Oregon symbolized the clean, cool edge, where one could fly free. But her mother had stopped growing at the same point and become increasingly embittered.

"Not me!" Justine had vowed. "I'm not going to have empty nest syndrome. I've already launched a new life."

She had long since dropped the wife role and recently let go of the original family house. Its many bedrooms were a continuing lure to her grown children. With the erosion of her servitude worn into the wooden step between kitchen and dining room, a reminder of obligatory holiday meals, that house was both the symbol and structure of her matriarchal role. She had thought selling it would free her. But still she felt burdened and unable to find her own voice. Why?

She had created an "office house" and filled it with other therapists, to whom she was on call as "mother," the one who fixed everything from the plumbing to professional rivalries. Justine finally recognized the repetition of her pattern. She was playing the matriarch all over again because it was a role she knew how to play well. The therapist had to tell herself: *Let go of the caregiver/matriarch identity; it's the only hope you have of recovering any part of that girl whose creativity was suppressed.*

And so, at 50, Justine escaped to the Oregon coast—the clear, cool edge. There, on the rugged ocean cliffs, she built a house with a view of her own where she could write a book and worship nature and explore her inner life. There are no bedrooms for children; that is key. The woman I found there, at 50, with huge fig-colored eyes and a froth of gray hair, looked prettier and far more energetic than the tired, stooped workhorse she had been at 19. Whom did she feel she had to please now?

"Nobody!" she exclaimed. "It's so wonderful. I have no lover. My kids write me notes saying, 'You're my hero.' " She is fiercely committed to making an impact by writing a book. She has found her voice. But the awe in her voice is reserved for the evidence of progress from one generation of women to the next: "I'm living the life my mother valued but was afraid to attempt herself."

Passion (outside sex) is something many women are afraid to embrace when they are younger. It takes time away from their children, their husbands, their homes, their income-producing activities. Some have kept special enthusiasms alive but on the back burner. These are the women who will travel, write, and perform poetry, take up the marimba, enter politics. And predictably these are the women who will have the most exciting and satisfying Second Adulthoods.

Other women find it very difficult to define what it is they can feel passionate about at 50. Thinking they had no right to ask that question during the extended parental emergency, they may have been deadened to the realm of their imaginations for a long time. But to create, one cannot be constantly other-focused; the energy must come from an inward place.

"The house on the coast was that for me," says Justine. "It was a space outside the role of caretaker, which doesn't allow much room for an inner life. When you're past the roles, you have the time to get lost in something. And that's what passion is about: allowing yourself to get lost in something."

Remember the Time Flies Test described in the Prologue to Book Two? What activity do you enjoy where time goes by without your even noticing it? (Sleeping doesn't count!) The more you focus on an activity you like, and the more time you give it, the more likely you are to become passionate about it.

"If you've clung to the creative spirit somewhere in the soul," Justine believes, "you can still regain it, even after the long period of servitude."

Justine has created several different sanctuaries, one where she paints, one where she makes wood carvings, and finally the hallowed computer room where she writes. "What's so freeing about being in one's fifties is to know the world wouldn't come to an end if you got lost in your writing or painting or marimba, and your house didn't get painted for six months, or you ate only macaroni and cheese," she says guiltlessly. "No one else is going to be severely neglected."

Most of us, of course, have to go on generating income while we're building our towers of dreams in the sky. The fickle business climate and the fact of age discrimination may threaten to short-circuit our power surges. Justine, too, recently became a casualty of shifting economic forces. Today's marketplace is inundated with female psychotherapists, even as insurers and HMOs are severely restricting the pool of patients and covering them for fewer and fewer sessions.

"They're putting me out of business!" Justine wailed at first. But she has learned by now not to waste time wallowing in victimhood. The handwriting was on the wallboard: *I can no longer support myself as a psychologist.* Justine challenged herself: *My life energies are precious. Do I have the courage to seek out what I love to do and also find a way to support myself?*

By our final interview, two years after Justine had relocated in her dream house on the Oregon coast, her solution was in place. It combined some rusty skills and a solid commitment to hauling herself and her computer into the interactive age. She had always loved trading stock, having managed money for various family members. "It was one of those things I knew I could be passionate about, but I'd never had the time to give to it. So last fall I sat down at the computer and tried to figure out how to use a modem to download the database and learn how to do technical analyses of stock." She rolled her eyes, remembering several months of total frustration. She told herself, *Okay, Justine, sit there and let it take as long as it takes, until you learn what you need to know.* She gobbled up software magazines and technical books and invested in more speed and megabytes for her new partner, the computer. "I vowed I was going to transform myself. And I did."

Ah, mastery . . . what a profoundly satisfying feeling when one finally gets on top of a new set of skills . . . and then sees the light under the new door those skills can open, even as another door is closing. For Justine, the solution is to conduct financial seminars for women. This self-created position allows her to combine her love of psychotherapy with her passion for money management. An added pleasure is to be able to act as a mentor who can teach women how to take power back by becoming financially astute. To satisfy the creative urge to write, she intends to do a book about women and money.

I asked her: Since she had let her creative self languish for so long, were there fears it wouldn't be there anymore?

She was totally honest. "There's always a nagging fear, even if I give it my all, I might realize I've been fooling myself all along." She caught herself taking only running starts at writing. But the only way one learns how to write is by writing. She would have to give up her procrastinations and throw herself into the effort.

"It feels like a trapeze act. You're hanging and swinging, and the trapeze goes higher and higher," is how Justine describes the sensation. "You have to drop the safety bar and fly forward. It's all dependent on faith in yourself, that you're not going to hit the rocks below and tumble into the abyss forever. You absolutely cannot get to the other side unless you let go."

9

WONDER WOMAN MEETS
MENOPAUSE

*M*enopause used to be a pit from which many women never emerged. The conventional script for a woman in the "Change of Life" was to become "difficult," or to be dumped by her husband for a "younger edition," or to disappear while friends whispered, "She's having a nervous breakdown." Fear and ignorance kept women in the dark about a passage as universal as puberty. Even a woman as strong and resilient as Barbara Bush fell into a despair so deep she flirted with the idea of suicide.

The Bushes had just returned from an ambassadorial year in China. It was the mid-Seventies, the women's movement was in full swing, George Bush was caught up in his new job as CIA director, and Barbara Bush was out of a job. All her children had left the nest. At one point she had stopped dying her prematurely gray hair. In an interview with Mrs. Bush I asked why, at a stage when women so often redouble their efforts to remain sexually attractive, she let her hair go.

Her reply was tinged with sadness. "George Bush never noticed."[1]

By the time Barbara Bush hit 50, she had plunged into a tailspin. "I was very severely depressed," she writes in her memoir.[2] "I hid it from everyone, including my closest friends. . . . *I felt ashamed.*" Like so many women of her World War II Generation, she kept silent. "My 'code' told me that you should not think about self, but others," she writes. "And yet, there I was, wallowing in self-pity. I knew it was wrong, but I couldn't seem to pull out of it." She never mentioned the *m* word. She never even associated hormonal changes with her dismal moods.

"Night after night George held me weeping in his arms while I tried to explain my feelings. I almost wonder why he didn't leave me." Her husband's suggestion that she see a psychiatrist drove her only deeper into gloom. Alone in the pit of menopausal malaise, she admits that she sometimes had to pull her car off the highway to stop herself from deliberately crashing into a tree or an oncoming vehicle.

Only today, almost twenty years after the fact, is Barbara Bush able to give that brief torment a name: "It seems so simple to me now: I was just the right age, fifty-one years old, for menopause."

Until very recently, almost all American society was in denial about this momentous passage. Doctors were not trained to deal with it. Scientists ignored it. The media recoiled from it. And women feared that by acknowledging it, they would be rejected as invisible, powerless, sexless, without value. If they were bothered by symptoms, most either blindly accepted medication or turned to tranquilizers or alcohol or tried to be good soldiers like Mrs. Bush and move on. Yet family life was routinely disrupted, because nobody could figure out *what to do about Mom.*

Then along came the first of the Boomer women who refused to take a one-size-fits-all prescription or a pat on the head for an answer. It was only in October 1991 that *Vanity Fair* boldly published my article on menopause.[3] People were shocked. Even to utter the word in polite company was new and uncomfortable. After publication of my book *The Silent Passage,* I was asked to appear on *The Oprah Winfrey Show.* The producer announced she had an easier time booking guests to talk about murdering their spouses than about menopause. In jest I said, "Why don't you have them on the same show? They're probably the same people."

Books by major authors like Germaine Greer and Betty Friedan appeared simultaneously, dissecting the subject with widely divergent views. (See Appendix V for list of current books on menopause recommended by women's health centers around the country.) Newspapers and magazines discovered the subject of menopause and made it the "hot" issue of 1992. TV held back because sponsors didn't want to be associated with "old" women—meaning any audience over age 40. That taboo, too, washed away once the marketing and advertising geniuses read the demographics:

Forty-six million American women are in or past the age of menopause today (over age 45).[4] And their numbers are growing by legions. More than one third of all women in the United States have already passed their fiftieth birthday.[5] And before the end of the century the target age-group (45 to 54) will increase by *one half.*[6]

Marketing menopause has become big business.

Menopause may be narrowly defined as the end of menstrual cycles and the cessation of a woman's reproductive life, but it is also a deeply meaningful psychological and spiritual passage. Anthropological accounts have revealed that cultural assumptions about aging and femininity can operate to magnify or ameliorate the physical symptoms.[7] The Chinese, who revere age, for example, do not even have a word for "hot flashes." Menopause is not an issue in China, according to Dr. Jane Porcino, who attended the first Chinese-American Women's Conference there in 1990.[8] "The women there all exercise, have a low-fat diet, and they take natural herbs for any discomforts." In contrast, for millions of women in Great Britain the Change is still the last great taboo. Only one in ten British women confides in her husband her apprehensions about approaching menopause, and few even discuss the matter with their doctors.[9] But in the United States women wield enough influence as scientists, physicians, nurses, legislators, journalists, and magazine editors that when they threw their weight behind opening up this subject in Congress and in the media, a huge wave of interest in menopause spread through society. We all seem to have discovered at the same time that we had an appalling lack of basic knowledge about this universal female transition. More pointedly, we had almost no hard data on the safety and efficacy of the hormone therapy routinely prescribed to millions, perhaps the largest *un*controlled clinical trial in the history of medicine.[10]

The lack of data at our National Institutes of Health was brought to public attention by government employees like Susan Blumenthal, who became the first assistant surgeon general appointed by the president as a watchdog for women's health.

"It's shocking that it's taken until 1994 to launch the first major study of estrogen replacement therapy, through the Women's Health Initiative," says Blumenthal.

Women have begun to let their doctors know they want a *dialogue* about menopause—a safe environment to ask questions and explore options—not to have hormones thrown at them. Physicians and medical centers have responded. More than a thousand women's health clinics have sprouted across the United States. Doctors (125,000 of whom are women today) are fighting over which specialty is best able to treat this newly identified and lucrative patient group. In 1991, while serving as head of the NIH, Bernadine Healy marshaled the government's backing for the Women's Health Initiative (WHI). Now well under way, with women volunteering by the thousands, the largest clinical study of women's health in American history is investigating whether women who use artificial hormone therapy for many years are actually better protected or at greater risk from such post-menopausal health hazards as heart disease, breast cancer, colon and rectal cancers, and fractures from osteoporosis.

As a member of the advisory committee to the Women's Health Initiative, it is my privilege to serve with some of the most prominent physicians and scientific researchers in the field of menopause today. Even though the earliest results from WHI will not be available until the year 2000, the pooling of professional experience and probing questions generated by this group are already helping to raise the level of awareness within our scientific establishment. In the meantime there are promising results from a three-year government-supported study of 900 women, known as the PEPI study (Postmenopausal Estrogen and Progestin Interventions), which has already changed significantly the way hormone replacement therapy is prescribed. (Results will be reported later in this chapter.)

Look how far we've come! In less than the last five years, we have emerged from the Dark Ages and moved light-years toward a new way of living through and beyond menopause. But along with this enlightenment, fueled by a new generation of women who have always been more at home in their own bodies, comes a new set of expectations. Contemporary women are accustomed to birth control and fertility control. Most expect to take control of this annoying little disruption called menopause.

Now what happens when we run into something that we can't control? Nobody has any magic against aging and certain inevitable changes that accompany it. When those expectations are not met, it results in rage.

"I'M OUT OF ESTROGEN, AND I'VE GOT A GUN"

I watched a brilliant, accomplished friend of mine, Dr. Ellen McGrath, race her motors and almost crash and burn as she went into combat with menopause. Her fierce determination to deny she was in the dread passage is typical of today's high-achieving woman in the Vietnam Generation.

But who could blame her? She was 47 years old, married, with two young children and a demanding private practice as a clinical psychologist in Laguna Beach, California. Having put in many years of academic training to reach the top of her field, having postponed marriage and motherhood until her late thirties, she saw herself in her mid-forties as a high-energy, high-performance engine primed to take off. Armed with all the professional and people skills she had spent decades developing, she fully intended to fly!

Weeks before she was about to set off on a whirlwind publicity tour to promote her first book, her body backfired on her. The blood flow was absurdly heavy. She was jumpy and irritable. A dead weight of sadness descended on her. Even picking up her son from preschool and sharing a picnic with him on the floor of her office didn't revive her usual ebullience. With the command performance of her career around the corner, suddenly she couldn't remember her own material. Chunks of it would fall away, as if the dense forest of her axons and dendrites were defoliating. *What's happening to me? Am I losing my mind?*

I had shared some of my research with Ellen while writing *The Silent Passage,* but as she said, "I never thought it would apply to *me.*"

She found the best gynecologist and demanded that he give her something to take all this away. She was given a megadose of estrogen by injection. A magic bullet. Within forty-eight hours her symptoms vanished. The doctor told her the injection would hold her for three months. Beautiful. All her symptoms could be blamed on the stress of the upcoming book tour. The doctor's other words, the "death" sentence—"You are in full menopause"— dissolved right out of her mind as she resumed her denial that anything had changed and flew off to take her bows as Wonder Woman, the author.

Three months later, when the predictable crash landing took place, I happened to be visiting Ellen. I was lying on the floor in the guest room, taking a yoga break, when she burst in upon me in a purple fury.

"Great, these doctors say my system is all screwed up, and I have to come off all hormones. I'm going to feel like shit, and then I'm going to bleed to death."

After the book tour her body had had a reaction to the heavy medication, and she'd begun to bleed very heavily. The megadose of estrogen was creating havoc with her own hormonal system. She began to look for information on menopause, but the more information she had compiled, the more frightened she had become, because she wasn't getting the answers she wanted. I sat her down on the floor and tried to talk her out of her agitated state.

"You know, none of us really believes *we* are going to hit menopause. And it's the women who are the busiest and brightest, like you, who are angriest about it."

"I'm *really* angry." She seethed. "I don't have time to deal with this."

"Of course. You're losing some of the control you've fought so long and hard to gain. The faster you're flying, the harder the impact when you hit this bump. But, Ellen, listen to me. You can't run away from it. What you have to do at this stage is go home. Listen to your body. Take the pause; you've earned it."

She looked at me with hard-glazed eyes. This was not the answer she was looking for. I knew that look. I recognized in it exactly where I had been myself only a few years before. Denial, rage, unrealistic expectations lead so many of us to the fantasy that if only we can find the right information, the right doctor, the right support group, the right understanding husband, the right pills or roots or herbs, it will make menopause go away. The answer Ellen wanted is the one we're all looking for: Tell us about a magic solution that will make us feel just as we've always felt, with the same energy, the same quality of orgasm, and no side effects.

Ellen had to interrupt our conversation to answer a call from a newspaper reporter seeking her out for her wisdom. The irony made us chuckle. At the same time her husband arrived, sounding very concerned from the doctor's latest diagnosis that she might have some terrible disease. "Ellen is different from other women," he said. "She's made it her business not to be stopped by any of the stuff society throws up against bright women."

Don't most women of her generation feel that way? Ellen's husband needed reassurance that *his* life wasn't going to be made hell by menopause. They had a solid marriage with shared intellectual interests and strong sexual chemistry, but this was just one more demand they hadn't counted on. "She springs me with this crisis and tells me I have to take over the kids and carpooling," he recounted. "Okay, I'm the one who takes care of crises, but I can't do it on a dime. So that proves to her I'm not there. She tells me this morning she hates me. I said, 'I hate you,' right back. We're acting like children."

I admitted that I'd been pretty impossible with my husband at the beginning too, swerving from weepiness to defiance in the space of minutes: "I just can't handle it anymore" to "Never mind, I can do it! I'll just take another exercise class." I told Ellen's husband that she would probably go through a phase of volatile hormone swings, and since she had to switch medications, she would probably feel a little depressed. Ellen reappeared, still angry.

"Do you get anything good out of this on the other side, besides survival?" she wanted to know.

"Yes, you do," I said with the full confidence of being in postmenopause. Menopause is a biological marker that demands women recognize where they are in life, I told her. It's an initiation into your Second Adulthood. Women who take the time to evaluate where they are, physically, psychologically, spiritually, are the ones who will move ahead; they'll be more balanced and productive in their fifties and sixties. "Think of it this way," I said. "You're going to live another thirty or forty years inside this house called your body. Don't let it fall into ruin. Start renovating now!"

Ellen looked bored. But her husband got the message.

"So that's why women live longer than men. Men don't have the pause." Ellen's husband brightened up. "Maybe I can learn from my wife's menopause."

I talked about how this marker reminds us that now we need to be conscious about how we eat, how we breathe, how to give the body regular exercise, and how to build in time for deep relaxation. "You can't take the body for granted anymore. Any more than a man can. When the muscles fire in an eighteen-year-old boy, he takes off like an antelope. If a man of forty-six tries that, he can rupture his Achilles tendon. Look at Al Gore. We all have to learn how to husband our bodies as we get older. If you don't give your body the feeding and breathing and movement and stretching it needs every day, it's not going to be there for you when you want to tax it."

"I don't want any peaceful meditative stuff," Ellen scoffed. "I've worked incredibly hard all these years to get a wide range of life skills so I can do the things I really care about. Now I want to *use* all that." She jumped up and began pacing. "I don't want to eat just vegetables and get a massage every week and do yoga aerobics and take a nap every day. Forget that! I need to consolidate my energy so I can focus on the contribution I want to make." She whirled around. "I want postmenopausal zest!"

It was a wonderfully absurd outburst. In mock innocence I said, "Um, I think you have to go through menopause before you get that."

She laughed at herself.

"I hear what you're saying," I said. "I was exactly where you were." I tried to explain that what she was going through was the beginning of the death of youth. It's painful. Nobody likes to go through a little death. We all resist it. We lash out; we feel angry that there isn't a cure-all. But if we take this pause to cultivate our inner resources, if we learn how to draw our energies from a deeper, disciplined place, if we honor this passage rather than fight it, I said, we definitely get something for going through it. "I promise you, Ellen, do that, and you will come out the other side with more force and focus than you ever had before. That's what postmenopausal zest is." With my last shot I urged her, "Just fly low for a while."

My friend did not buy my argument, not then anyway. She had a right to her anger and denial. These are normal, predictable reactions to the first phase of the crisis of menopause. It is especially predictive behavior for the achieving women of the Baby Boom: You will be angry, embarrassed, impatient, and incredulous that this could happen to you. You've been out there running a marathon and nobody told you that you'll probably hit a wall in your late forties—splat! You will be sure that if you do give in to menopause, your identity will disintegrate along with your body, and you will turn into a dried-up old crone overnight.

You are not alone. Scores of women I have interviewed feel the same way at the outset of this passage. It may be a bumpy ride of highs and lows for several years, but this, too, shall pass. The worst of the "pit" phase usually lasts no more than six months to a year.

One often comes out of it as abruptly as one falls into it. Looking back on her menopausal depression, Barbara Bush writes, "I wish I could pinpoint the day it went away, but I can't. All I know is that after about six months, it just did."[11] She adds that if she had it to do over again, she definitely would seek help.

You say you don't have time for menopause. Guess what? Menopause has time for you. The question is, Who will have the upper hand? The sooner you become willing to accept the passage, the easier you will find it to become the master of your menopause.

Today, you can plan for your menopause the way you planned your pregnancies. This is a whole new way to think about the Change. You can start by searching out information from mentors who are older than you, from books and magazines, from the women's health conferences that are now routinely held in most communities. You can also begin to establish a life-long relationship with a doctor who has a genuine interest in mature women and who understands the necessity of treating them as partners.

Menopause can be broken down into three broad phases, each of which creates a very different hormonal milieu, makes different demands, and offers its own liberation. This chapter will offer a brief review of each phase.*

PHASE ONE: THE PERIMENOPAUSE PANIC

Almost all women experience some menopausal symptoms, but few have severe problems. An estimated 20 percent sail through with little difficulty,

*For more detail and up-to-date information on hormonal and nonmedical treatments, see the revised spring 1995 softcover edition of *The Silent Passage.*

and another 10 percent or so are temporarily incapacitated. In between are all the rest of us—70 percent of women—most of whom probably don't know that the peak of hot flashes, emotional symptoms, and bleeding problems occurs over the months or years *before* the actual event of menopause.

This first phase, *perimenopause,* is the least understood and potentially most confounding part of the menopausal passage. Perimenopause is a lot like puberty. Surges and dips in hormones are the most severe and unpredictable. Estrogen is involved in at least three hundred bodily processes. Thus, when it dips below levels the body has come to depend upon for thirty years or more, predictably the body is thrown out of balance. The brain's brain, the hypothalamus, cannot coordinate many functions with its usual precision and may play havoc with your sleep, temperature, appetite, libido, menstrual cycles, and mood, making you feel temporarily estranged from your body.

When does it happen? Researchers admit they have underestimated the number of younger women who experience all the symptoms of menopause, even though they still have periods.[12] The latest surveys reveal a surprising number of women in their *early forties* are perimenopausal.[13] The first thing you need to know is this:

> Menopause is as individual as a thumbprint.
> No two women experience it alike.

The spectrum of signs and symptoms in perimenopause is bafflingly broad. One woman will brush it off—"I feel hot for a few seconds a couple of times a day, but not enough to bother me"—while another is terrified that she will flare purple and start leaking drops of perspiration during a business conference or forget phone numbers she just looked up. A third woman, who complains of waking up four or five times a night, swamped in sweat, changing nightgowns, having Thermostat Wars with her husband, is mistakenly diagnosed as being in clinical depression. In truth she is suffering from the effects of serious sleep deprivation.

It hardly seems possible that all these people are talking about the same organic process. Even when discussing the most commonly shared symptom of perimenopause—erratic bleeding—women in their forties should be warned, "Your cycle will get longer or shorter, lighter or heavier, closer together or farther apart."[14] All these eccentricities are age- and hormone-related. Most often they are perfectly normal. But maddening! Johns Hopkins epidemiologist Trudy Bush, Ph.D., predicts that perimenopause is bound to become a serious public health issue: "When Baby Boom women reach their forties and fifties and begin to experience embarrassing symptoms like hot flushes and excessive bleeding in the workplace, they will demand that more attention be paid to perimenopause!"

Dr. Patricia Allen, the New York obstetrician-gynecologist, is on the receiving end of those demands. "Baby Boom women come into my office now in an information-feeding frenzy. The silence about menopause has turned into an obsession. They want the perfect treatment without consequence." A gifted and intuitive practitioner, Dr. Allen reassures her new patients that they are doing the right thing by looking for guidance. It is much healthier to be conscious of the need to evaluate their lives at this point and to understand the passage, as opposed to just wandering through it, having up days and down days, and fearing the worst. She tells women, "It is important that you make informed choices. But you also have to recognize that everything we do, or don't do, has some price."

The mood swings characteristic of perimenopause may bring on sadness, malaise, mild depression, irritability, poor concentration—in general, the feeling of being on a roller coaster.[15] Western medicine still fosters the erroneous assumption that these *temporary* mental symptoms herald a marked deterioration in the mental health of postmenopausal women. Exactly the opposite is true. As previously cited, studies now show that women in the *post*menopausal years show *less* evidence of any psychological problems than younger women. It is women in their mid- to late forties who manifest a peak in minor mental symptoms in the five years *immediately prior* to the end of their menstrual cycles.[16]

Stress has been shown to increase the severity of symptoms in Phase One of menopause and may even precipitate it prematurely.[17] Nine months after Ellen McGrath's initial skirmish with the symptoms of perimenopause, she was still angry. Like many women who have worked hard to develop confidence in their own abilities to use their knowledge and creativity to make a difference, she was frustrated whenever the fatigue and fogginess of early menopause threatened her performance.

"This is like the female version of midlife crisis," she told me. She had seen herself as the butterfly, flying high, alighting on all sorts of sweet new places. "Suddenly it feels like I'm back in the cocoon, as though I have cotton in my head. That's my daily reality. And I feel so fat." A beautiful and normally seductive woman, Ellen began wearing big, sloppy shirts and long, baggy shorts. But against the drizzly scrim that seemed to separate her from

Women Entering the Age of Perimenopause
Women aged 40–49

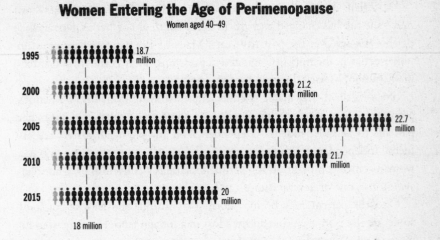

1995 · 18.7 million

2000 · 21.2 million

2005 · 22.7 million

2010 · 21.7 million

2015 · 20 million

18 million

the usual sunniness of her nature, she also found there were "moments of shining," when she felt suffused with light—light with a focus. These moments of shining are a glimpse of her postmenopausal future, but it's almost impossible for a woman in early menopause to project that far. Then the hormonal waves come on, and "it gets gray again and foggy," was how Ellen described the sensation. "It feels like it will be this way from now on, indefinitely, although I know intellectually that can't be true."

Resistance to accepting that one has entered the long passage leading out of youth and fertility and into unfamiliar territory is perfectly understandable. But remaining resistant to that reality blocks a woman from entering her Second Adulthood. Here is where Ellen and many busy active working women like her may trip themselves up. None of these women have any idea of the mess menopause can make of their lives if they remain in denial or rage, any more than most of us knew what years of sunbathing with baby oil and iodine would do to our skins by middle age.

Each woman does have to reinvent the wheel.

That is the observation of Dr. Allen, who by now has seen well over a thousand women in various stages of menopause. "Patients seem to appreciate, as we begin to analyze their thumbprint, that it may take awhile for us to collect all the information we need to make a proper risk-benefit analysis and arrive at a treatment plan that is right for them—for the moment."

Dr. Allen, my own menopause mentor and physician, recognizes how much she too has changed and grown in the subtleties of her understanding of this passage over the past five years. Many of her patients first show up in her office in the midst of agitated depressions. They come from California, Chicago, Mexico, looking for the magic.

She tells them that magic is ephemeral: Just as we don't know when it's going to appear, we don't know when it's going to go away. She wants her patients to be independent. "Dependence on any physician fosters resentment. Independence promotes growth." Dr. Allen believes that when a woman's chief complaint in the perimenopause is a collection of emotional symptoms, one of several things can be going on.

One, the patient may be in a normal transition. She feels rocky, as if someone else is in her skin and she's lost in a foreign land. She may need no medication. What she needs in this early phase is information from books and magazines and a human guide, which may come in the form of a doctor, friends, a husband, a mother, or an older sister.

The second possible explanation is that her emotional symptoms are primarily the result of hormonal upheaval. This woman may benefit from the use of low-dose birth control pills. They suppress her own hormonal fluctuations and provide a stable hormonal milieu in the perimenopause phase.

A third primary cause could be a full-out midlife crisis. In this case a woman has unresolved psychological conflicts or traumas that must be addressed before she can move ahead. Dr. Allen frequently suggests she see a female therapist, one who is old enough herself not to be threatened by menopause and can function as a successful role model as well as a guide and therapist.

The least frequent possibility is number four: a biochemical problem causing the woman's depression and agitation. "Often these patients are the angriest and most confused," she observes. "They believe they couldn't be depressed unless they can't get out of bed, lose their appetite, and have suicidal thoughts. The agitation masks their depression and confuses the issue. These patients may display a manic intensity. And for them, hormone therapy is the wrong treatment. These patients need evaluation by an expert trained in psychopharmacology."

While Dr. Allen uses this somewhat arbitrary approach in evaluating her patients in menopause, she is convinced that there is no simplistic diagnostic magic either. Nearly always, she suspects, some element of all four factors is involved. Dr. Estelle Ramey, professor emeritus and physiologist at

Georgetown University, drawing upon forty years as a pioneer hormone investigator, offers a scientific hypothesis for this interplay.

"The human nervous system (the brain), the endocrine system (the hormone regulator), and the immune system are a package," she says.[18] "There is more and more evidence that they work interactively. And it's now beginning to look like the central endocrine gland is the brain, which may secrete as many as a hundred hormones. We're a very complicated organism. As researchers we've only just scratched the surface."

PHASE TWO: OVER THE HUMP

In the intermediate phase—the year in which a woman's menstrual cycle stops—prominent changes take place in the body:

- Blood vessels begin to lose the natural protection provided to women by estrogen. The rate of heart disease rises sharply during a woman's fifties and sixties.
- The vagina is no longer naturally lubricated and begins to atrophy. This may make intercourse uncomfortable, and sexual desire may flag.
- Muscle mass begins to decrease, and fat cells take its place, resulting in a more sluggish metabolism and weight gain.
- The hidden thief of osteoporosis goes to work on the lacelike structure of the skeleton. In one third of women, bad cells (osteoclasts) cut up the lacelike web of bone matter faster than the good cells (osteoblasts) can rebuild those webs. One doesn't feel a thing. By the time one feels the symptoms of osteoporosis—usually in the sixties, when simply stepping off a curb can create a stress fracture or when a fall causes a broken bone that won't heal properly—it's almost too late to correct.

But the good news is that osteoporosis and heart disease take decades to develop. That means a woman has many years and more than one opportunity to decide to intervene—hormonally or with serious modifications in diet, exercise, and mineral supplements—before deterioration becomes irreversible.

The most obvious change in the intermediate phase is that a woman's reproductive life comes to a thudding halt. This presents her with a psychological hump that may take quite some time to get over. A gray-haired, prematurely gone-to-plump woman stood up before an audience of two thousand at one of my speeches on the Silent Passage to say, "My children are grown up and already left home, and I never thought of wanting more, but now that"—her voice broke—"now that I'm in menopause, I find myself—I know this is crazy—wanting to do it again, *wanting a baby*. Is this hormonal?"

The audience laughed, but mirthlessly, a laugh of self-recognition. The speaker had touched a raw nerve. I felt a twinge myself. Giving up the magic of fertility is bittersweet for most women, especially if they have loved giving birth and being mothers. It is especially poignant for the woman who has given birth in her forties because the experience is still so close, so palpable. Even when we are satisfied with having completed the family we hoped to have, surrendering that magical power is a momentous metaphysical loss, and it needs to be mourned.

"When I turned fifty, I cried a lot," says a devoted mother and successful shop owner. "You have to grieve, and then, when you come out on the other side, it feels very liberating."

But that sense of loss comes and goes in waves. This is the time when women come up against the wall of ageism and sexism, and it makes even the strongest feel very vulnerable. While you are feeling the loss of a former identity, and before you get to the other side where you can feel mastery, there may be a lengthy period of mourning.

Singer-songwriter Joni Mitchell describes another variation on the pits-to-peak passage. When we first talked in Los Angeles in 1991, she was a mere babe of 48. Nervous and edgy, still chain-smoking, she wore a black beret over her braided silver blond hair, and her skin had the fragility of parchment. She acknowledged that doing a lot of drugs "dries your juices right up; it really ages you." Asked if she knew how to be 50, she answered mystically, "It will make itself known." Two years later I went back to her to find out.

"I worry differently," she said. "I went over the hump of the middle-life crazies. There is a kind of mourning period; you go into grief for those things you can no longer do. But then something happened of its own accord. You can feel it created by a chemical change in your body, as you go over that hump. Things don't bother me for as long. You weed them out. You have a greater ability to let go and say, 'Oh, I don't want to think about that now,' which is the thing I always admired about men."

It is particularly impressive to hear someone who has battled illnesses and depression all her life, as Joni Mitchell has, describe coming out into the clear at 50. An intriguing bit of biological research might validate her artistic intuition about the chemical change. Between 40 and 60, people may actually lose cells in the part of the brain that responds to stress, the locus ceruleus.[19] So after menopause we aren't made anxious nearly so easily as when we were younger—another liberation.

SHOULD I TAKE HORMONE REPLACEMENT THERAPY (HRT)?

This is a question of overriding importance for most women. There are a few basic points that should be made. *Point one:* estrogen is good. Taking estrogen to replace what her body makes is not for every women. But it *is* for every woman to consider.

Point two: If you elect to use hormone therapy, you should do so for a good reason. So often women tell me they're taking estrogen only because their doctor handed them a prescription on the way out the door. A whopping 75 to 95 percent of American obstetrician-gynecologists surveyed, according to *Hippocrates* magazine, said they would prescribe hormones to most of their recently menopausal patients.[20] But many women say they're uneasy about taking drugs for something that is natural, not a disease. And they're right about that. Just because a woman has some normal menopausal symptoms is not a good enough reason to rush out and buy drugs.

Point three: It is also not "natural" to live much beyond menopause. Most of our grandmothers did not live long enough to have to deal with the debilitating consequences of bone loss or chronic heart disease. Nature never provided for females who would *routinely* live three or four decades, in an estrogen-deprived state, past the point at which they had made their genetic contribution. We therefore have to provide for ourselves—intervening hormonally or with dietary modifications, exercise regimens, vitamin and mineral supplements—since we cannot assume that aging will go smoothly.

Point four: Each of us has a specific health profile that needs to be researched and written out before we can consider the question in an informed way—each woman with regard to her particular risk/benefit equation. My advice to women is this:

Custom-design your approach to menopause.

A running suggestion throughout this book is that you take a custom-designed approach to mapping your adult life cycle. If you haven't begun making a new life plan already, menopause is an ideal place to start.

Point five: You don't have to make a decision for life. You make a decision that addresses the phase of menopause you are in right now. When you review it again next season, predictably you will need custom tailoring as routinely as you let your skirts up or down or in or out. If you decide to try HRT, *expect* the first year to be trial and error. Choose a doctor who recognizes the need to readjust the dose and regimen constantly until your body chemistry responds optimally.

Hormone replacement therapy is taken by 27.5 percent of women age 45 and over who are menopausal, a significant increase over the last several years. Sales of estrogen products were up 11 percent in 1994 and are now nearing a billion dollars a year.[21] Yet surveys show that almost two thirds of postmenopausal women have never had any doctor explain to them the risks or benefits of HRT. Among those women who are given prescriptions for HRT, fully half of them either don't take the hormones as prescribed or throw out their pills within less than a year. Why?

The two main reasons women resist or discontinue taking hormones are weight gain and fear of breast cancer.[22]

THE BREAST CANCER PHOBIA

If there is any thought that estrogen might increase a woman's chances of getting breast cancer, no matter what other obvious benefits it might have on her health, she is usually reluctant to run the risk of taking hormones. What do we know about the risks? Not much.

The general world consensus from the best studies indicates that there is little or no danger of increasing the risk of breast cancer by taking estrogen for up to five or six years. Some studies cite no increase for up to ten years. The PEPI trial found no hint of an increase in breast cancer, although a three-year study is not long enough to make any claims. Dr. Elizabeth L. Barrett-Connor, a principal investigator, is cautiously optimistic. "I think estrogen is safe for five to seven years," she says. "After that, I don't know."[23] Menopausal women are already following roughly the same yardstick: The average length of time that women continue on HRT is 4.6 years.[24] The risk of breast cancer does increase after ten years on HRT, but just how much has not been reliably determined; it ranges from 10 to 25 percent. But although there is an increase in *diagnosis* of breast cancer after ten years in women on HRT, there is no increase in *death rates* from breast cancer, compared with women who have never used hormones. In fact, studies of middle-class American women who take HRT indicate they live longer—with a 20 to 40 percent reduction in mortality rate from any and all causes.

So why do women back off?

"Women are very well aware of the one in nine statistic for breast cancer," says Dr. Trudy Bush. "We have to teach them that it's a six in nine risk for getting cardiovascular disease."[25]

It is a well-established fact by now that heart disease kills four times as many women as breast cancer does. There are, however, women whose family history or lifestyle puts them at much higher risk for breast cancer. Among those risk factors are premenopausal breast cancer in one's immediate family; early menarche; first pregnancy at a late age, or no children; a habit of more than seven alcoholic drinks a week; low levels of vitamin A from a diet poor in green leafy vegetables and beta-carotene; and high fat intake. International health statistics point to a much higher incidence of breast cancer in countries where women eat high-fat diets.[26] Also, as a generation Boomer women, having been the first to use both oral contraceptives and estrogen therapy, carry an increased estrogen load. If you are still premenopausal, I would urge you to consider your lifetime "estrogen budget"—counting your periods from how early you entered menarche, adding the number of years you may have taken birth control pills and the high doses of estrogen you may have added if you ever took fertility drugs, and subtracting for the number of pregnancies you have supported.

THE WEIGHT GAIN FALLACY

Women invariably blame hormones for whatever weight gain occurs over the next few years once they start taking HRT. The number one side effect named in a survey by *Prevention* magazine was weight gain, reported by 60 percent of women who took hormones.[27] What most of us don't understand (or don't want to accept) is that a dramatic change in metabolism takes place in both women and men in middle life. In women that change coincidentally corresponds with the menopause transition, which usually gets blamed for it.

"Women preserve their fat-free mass quite well, relatively speaking, up to about age forty-eight or forty-nine, with little age effect," according to Eric Poehlman, Ph.D., associate professor of gerontology at the Veterans Administration Medical Center in Baltimore, who has studied hormonal changes related to food, diet, and exercise in many different populations.[28] "But there's a significant change after age forty-nine, about a four or five percent decline in fat-free body mass. And that is in healthy women *not* on HRT."

The PEPI study confirmed this conclusion. The women who gained the most weight during the three-year trial were those who took no hormone therapy at all.[29] And over large studies it has been found that women who take estrogen tend to weigh less and be thinner than women who do not.[30]

The good news is that a woman can wipe out the age effect on her weight with exercise. Resistance training (with weights), if started before she enters menopause, can prevent or at least blunt the age-related decline in her resting metabolic rate, says Poehlman.

On balance, hormone replacement looks like a good way for most women to support longer, healthier lives. But so do exercise and diet modification: eating lightly, concentrating on low-fat foods, exercising an hour a day at least four times a week, and using soybean products (which are high in natural estrogen).

Ellen made this discovery a year and half into menopause. "I've refocused," she told me. "I've started to do more exercise. You were a role model for me because you were running every day. So now I get up earlier and jump on my Exercycle every day for thirty minutes. It's been rewarding because I can also read two newspapers while I'm pedaling. Then I get the kids up and out." She was also forgoing her lunch hour for a yoga class once or twice a week.

As Ellen approached her forty-ninth birthday, even though she was two years older, she was down from a size 12 to a solid size 8. "I can now wear shirts tucked in!" she exclaimed. "I don't feel fat anymore. I'm not using food to fight stress. The morning pedaling and the yoga is whittling down my body. I'm still struggling to find a new identity. It's really interesting to be caught in the middle—you can *see* the other side, but that doesn't mean you can get there as soon as you'd like to."

Yet all that mourning and anger can push us to attempt more meaningful work and more emotionally honest relationships. The results can be exciting. Ellen, for instance, had harbored a dream for many years of becoming a media psychologist, one who could reach and empower millions more people than the patients in a private practice. Her efforts were finally rewarded when she was invited on *The Oprah Winfrey Show* to discuss her book on depression. In the process of empowering others, she felt a surge of new power in herself.

"But the way you get there," she conceded, "is by going through that dark passage, the temper tantrums, the sloppy-shirt period, all the rest of it." She laughed at herself. "You begin to think maybe it's not such a bad thing to be an adult—at forty-nine—because now you have a chance to really do your dreams."

PHASE THREE: POSTMENOPAUSE

How long should I take hormones?

This is probably the second most pressing question for women concerning HRT. The answer differs widely, according to a woman's menopausal thumbprint and the phase confronting her. When a woman is in a raging perimenopause, calming the hormonal swings may be worth any perceived price. "If a woman is using HRT to relieve symptoms, two or three years on hormones are probably all she needs," suggests Dr. Allen. "Once she has settled down, she may want to take a few months' break from hormones and see how she feels, then reevaluate her risk/benefit ratio again."

But this covers only Phase One or Two. What about the health of the rest of her life? The majority of women regard menopause as a short-term event, according to national surveys. They do not relate the Change to long-term health problems such as bone loss, heart disease, or the effects of estrogen deprivation on the brain and memory.[31] The briefest review follows of HRT's effect on these long-term consequences of aging.*

Heart: If your goal is to lower your risk of heart disease, you may want to take hormone therapy indefinitely. Estrogen's protective effects on the heart are multifactorial. Besides reducing a woman's total cholesterol, it has a direct effect on the wall of the blood vessels, smoothing muscle cells and causing whole vessels to relax. It also blocks the buildup of plaque, fostering good blood flow.[32] The recently reported PEPI trial adds to the already impressive evidence from the Nurses' Health Study: Estrogen has cut the potential of cardiovascular disease among women in *half.* It also reduces by 50 percent their risk of dying from a heart attack. For women who have had a hysterectomy, the most beneficial postmenopausal therapy is using estrogen alone. At last, after a half-century of conflicting data, Dr. Healy confirms, "We can confidently assert that estrogen reduces key cardiovascular risk factors in women at a time when they become especially vulnerable to heart disease, namely, after fifty years of age."[33]

Uterine cancer: Results of the PEPI study suggest a woman is in almost no danger of uterine cancer if she takes combination therapy: estrogen together

*Again, see the revised spring 1995 softcover edition of *The Silent Passage* for details.

with a natural progesterone or a synthetic progestin. But using estrogen alone *is* hazardous for a woman with a uterus. A surprisingly large number of the subjects given unopposed estrogen had to be taken off this regimen, because of precancerous changes in the lining of the uterus. But Dr. Bush passed on relieving news for women who have been taking estrogen alone (often in contradiction to doctors' advice). Two months after progesterone was introduced to their regimen, the lining of the uterus returned to normal.

Uterine cancer is a somewhat overrated concern, according to clinicians advising the Women's Health Initiative.[34] Even women who do get endometrial cancer, and have appropriate treatment, live longer than women who *never* took estrogen and *never had uterine cancer*—a startling statistic.[35] Nevertheless, using *combined* hormone therapy can diminish the concern of uterine cancer from the start. And annual sonograms are quite accurate today in detecting any irregularities in the uterine lining. To be absolutely certain, an endometrial biopsy can be performed with minimum discomfort.

The problem has been that women given the standard treatment of 10 mg. of Provera (synthetic progestin) for ten days along with their Premarin (estrogen) are often startled by feeling unpleasantly premenstrual and having their periods start up all over again. A typical reaction is that of a busy New York publishing executive: "When I first started with Provera, I was a basket case—bloated, crampy, headachey, I felt awful. I thought, *Why am I going through this for ten days a month? Who needs it?*" Such women frequently call their doctors and say, "Why did you give me that stuff?"

When women are given no other choice than this combination, they often bag the whole idea of hormone replacement, or, more dangerously, simply drop the protective progestin altogether. Osteoporosis experts, like Dr. Robert Lindsay at the Helen Hayes Bone Center, fret that "many people who would gain in healthy active years on estrogen replacement are turned off by the required addition of a progestin and the continuation of periods."

For the first time, other alternatives are appearing.

The PEPI study found a woman doesn't need the "elephant gun" dose of progestin routinely prescribed. Instead, a much smaller dose of a progestin—2.5 mg. taken daily—protected the uterus. The FDA has now approved at least two options of hormone replacement therapy. One is the old cyclical regimen (Premarin for fifteen days alone, 10 mg. of progestin added for the last ten days of the month). The other is the newer continuous regimen that proved itself in the PEPI trial (a daily combination of Premarin and 2.5 mg. of Cycrin, which is the same as Provera).[36]

An even more promising, but elusive, alternative is on the horizon.

In the first edition of *The Silent Passage*, I reported that new-generation gynecologists and research scientists, such as Dr. Jamie Grifo at New York Hospital–Cornell Medical Center, believed the wave of the future to be natural micronized progesterone. It is widely used by European women. But American physicians have been reluctant to prescribe it because it doesn't have FDA approval. Our medical-pharmaceutical establishment persists in fostering suspicion of any "natural" compound that might alleviate symptoms, a shaky position, given the many "natural" plants and tree barks from which major drugs like digitalis and even aspirin are derived.

The PEPI study investigators did not share this outmoded view. "We were going out on a limb [to test natural progesterone], but I'm glad we did," say principal investigators for PEPI Dr. Trudy Bush and Dr. Elizabeth Barrett-Connor. Their boldness paid off in good news when the results of the three-year study were announced in late 1994. Estrogen combined with *natural micronized progesterone* turns out to be the best regimen for a woman with a uterus.[37] Natural progesterone is made from soybeans or from Mexican yams. *Micronized* means that the particles are finely ground and thus more completely absorbed. The natural form does not significantly blunt the healthful effects of estrogen on the heart, as synthetic progestins may do. Natural micronized progesterone also stimulates the libido. The other great benefit is that natural progesterone presents fewer unpleasant side effects in most women, compared with the synthetic version.

There was only one problem. American women can't get natural micronized progesterone.

Schering-Plough, the German company that supplied it to the PEPI trial for experimentation, sells the product in Europe but did not apply for FDA approval and thus cannot sell it in the United States. At present, the only way a woman can get hold of this promising compound is if she knows the names and numbers of the few pharmacies in the United States that sell it, and can persuade her doctor to write a prescription for it. (For information on how to order this product, see end note.)[38]

Intelligent and influential women reacted with anger and disbelief to this Catch-22. Why should patients and doctors have to use an underground network to obtain a natural product when a government study, supported by their tax dollars, suggests it may be the safest and most effective choice for combined hormone therapy?

I called the FDA. I was told the agency had no applications from any drug company asking to test natural micronized progesterone, end of story.

I turned to Ruth Merkatz, who heads the new Office of Women's Health at the drug regulatory agency. Her job is to make sure the FDA is proactive in bringing products to market that will promote women's health. Why, I asked her, if this natural preparation has all the positive benefits one looks for and few of the negative side effects of Provera, doesn't it have the FDA seal of approval?

She promised to get back to me. And ten days later she did. But a lot had transpired in those ten days.

"Big drug companies have been encouraged to submit applications to us for testing natural micronized progesterone," she reported, "and we will accelerate the process." Dr. Sol Sobel, head of the FDA's division of Endocrine and Metabolic Products, added his own hopes: "It's quite possible, if proper doses of micronized progesterone are presented to us, we may be able to establish the lowest effective dose to protect the endometrium and get that drug on the market—in a year or so."[39]

Bones: If your major concern is osteoporosis, researchers now recommend taking HRT for at least seven years.[40] This is because bone loss is accelerated over the menopausal transition, before it settles back down to the normal attrition with age. Estrogen protects the bones. Natural progesterone may even help rebuild bone already lost. John Lee, a Harvard-educated M.D. with a family practice in Mill Valley, California, claims that osteoporosis is *not* irreversible.[41] He has been treating women over 60 years of age with natural progesterone and claims that all those who have been in his program for at least six months have shown an increase in bone density.[42]

Brain: There is mounting evidence that estrogen has a critical impact on the activity of the human brain—in both women and men—throughout the life cycle. It is now possible to report confidently that estrogen has a definite effect on cognitive functioning, according to Dr. Barbara Sherwin, a professor of psychology and obstetrics-gynecology at McGill University in Montreal.

Dr. Sherwin has been doing studies over a period of nearly ten years on a total of several hundred women in all stages of life. They are given standardized neuropsychological tests when they are in an estrogenized state and when they are in an estrogen-deprived state.[43] The results are clear, says Dr. Sherwin. "Estrogen helps maintain verbal memory and it enhances a woman's capacity for new learning."

Estrogen also spurs the production of an important enzyme in the brain that helps the connections between brain cells to flourish, making it quicker and easier for messages to leap from one neuron to the next.[44] The inside of a robust estrogenized brain might look more like the dense telephone wiring in an urban telephone terminal box, while the brain of an older estrogen-deprived woman or man might look more like the sparse wiring of a rural telephone substation.

Estrogen has recently been posited as a woman's best defense against organic brain disease in later life. In a study of 2,418 women by Dr. Victor Henderson and Annlia Paganini-Hill, both of the University of Southern California, those on hormone replacement were much less likely to develop Alzheimer's disease than women who never took hormones.[45]

CALL OF THE WILD GIRL

The best gift for making a conscious, disciplined trip through menopause is *postmenopausal zest*. This is a special, buoyant sort of energy, fueled in part by the change in ratio of testosterone to estrogen. When my mentor anthropologist Margaret Mead coined the term, it was on the basis of her observation of women across cultures. Given further evidence of the cross-cultural phenomenon of postmenopausal zest, the surmise must be that it is not about socialization. It is part of the evolutionary wiring of being a woman.

Once a woman has come through the menopausal passage, she can say good-bye to pregnancy fears and monthly mood swings. Now that she is no longer confined by society's narrow definition of woman as sex object and breeder, she is freer to integrate the masculine and feminine aspects of her nature. She can now claim the license to *say what she truly thinks.*

Often, when I interview women in their fifties and urge them to recall the girls they were at 10 or 11, they begin to cry. The wrenching change from the freewheeling, funny, even fearless tomboys they once were, before being initiated into what Anna Quindlen calls the "cult of the nice girl," is revived in all its painful intensity, and for perhaps the first time the awful price is calculated.[46]

TV producer Linda Ellerbee was warming up as a girl to play third base for the New York Yankees. Told she would have to be very good, she said, "I'll practice." Told she would have to grow up, she said, "I'll wait." At 12 or so she was given the real reason: "You have to be a boy."

Most preadolescent girls show just as feisty a Seeker Self as do boys. My interviewees describe themselves, before their periods started, as loving to climb trees, make forts, gallop horses flat out, play touch football, explore other neighborhoods, express loud opinions, challenge rules, and fight back with boys. But something changes drastically around the ages of 12 and 13. Studies show those ages mark the start of problems such as teen pregnancy and destructive behavior by boys.[47] Girls have been found to be more vulnerable during this transition than boys, since it hits them in mid-puberty (typically boys don't mature sexually until two years later).[48] Through TV and magazines, movies and street behavior, the culture bombards the developing child-woman with instructions for how a girl should look and act. What happens to her voice? She loses it.

"Girls dummy up at twelve," affirms model Lauren Hutton. Most of my interviewees agree. Writer Linda Francke was a horseback-riding hellion at 11 and 12 and very comfortable with herself. The hormonal turning point did not occur for her until she skipped a grade and entered boarding school at 15. Plunged into an unfamiliar world of sophisticated tenth graders, she recalls, "All I wanted to do was study the girls who knew how to curl their hair and what sweaters went with what. Social acceptance was all that mattered—everything else fell away, everything."

A groundbreaking five-year study by Harvard psychologist Carol Gilligan and Lyn Mikel Brown at a Cleveland girls' school pinpointed the collapse of the Seeker Self. Girls between 7 and 12 were "candid, confident, psychologically astute and shrewd" (if they hadn't been abused). But under the weight of societal pressures to be "nice" and "fit in," that outspoken and purposeful personality was self-censored at 12 or 13, and gradually girls stopped trusting their own perceptions. They began to *falsify* what they knew and saw and felt. The persona that emerged modeled itself "on the image of the perfectly nice and caring girl."[49]

Be prepared for a comeback of the wild girl. A lust for adventure and often a resurgence of athleticism become apparent as patterns in the activities of women experiencing the Change of Life. I wish I had a penny for every postmenopausal wild girl who's told me she's off to track gorillas in the Congo without her husband, or she's setting off with another woman friend to climb mountains, or she's resuscitated her tennis game and is now entering tournaments. Risk-taking in their careers and love lives is also more likely.

I asked Linda Francke if there was any correlation between the way she acts now, at 50, and the wild girl she left behind. "Yes, when I was 45 I had a hysterectomy, and that completed the new passage. It returned me to the more gender-neutral and focused self that I'd inhabited as a young girl. What I'm doing now is more of a mirror of what I was doing when I was eleven or twelve. Hormones take up so much of the time in between!"

10

FROM PLEASING TO MASTERY

At the height of my research on women in Second Adulthood, I felt the need to share ideas about common themes in our personal journeys to the midcentury mark with some of the thoughtful women I'd interviewed over the past several years. It would be a brunch in celebration of our Flaming Fifties. I started by calling up singer Judy Collins.

"I wouldn't miss it!" she exclaimed, then groaned. She had a concert the night before three thousand miles away in California. "Could you change it from brunch to a linner?" she asked. "A combination of lunch and dinner?"

"You've got it," I said.

Judy promised to join us even it meant taking the red-eye. "And I haven't done *that* in fifteen years."

The next half-dozen women I phoned all sounded just as intrigued. Congresswoman Lucille Roybal-Allard, the first Mexican-American woman elected to the House, vowed to break away from debate on the president's tax bill. Judith Jamison, artistic director of the Alvin Ailey American Dance Theater, was enthusiastic, as was Linda Ellerbee, who had a refreshing concern. The TV anchorwoman turned essayist and producer wanted to be sure I knew she was only 48. Would that disqualify her? Hardly. She sounded genuinely flattered to be invited to a celebration of the Flaming Fifties—a good sign.

Within hours an all-star team of nine women had eagerly accepted my invitation. Stunning in its absence was any hesitation among the invitees about going on the record about their ages. Before they arrived that Sunday afternoon in June, I reviewed my notes on their lives.

"The first half of my life has been an attempt to get over the hurdles of motherhood, divorce, and trying to get the right to be an artist," Judy Collins had told me. "The most difficult thing to remember is that *this is what you're supposed to be doing*. It's almost a daily struggle."

Next I recalled the poignant voice of author and *USA Today* columnist Barbara Reynolds, who had told me the story of her struggles as a black woman rejected by her own mother.

"The pain caused by a runaway mother cuts deeper than incest," Barbara said. She had endured both. Growing up with her grandmother in Columbus, Ohio, she'd hidden the fact that she had the highest IQ in her junior high school, just as now, at 48, she was hiding inside excess weight. Barbara described feeling that she had no ego: none in her twenties, even less in her thirties. As a reporter at the *Chicago Tribune* she had been awarded a Nieman Fellowship. But when she went to Harvard for the interview, "I couldn't speak. I couldn't even lift a glass," she recalled. "I started shaking uncontrollably, because my mind and heart said I didn't belong there." I'll never forget her sweet, wounded expression as she stared into the past at the refuse of various addictions she had overcome and began to tell me about the new life she was building for herself.

Judy and Barbara, Judith Jamison, Congresswoman Roybal-Allard, dry-witted Linda Ellerbee—what common ground, I wondered, would they find with my friend and literary agent, Lynn Nesbit, who works seventy-hour weeks, wears power red Chanel suits, and studies religion? "With professional success, you feel a little more relaxed, you enjoy things more," Lynn says. "As I've become older, it's such a relief not to have to prove yourself." Now her inner voice whispers, "Let it happen, don't try to be so controlling, and all things will work out more easily."

None of these East Coast sophisticates, I knew, would be able to resist Mary Ann Goff, whose first forty-nine years had been circumscribed by Newark, Ohio. Now 60, having escaped to the South, she dates avidly and has a drawerful of sheer teddies that her children find appalling. I took pleasure in anticipating the other guests' shocked looks when Elizabeth Stevenson, a Jungian psychoanalyst from Cambridge, Massachusetts, a woman who would strike them at first glance as the soul of propriety, shared her far-out dreams, or when Ginny Ford, a Rochester businesswoman, told the story of running away from her husband and coming back to start a career at midlife.

This gathering was the perfect excuse for me to see all of them again and watch them discover and draw strength from one another. Would they recall their lives as narratives of female decline, the kind one has traditionally found in novels like Doris Lessing's *Summer Before the Dark,* Joan Didion's *Book of Common Prayer,* and all of Jean Rhys's and Anita Brookner's books? Or would these women tell their stories as narratives of progress? An important part of the transformative work in middle life, I was convinced by now, is to revise our own stories, forgiving the failures and composing our idealized selves with our real selves.

On the Sunday of the gathering, as I went out to greet my guests, I found the early arrivals already on the floor in starfish postures, enjoying a yoga session with instructor Jaki Jackson. As others arrived, we naturally fell into a circle. It called to mind the sacred stone circles in Ireland that have witnessed five thousand years. Perhaps we would feel some connection to the ancient Wisewomen who created rites of healing around those circles.

ON THE PRIVILEGE OF BEING 50

"I just turned fifty," Judith Jamison, dancer-choreographer, announced proudly as she arrived and greeted everyone. She materialized in the entrance hall like one of the stone colossi in the temples at Luxor, an extraordinary presence, tall and beautiful with tight black-and-gray cornrows twined close to her scalp. As she descended the stairs, I remembered the grace and terrifying power she brought to *Cry,* in the role Alvin Ailey created for her as a tribute to black women.

"Nobody ever tells you about how great it is to be over forty-five," Judith told me a few years back. "I can't wait to be fifty!" So was it what she'd expected? "As a dancer, it has always been about survival," she told the group. "And I still jump on the stage with the kids at Christmas and perform."

Mary Ann Goff, the escapee from southern Ohio, looked quite frisky in her navy sailor dress and light feathered curls. She spoke of another voyage, when she turned her life around by driving for the first time on an interstate highway at the age of 53.

"My parents were alcoholics, so I got married at nineteen to get away from it all," she told us. All four of her children were well along in school when she started college; typically she was 38 before she took her own life seriously. "My ex-husband just put me down and ridiculed me. He didn't have the education that I was pursuing, so he was very jealous. 'Why do you need this schooling?' he'd say. I thought, *Do I go on being passive, or do I say, 'This is my life too?'* "

Her husband had prostate disease, and soon their sexual relationship, which had been highly charged, began to disintegrate because of his condition. Mary Ann hungered for the lapsed loving and touching. She urged her husband to see a sex therapist. He refused and eventually lost his sex drive. Naturally she blamed herself; her weight, her age.

"So I went to counseling, and I found out it wasn't me who was crazy." Her husband eventually saw a therapist, who treated his problem, but the relationship failed anyway. However, because she had four children, she waited until she was in her fifties to get a divorce.

"I picked up all my life—I'd never been out of state—and moved to Charleston," she said, her slow-paced speech picking up speed. "It was really scary. I had a lot of stumbling blocks, and no one to depend on, but I started all over again." Her smile was benignly defiant. "It made me very, very independent. And I felt so much younger!"

I recalled my own fiftieth birthday: "My daughters gentled me through it. They said, 'Can't you accept and enjoy what you've already done? You made us, and we turned out pretty well. You have work you can be proud of and a wonderful marriage. *Own it.* Honor it.' That was such a wonderful birthday present."

Barbara Reynolds had chosen the oversize wing chair, and her position expressed the duality I had always sensed in her. At first she sat firmly and solemnly, her eyes penetrating all of us with fierce honesty. The other, more vulnerable side of her became apparent as she sank deep into the embrace of the chair, still needing to be sheltered, healed.

"I have to be truthful with you," said Barbara. "Not everybody can face turning fifty with courage." Her mother, she remembered, had lied about her age. This vanity exacted a painful price from the daughter she had abandoned.

For fifteen years, from the time she was 2 years old, every time she looked out her window, Barbara longed to glimpse the mother of her dreams in the flesh. She wanted her mother to look up at her and make her real. Finally she could bear the yearning no longer. At 17 Barbara persuaded her grandmother to let her go visit her mother for the first time.

"I walked in, and the first thing I saw, on her piano, were pictures of her other four children. But not me." Barbara's voice throttled down from its normal resonance to a whisper. "I said, 'Mother, you have *five* children.' "

"Well, I have to talk to you about that," her mother said. "You see, I put my age back." She didn't want her friends to know that she had a daughter as old as Barbara.

"As I moved toward forty and then fifty," Barbara admitted, "I began to think, *Maybe I should lie about my age, too. Maybe something really is wrong.*" She looked around at the vibrant, sympathetic faces in the room. "But I'm beginning to feel better just by being here."

Judy Collins dashed in late, but the warmth of her personality bound her into the group right away. Her skin looked smooth and natural, and her sandy hair was caught up with combs in broad wings at the side of her face. She was no longer the fragile Sixties waif with a face swallowed up by her huge quartz eyes. The strength of her middle years was apparent in hands made powerful by years of playing the piano and guitar and in a body as taut as the black tights over her shapely legs.

Judy remarked that the real tragedy at this stage would be to deny your past. "It's important to own who you are," she said. "You're not all good, and you're not all bad, but the owning is part of the passage, I think."

Linda Ellerbee brought the group down to earth in one sentence. Sprawled in the deepest armchair, with her sneakers kicked off, hair clipped short, pant cuffs rolled up, she looked like a rambunctious kid as she peered through her gogglelike glasses to confront the group.

"I started out last year with breast cancer, so, although I'm forty-eight, to me the flattering thing about being invited to this dinner was that someone thought I was going to *live* to be fifty!"

Sensing the tension, she dissolved it gracefully with a joke. "I have never lied about my age, but I have always lied about my height!" I remembered Linda as perhaps the sexiest, earthiest newswoman on TV. Her commentaries were droll, straight shots to the heart of whatever she chose to dissect. Her voice had a great Dietrich huskiness; she seemed like a woman who could slam down a drink and laugh heartily with the boys.

Her face tensed slightly as she told us how she had left TV before she was told to go. "The networks feel that you can grow old on the air as long as you don't *look* old," she said. "And I wasn't blessed with the kind of face that was going to look thirty-five forever. So I started my own company to allow me to produce television."

Linda had other problems before the cancer: alcoholism, men—all our familiar vices. "But the whole last five years of my life—and this last year in particular—I truly have come to understand the words *state of grace*," she said. Her face relaxed, not a trace of makeup obscuring its clarity. "I have never felt quite so alive or quite as grateful or aware about everything. And I think a lot of that comes not from the close brushes but from this five-oh—coming up to fifty." The weight of her next words sent shivers through us all. "We've been somewhere; we *are* somewhere."

MOVING TOWARD MASTERY

We realized that we all had been defined in our First Adulthood by our relations to others: husbands, children, or the dominant fathers or mentors for whom we performed. Most of the women in the room had not been autonomous and had no idea how to find the voice of their truest selves until they reached early midlife. Most had made jailbreak marriages, moving directly from fathers to husbands. Even though all these women had turned out to be very successful, they had had to wrestle with all the obstacles and life crises that anyone might face. It was also reassuring to hear how late they got started being autonomous: One of the women said she hadn't earned her first paycheck until she was 45. Judy Collins hadn't written a check for herself until she was 42. That's late! But by the time they reach the Flaming Fifties most women have acquired the skills and self-knowledge to master complex environments and change the conditions around them. On one advantage of being in Second Adulthood women of all social classes seem to agree:

> I can now live by my own lights and stop trying to please everyone.[1]

"At last we can get started!" Judy Collins enthused. At the age of 54, for the first time, she feels clarity about herself as an artist. All our stories were testimonies to the fluidity of women's lives. They also illustrated that it is not merely affluence that determines whether or not one comes out well in the fifties. It is the way one goes through the passages on the way to Second Adulthood.

The fundamental shift for women entails moving away from dependence and trying to please everyone else toward repossessing their intellectuality and originality of thought, sharpening their instrumental and critical skills, and mastering the complex environments where they now hope to operate. Mastery is an accumulated inner strength, not dependent on immediate outer conditions or the approval of others. Or, as Judy Collins expressed it in shorthand, "Mastery is an inside job."

"Fifty for me was a time when I really for the first time owned my body," said the Rochester businesswoman Ginny Ford, whose blond hair and dimpled smilingness evoke Doris Day movies. "I had been very ashamed of my body, and now I love it."

Her remark illuminated the intimate connection between the state of a woman's psychological vitality and her body image. In her thirties and forties Ginny had great legs and could wear a size four off any rack. She favored slinky spaghetti-strap gowns for when she and her husband, Bob, went dancing at the country club. They were Rochester's Perfect Couple, sexy and successful.

The story behind this façade was classic.

"I was a traditional housewife and a community volunteer," Ginny said. "My husband gave me cash to manage the household, but none of it was ever my own. When my youngest went off to college, I drifted into the work world." Starting at 42, she worked up to president of the Junior League and took a seat on every board in town. "I felt I was on a pedestal, in the eyes of the community and my family. But inside I was crumbling. I needed to get off."

She pulled a midlife adolescent rebellion. Threw some clothes in the back of her car and disappeared into a yearlong romantic escapade. "It was as if I had to kill off that earlier self," she said. "I brought a different person back—more open and fun-loving and financially independent for the first time." Reuniting with her husband was not the hard part; giving up her own apartment was.

But shortly after her rebellion she discovered that she could fulfill her own dreams. While rebuilding her marriage, Ginny became a founding partner of a market research firm, which she helped transform into a multimillion-dollar business in less than ten years. In 1986 she cashed in, keeping sole ownership of one division. She proceeded to tell us how her body had instigated—as if with a will of its own—a life-changing period of self-assessment.

Ginny has always been a strong skier. A few years ago she took her husband on a dream vacation to Jackson Hole, Wyoming. In a disastrous accident she tore all the ligaments in her knee and spent the following year on crutches. During her time of healing she became a grandmother. The juxtaposition of these two life accidents—the death of her young, carelessly agile self and the birth of a new generation of family—initiated a period of inner questioning. (Life accidents, you'll remember, are those events we can neither predict nor prevent, and when they coincide with the start of a new stage in the life cycle, the passage is often accelerated.)

"Being slowed down by the crutches and bowled over by my grandchild, I did a whole lot of thinking. Instead of rushing at life and producing furiously, I wanted something more meaningful. The net result is I have taken a year off from my business and have given myself to the National Women's Hall of Fame. They honor women's achievements. I signed on, pro bono, as my legacy to my daughter and granddaughter."

Now fully recovered, she told us that she would be leaving on a hundred-mile hike across England from the North Sea to the Irish Sea, not the kind of vacation we once would have expected of a woman in her fifties. "When I think of the time I spent dealing with the whole packaging of the outward piece of myself," she said, rolling her big blue eyes. "Now there's all this inner stuff going on. I'm probably ten pounds heavier; my thighs are a little rumply; my arms have flab. Fifteen years ago I would have starved myself. But now I'm enjoying Bob's pasta. I exercise every day, I enjoy myself sexually, and I'm proud of this body. It really works!"

Mary Ann Goff recalled the mind-set of the 1950s, when we were socialized. "I came across a paper the other day I wrote in the twelfth grade," she said. "It asked the question, Can a married woman have a career? I'd written, 'Absolutely not—her place is in the home.' I couldn't believe it. Did I write that? This can't be me!"

"You really only came alive in your fifties," I reminded her.

"Oh, yes. Once I got on that interstate—"

Vicarious laughter erupted.

When she moved to Charleston, South Carolina, just being in her own apartment felt like a new world. Mary Ann dropped fifty pounds and took a younger lover and a job with the U.S. Air Force. She continued collecting credits toward her college degree. "The more you challenge yourself, the more you learn to do, the more your self-esteem really shoots up: *Hey! I can do this!* You're a success."

"Growing up, it was *never* me," said the quiet congresswoman, Lucille Roybal-Allard. Petite and dignified with olive skin and a shiny helmet of dark hair, she sat properly on the edge of the sofa. Her father, retired Congressman Edward R. Roybal, was the first Hispanic elected to the Los Angeles City Council. "It was always my sister, my brother, my mother, my father who came first, and then, in my adult life, my first husband and my children. I was always putting myself second."

When her father was elected to Congress, thirty years ago, "people in Washington, D.C., had no idea there was any such species as Mexican-American," she said. At the same time "some Latinos thought the Roybals were too swell.... *Mmmphh, that's Roybal's daughter.*" Feeling alienated from the white and even sometimes the Latino communities, she never really had a childhood. "We had to be the model, to prove that Mexicans could eat properly; we had to be careful of everything we said." She told us that she grew up scared to speak out and give her own opinions. What if it was the wrong thing to say? What if it could be used against her father or reflected badly on the Latino community? As late as six years before, when she was first elected to the California State Assembly, Lucille still had to fight off those childhood fears as she assumed a growing leadership role and fought for issues she believed in. "That's just the little girl in me," she tells herself, "who had to be real careful to keep her mouth shut."

All the women at the gathering described aspects of this transformation from pleasing to mastery. Ginny and Lucille are moving from pleasing as conventional wives to mastering the skills necessary to effect social change. Judith Jamison is moving from pleasing as the child performer to mastery as the teacher. Linda Ellerbee's commitment to mastery pits her against the despair of illness. "I live my life as if the cancer were never going to come back because nothing else matters. I *intend* to reach fifty," she declared.

Barbara Reynolds had never succeeded in pleasing. Divorced and child-less, she had adopted a son and was determined to become an ordained minister. Twenty years after being rendered speechless at Harvard by her own self-doubts, Barbara was gaining the courage to speak with her own voice, publicly, about the most important things.

FINDING ONE'S OWN VOICE

When Barbara entered the Howard University School of Divinity in 1988, it was not primarily for the degree but because she wanted to serve the God that had taken her from being a nobody to a somebody. In a worldly sense she is seen today as one of the most influential black Americans of her gen-eration. Pick up a copy of *USA Today* anywhere in the world, and her unique voice will be prominently displayed on the opinion page. Her bosses love her; they told me so. She is a TV essayist, a writer of controversial books, and a Du Pont visiting scholar at Shenandoah University. But I wondered, having turned 50, could she move beyond surviving to feel *worthy* of it all?

"I've just graduated from the seminary. I can *feel* myself becoming a minister," she said fervently. "I also feel I can at some point master the anxiety within me and lose weight; it's still not too late." Survival for Barbara, for so many women of color, always meant trying to fit in. Having found that impossible, she has made herself a professional "misfit" whose voice now counts. "Instead of getting angry, now I try to stop and teach," she said. By mastering her anger and honing her creative skills, she is able to give comfort and inspiration to those as powerless as she once felt.

"I'm very interested in your becoming a preacher," Lynn Nesbit said to Barbara. "No one talks about religion in New York; it's a word you can't mention. You can talk about sex, anything, but if you're religious"—she affected a look of shock—"people look at you suspiciously."

The literary agent does not function in a world where people spend a lot of time dwelling on the soul—unless it can be turned into a best-seller. Sitting in her office on Madison Avenue, as I did to interview her a few years ago, one could not imagine her finding time to think about such matters. With her arms tensely latticed around her waist, phones jangling, Lynn was tied up in a foreign auction on yet another big book. But even then she spoke about a new dream for her Flaming Fifties: "If I were to do something else right now, I know exactly what I would do. I'd get a Ph.D. in religious studies."

After twenty-three years of building a solid reputation at ICM, the huge, all-purpose talent agency, Lynn had a radical change forced on her when the male hierarchy there reorganized the agency and failed to offer her a policy position on the board. This disruption coincided with the departure from home of her two daughters, with whom she had deeply intimate bonds.

"Both events were more disturbing than I acknowledged to myself," she said. Nesbit joined in a partnership with another successful agent, Morton Janklow, forming what may be the dominant independent literary agency in the country. Even as these unavoidable changes impinged on the youthful illusion that one can control one's life, they stirred up her spiritual innocence. She realized that willpower alone is not enough to get one past life's pitfalls. It started her on the religious quest that has become the dominant theme of her delayed middle-life passage. "I'm taking one course a semester," Lynn said. "I find that centers me."

Mary Ann Goff, who was by now 60 years old with twenty hours left to go for her bachelor's degree, vowed fervently, "I'm gonna make it." She cocked her head and smiled. "Soon I want to be Dr. Ann—doing sexual education, like Dr. Ruth."

The group wondered how busy women like Mary Ann, Lynn Nesbit, and Barbara Reynolds found the time to go back to school. "I found the seminary a snap," Barbara said, "compared to what I had to do before. I had money, credit cards, a car. I didn't have to worry about boyfriends. All the pressures I used to have were over." She had to work, of course, as a columnist facing a deadline every other day. "But that was nothing compared to struggling for identity as a teenager."

I told them that I had found a desire to go back to school to be an almost universal yearning among women in middle life. "Many women go to complete themselves. Quite a few get turned on by using their minds and go on for their master's degree or doctorates for the sheer joy of it. What is it about us?" I mused. "Perhaps we sense we're just going to go on forever, so we change our perspective on time and on life."

In her liquid voice Judy Collins began a meditation on her own story. "I do think men and women in the middle years suffer these huge reorganizations of their psyches." Like so many women wishing for total acceptance from a parent, Judy has had to overcome the habit of driving herself toward the perfection she subliminally hoped might finally secure her father's love. A mythic figure to her, Judy's late alcoholic father hosted a popular Denver radio show. She was his "dreamboat." Though blind, he played the piano well, but Judy was expected to fulfill his dream of becoming a serious musician. He fully supported her as a performer, yet she was invisible to him as a little girl. When he demanded that she play a piano piece beyond her capacities on his show, the fear of failure made her wish she were dead. Her suicide attempt at 14 initiated a long battle with depressive episodes.

After the divorce and custody battles of her twenties, it became clear that she had a problem with alcohol. "This thing inside me—the talent—made me a prisoner, almost a hostage," she had told me. "The other side of me, the side who wants to have fun, was dragged along, fearful, always wondering, Can I do this?" Her career ruled her, and she became dependent on her record company to "take care of me." Reaching her late thirties, she was still acting like the gifted child. But by then "my act was a total disaster," she said. "I couldn't sing, I couldn't work. The next step would have been a locked ward." Elektra Records later dropped her flat.

She told the group that the day after she committed to sobriety, she met a man with whom she has achieved the first mature love relationship of her life. By now she has developed the discipline to go into a locked room every day, even on down days, to compose music or write prose. She describes her transformation as "catching up the inside with the outside." Affirmation came out of the blue when she was summoned by President Clinton to perform at his inaugural gala. There at the Lincoln Memorial she felt like part of American history.

"It's almost as though people are saying suddenly, 'Oh, yes,' remembering how I have permeated their lives personally, politically, socially for these thirty years. That's very thrilling to me. Because that's the visibility I never had with my father." The sightless, selfish, adored father. "In other words, suddenly they not only hear me but *see* me."

Judith Jamison spoke up, suddenly more vulnerable. "My fiftieth birthday this year was spent in total angst. My father had a heart attack and a triple bypass." She hesitated and almost visibly shrank. "I always feel like a child inside because all I am is a performing artist."

All I am is . . . the poignancy of those words reminded us all of parts of ourselves that we had necessarily set aside or lost to a sense of obligation, back when we made the decisions of our twenties.

"Whatever was assigned to me, I had to go over the edge with it," Judith told the group. "My mentors took advantage of my need to please." Murmurs of recognition. Discovered by master choreographer Agnes de Mille, Judith gravitated toward mentors and what she calls "spiritual walkers" (her phrase comes from Stevie Wonder). Alvin Ailey endorsed her talent, and she helped make the Ailey company famous by touring throughout the world nonstop for fifteen years. For Judith, First Adulthood was about enjoying herself as an artist as well as proving herself worthy of the love of her "spiritual walkers." She had no husband, no children, no inner life, and very little intimacy.

At 39 Judith had experienced a "little death" and retreated to a house in Connecticut where she spent the next two years alone. "I was mentally and physically exhausted," she had told me. She was meant to collaborate with Miles Davis on a new piece. "When I told him that I had been in the country, just kind of lying there for six months, he said, 'Oh, you just went to sleep.' He understood. In that period of life I needed to do that."

Jamison was 41 when she took up choreography. Ailey encouraged her to move on, easing her transition by providing his students for her experimentations. Their aesthetic marriage flourished into a partnership, and Ailey prepared Judith to carry on his legacy. She was 46 when Ailey died, in 1989, and within several weeks she became artistic director of the Alvin Ailey American Dance Theater.

Here, again, is the juxtaposition of a life accident with a major transition: Judith was wrestling with the shift from performer—the indulged, gifted child—to master, and was expected to be the artistic matriarch to a group dominated by boisterous males in their twenties who are always in her face, when she almost lost her father. Had the shock given her something to work with?

"Ten years ago, when I was dancing, I wouldn't have dealt with it," she answered. "Dancers are all about *my* leg, *my* foot. Now the whole thing is reversed. I have to play mother, nurse, mentor, policewoman. Now, it is 'How is *your* leg? How is *your* spirit?'"

Elizabeth Stevenson, the Jungian analyst, appeared to be all proper New England, wearing her original face, no makeup, and unfussed silvery gray hair. With her generous body wrapped in a loose crocheted sweater over a midcalf skirt, she sent off a strong signal of centeredness. "I may look like a nice middle-aged lady, but I'm not," she told the group with an impish smile. "I'm radical."

Our generation may have broken the trend, I observed. We're all becoming more radical as we age.

Elizabeth told us how abruptly her time perspective shifted when she was 35. She was telling her analyst about going to her grandmother's hundredth birthday party when he asked her the most important question of her life. "You mean you've got a grandmother who's a hundred years old?" the analyst marveled. "Wow! All those years left in your genes." Then, dead serious, he asked her: "What have you been doing with your life?"

"And here I was a floppy little housewife with two kids," recalled Elizabeth.

"And you still had two thirds of your life left?" I observed.

"Or more. My grandmother eventually lived to be a hundred and four."

"Did you start recalculating your life plan?"

"Oh, yes. That week I decided to become an analyst."

After a painful divorce and years of training, Elizabeth has a thriving practice in Cambridge, where she educates high-achieving women to honor the "feminine principle"—their naturally given gifts of expressiveness, interpersonal warmth, intuitiveness, and capacity for joy—so often forfeited in the fierce effort to ape the forcefulness of men.

"I think the place that women our age find themselves in is really fascinating," she said. "Men may be very powerful in the world, but emotionally
they're pretty starved. And we have a lot of life in us. I mean, look at this
decade! The 'networking' among women is a connective tissue that is very
much part of the feminine principle, and we are loaded with it, just *loaded*
with it. Men mostly are very scared of it. So women and men find themselves pretty far apart at this point, with the potential for a lot of envy."

FROM ANGER TO FORGIVENESS

As we gathered around the dining table to break Italian bread and pass
chicken tarragon, late-afternoon clouds began hurrying across the sky. The
talk turned back to our forties. Linda Ellerbee remembered a feeling she had
on her fortieth birthday: "How angry I was. At that age I was so tired of
waiting for men to get smart!"

Everyone howled.

We had come of age under the docile, prefeminist code of early Doris
Day movies. Our lives had been hacked open halfway through young adulthood by the discontinuity of social revolution. Too late for birth control
and the carnal nights of the Sixties, many of us did not take the license for
adolescent sexual exploration until much later, when we were supposed to
be settled. The costs were high: broken marriages, children cast adrift; for
some, years of alcoholic chaos.

"They changed the rules on us," I observed.

"And they kept changing them," said Linda. "How about the men in our
lives?" She talked about her partnership with Rolfe Tessem over the last
seven years. "We run a business together. And we live together." They haven't
married, she said. "If a woman marries a man more successful than she is, the
world congratulates her. But if a man is married to a woman more successful than he is, the world asks him how he's coping with it. After a while he
begins to think there's something to cope with. It's a major problem."

Others talked about the envy they feel from men in middle age, who age
differently and who often become more passive and emotionally dependent.

"I kept thinking things would get better someday," Ginny observed. "But
this is someday."

"You finally have the permission, in this pretty nasty patriarchy, to be
who you are," pronounced Elizabeth Stevenson. The Jungian analyst had

found the courage in her fifties to follow her own feminine instincts. "If you live from the center of yourself, if you live out of your feelings, they will flow like very gentle waves and direct you."

Linda marked our progress. "I attended a women's dinner in the Seventies where the main subject was food. If this dinner had happened in the Eighties, the subject would have been power. In the Nineties the subject is the journey and forgiveness."

"It's almost as if you have to forgive the things that happened in the first half of your life—the people who failed you and the ways you failed yourself—in order to go on for the second half," I said.

"And we have a lot to forgive people for!" Linda drummed the table for emphasis.

"We do indeed!" It was a Greek chorus.

"*Forgiveness* is a key word," said Barbara. "I have had to learn to forgive my mother." Struggling to rise above racism and sexism is easier now, she added.

"That's miraculous," Judy Collins said, contemplating something deep inside herself.

"But you have to forgive." Barbara repeated it like a hymn.

It moved Judy sufficiently that she shared her own private agony. "You have forgiven your mother. I have to work on forgiving myself," she said. "I lost my son last year to suicide."

The room hushed. No one moved.

"I *know* we don't cause other people to kill themselves," she hastened to add, "but sometimes you can't help blaming yourself." Judy sketched in just enough of the story that we knew she sometimes blamed herself "because of the chaos of my background, the alcoholism.... I was fifty-two when that happened. In the middle of all the wonderful things of my life, this terrible thing, the worst possible thing that could happen... It changes you. There is a point where nothing matters, but everything is okay. It's mysterious. There's a kind of surrender. Catastrophe opens a space in your life, a silence, if you let it, which I believe can be a transformational place."

Today the artist in Judy Collins is able to open up those trembling places in her concert audiences when she sings "Amazing Grace." Considering the experiences of Barbara, Linda, and Judy, the group had been confronted with three of the most inconsolable losses a woman could endure: a parent, a breast, a child. But they also took us to the next place on the journey.

Linda recalled her teeth-gritting resistance to the miraculous when she went into recovery. "I said, 'I'm going to get sober, but I'm certainly *not* going to find God,' and then one day, 'Oh, shit!' "

Honks of laughter. "I have come to a spiritual place on this journey in the last few years," Linda acknowledged. "I think it has a great deal to do with my age."

"Right," the women murmured.

"I read something in the Bible that helped me," offered Barbara. "When Jesus told Martha to roll the stone away from Lazarus' tomb—a lot of us won't roll that stone away." She confessed, "I can say that it's only been in the last three years that I've begun to be able to forgive my mother."

The intense empathy around that table created what felt like a magnetic field, a circle of healing. As we lifted glasses to toast ourselves, I told the group they reminded me of the Stone Age women who sat on great limestone slabs, holding crystals, to conduct their sacred rites. "This is archetypal."

"If there's a picture here, it's an old-fashioned one," said Linda. "It's the gathering of women around a quilt. Because a quilt is made up of broken pieces of many things, put together into some pattern lovelier than the whole."

"Also, we can finally *see* the pattern," I added, "and that then becomes our guide."

"Of course, I can't sew a stitch." Linda laughed.

"That doesn't matter," Elizabeth said. "It's a beautiful image."

If you are aware of the fact that the fight of life is taking you somewhere, you can not only make the journey better but also be more determined and resilient during the many battles. The impact of the dinner had been to make us all *conscious of the quest*, the realization, upon reaching this point in life, that this is what the struggle has been about and that we can take the rewards forward with us.

It seemed the most natural thing in the world to join in a sacred moment with a simple prayer. Eyes closed, our hands clasped firmly together in a ring of friendship, we offered up a final thanks for reaching this place and time. Barbara began in the rolling cadence of the wise old preacher lady we could all imagine her becoming:

"God, whatever strength is in this circle, let it not be broken. Whatever strength is in this circle, let us know where we got it from. Give us the strength to continue forgiving. The hurt's gonna be there, Lord, but the power to forgive will get us through it. Let us be a friend to each other and an example for all the world to see, whatever it's about, Lord, that when people look at us, they can see you. Amen."

. . .

We all hugged and my guests left, but the event did not leave us. Over the next few weeks almost everyone called me with reverberations. We agreed that an annual Flaming Fifties linner would be a welcome thing.

But it was Barbara's call that crystallized the alchemy that had occurred. She couldn't sleep that night, she said. "There are certain life-changing experiences, and this gathering I would put in that category. I don't feel ashamed anymore. I feel healed. It was like something moved away." Even her voice sounded lighter. "When Linda told us she was so glad to be able to look forward to fifty, I realized that fifty is not something to trudge through like a mud ditch. Fifty is a gift."

Part Five

FLAMING FIFTIES: MEN

11

THE SAMSON COMPLEX

Creon to Oedipus: *Do not seek to be mastering everything, for the things you master did not follow you throughout your life.*

—SOPHOCLES, *OEDIPUS THE KING*

*W*omen must deal. Men don't have to.

Although 50 represents just as significant a crossroads for men, it is not as clear whether or not theirs will be a passage to the Flaming Fifties or to flameout. Women have a biologically timed BOOM—menopause—that forces them to acknowledge they are changing. Once they navigate through the many layers of that profound change, most come out on the other side of the sound barrier.

Men don't have to face aging. At least not as early as women do. In their First Adulthood most men are on more singular achievement tracks than women are. The tracks are made for them; they know all the stops; they are very aware of whether they're racing ahead or falling behind. Most pour out tremendous energy and often dangerously suppress their emotional needs. At least until their forties men can gain strong personal identities and a sense of self-worth simply from engaging their aggressive instincts in a struggle for dominance and position in the social hierarchy.

But these aggressive instincts are an appetite, like the sexual drive. They build up, a man satisfies them, and they build up again. By the time a man reaches middle life, however, he is not as easily filled up merely by engaging in the competitive struggle. Simultaneously he is being challenged by younger men and women whose aggressive instincts are still raw and uncontrollable. His body doesn't work quite the way it did. His job may not be as secure as he thought it would be. Even the most successful men of this age almost inevitably feel some ebbing in the thrill of the chase, a want of meaning beneath the mask of invulnerable masculinity.

Such men often meet the crossroads at 50 with the involuntary reflex of Samson, expecting that they must continue to show the same extraordinary physical strength and implacable emotional veneer they prided themselves on in youth. This effort can drain important energies away from the more important task of developing their inner resources. But since they haven't had to face inexorable limitations before, they don't think there is anything they can do about aging, except to ignore it.

What most men want to do at 50 is to stay where they are, to keep what they've got. They don't want to make a passage. And there is no finite marker that tells them when they must. There is an untold story here, however. It has traditionally been assumed that aging is kinder to men. A different truth comes out in personal interviews. I found far more uncertainty among men in middle life than among women; indeed, they often appear to be going in opposite directions. Even though most of the financially secure Professional Men I studied are much happier than when they were younger, as many as one third have arrived at the doorstep of Second Adulthood in disillusionment about themselves or having adjusted their aspirations downward.

In middle life a man's suppressed emotional needs usually come to the surface. Yet even as his emotional life is becoming more important to him, his surly teenage children are probably rebelling, his older children are leaving home for good, and his wife is becoming more assertive. If his wife is roughly the same age, she is likely to be either bouncing off the walls with menopausal mood swings or soaring with postponed ambitions, joining nonprofit boards or political campaigns and paying less attention to him than to saving refugees. With all these fears and losses on their minds as men approach the passage to the Age of Mastery, what do they worry about first?

Losing hair.

THE MALE VANITY CRISIS

In almost all the group interviews where men gathered with me to discuss the ups and downs of middle life, the conversation began with their hair. In the Louisville group a silver-haired manager in his early fifties opened the subject.

"I keep asking my barber every time I go in, 'Is it stopped yet? How much more?'" confessed Jerry Krupilski. "And my barber, bless him, will say, 'Looks like it might be ending.' He tells me hair loss slows down at about fifty-five to sixty, so if you're not totally bald by then, you will not be. So there's hope."

Other men laughed nervously.

A highly fit specimen of 59 told the Louisville group, "I am really proud to be my age. If I wanted to, I could train right now and run a mini-marathon. But I hate my hair! I pull it down, I curl it over, I can't do anything with it—it makes me feel goofy." He demonstrated his comb-over. "There's nothing I can do. It's an indelible mark of aging."

A silver-mustached salesman of 48 extended the metaphor. "It's a matter of control. I don't know what fifty is going to hold, but part of that whole aging process and fear of losing control is losing hair."

Krupilski described it as his biggest problem. "You can look really great indoors. Then you go outside and it's windy. Your hair flies up, and all the bare spots show, and you think, *God! I hope no one sees me.* It's humiliating."

His wife consoles him by insisting that she is turned on by balding men. An executive in the group pats the shiny saucer of whiteness on top of his skull that has become a standing family joke. "I explain to my son—he's fifteen—that this is really a solar panel for my sex machine."

An older, balder man sneers. "There's a whole lot of rationalizing going on around this table."

It would seem, from the intensity of their concern, that losing their hair is for men the first public sign of weakening, almost like walking around with an exposed ego wound that everyone can see, as if hair were what Samson believed it to be: the symbol of a man's power and sexual prowess.

The other subject that inevitably provoked frustrated confessions in the men's group interviews was their ability to do sports. Almost universally men note the ebbing of their youthful physical strength as another of the first signs of encroaching middle age. The struggle over relinquishing physical dominance is, for men, as fierce and painful as the struggle over surrendering their youthful beauty is for women. And those who have been the most athletic in their youth feel the loss most stingingly, as was plain when the Louisville group changed the subject to physical prowess.

THE AGING ATHLETE, AGE 57

"I knew I was getting old when my boys wouldn't ask me to play ball with them anymore."

His paid vocation is director of education and training for a large regional health care system. But where this man *lives* is inside the body of an aging softball player. Tall, proud, lantern-jawed, he combs his silvery hair forward. He exudes presence.

"I've been an athlete all my life," he said by way of introduction. He started noticing major changes in his mid-forties. "Playing against the kids got a lot harder. In quickness and speed the kids were just a little more aggressive than I could be anymore. And I'd *really* been aggressive." The muscles jumped in his forearms as if to emphasize his point. "I knew I was getting old when my boys would play softball, but they wouldn't ask Dad anymore. Now I get, 'Would you like to *coach*, Dad?' Not 'Would you like to *play*, Dad?'"

The other men nodded empathetically at this story.

"I've passed fifty," said David Allen, the physician in the group. He had always found pleasure in skiing with his kids, but he too saw the first sign of a massive shift in his concept of himself in his mid-forties. "I noticed a change in the excitement of skiing down the double black diamonds. I was not enjoying the envelope between high tension on the fun side and tension from the threat of bodily injury that could happen in a fraction of a second."

The salesman made a telling slip. "I think you reach a point in your life where you start to realize your own immortality."

"*Mortality*," the former ballplayer corrected him.

"That's right, I mean . . ." the salesman stammered, "yes, your own mortality, thank you."

But there is something other than mortality that stands in the way of a man's satisfying the emotional needs that are surfacing at this stage. It is the drive to retain dominance by the same means he has always used: the Samson Complex. This effort can drive a man to extremes as ridiculous as they are poignant.

A father of 46 told me the story of his last stand over his rebellious 16-year-old son. When the son refused to carry out an order of the father's, they engaged in a shouting match. Back and forth it went, until the frustrated father declared, "Okay, we're just going to have to fight this out." They started wrestling. Though heaving and puffing, the father managed at one point to pin down the son. "It took all of the strength I could possibly muster to hold down this strong colt," he later admitted. But in those few fleeting moments that he was able to maintain his physical dominance over the boy, the father threatened him: "And just let that be a lesson; you can never defy me again!" He then quickly released the boy.

Later, telling the story, the father had to laugh at his farcical behavior. Within months or a year that same boy would be a young man who could never again be forcibly subdued by his father, physically or otherwise. Yet the father had to play out his last moments as the dominant male with all the vehemence of a top baboon.

The Samson Complex is particularly acute for men of the Silent and World War II generations, who were socialized to fulfill instrumental roles and reject all that fuzzy-wuzzy stuff about feelings. Let their wives worry about "relationships." Their domains were work and sports, which often became the exclusive sources of male identity. Anyone who listens to older men today should know that most of them are confused and floundering to find new definitions of masculinity and sources of emotional security. And why not? Just about everything that they have been conditioned to believe defines their masculinity has come under attack. In my men's group interviews I always asked how they defined masculinity.

When I was growing up . . . men were into control and one-upmanship.

—STEVEN ZUCKER, AGE 53, PSYCHOTHERAPIST,
SANTA MONICA, CALIFORNIA

When I was in my early twenties, being a man was to feel only two feelings: either anger or sexual desire. All other emotions were feminine and therefore weak and to be abhorred.

—HAROLD WAHKING, AGE 62, FAMILY THERAPIST,
ST. PETERSBURG, FLORIDA

Being a man was being an athlete. All I did growing up was play baseball, and I still do. I used to be one of those Monday to Friday absent fathers as my kids were growing up.

—ROB TAYLOR, AGE 58, BUSINESSMAN, DALLAS, TEXAS

Growing up in the Forties during the war years, you were supposed to eat all your eggs and meat and potatoes, and all my heroes smoked cigarettes: John Wayne, Humphrey Bogart.

—BOB FOWLER, AGE 54, AIRLINE PILOT, DALLAS, TEXAS

It was my duty as a man to protect women, to do for them what they couldn't do for themselves, and in return it was expected that they do domestic chores.

—TOM DRIVER, AGE 68, SEMINARY PROFESSOR, ON HIS
UPBRINGING IN THE AMERICAN SOUTH

These familiar descriptions of the traditional masculine ethic have all undergone a barrage of attacks and ridicule, not to mention stringent new laws and behavioral taboos. But it is not just man's dominance in the workplace or in the family hierarchy that contemporary men are struggling to hold on to; they are being asked to fight against their own natures. The instincts that make them aggressive, those very competitive qualities that were necessary before the computer age for the survival of the species, are now held up as the scourge that makes our streets violent, our corporations inhumane, and every date a potential rape.

Certainly, long-standing male abuses of physical, sexual, and institutional power cried out for a new awareness and overdue reforms. But the tremendous increase in confidence on the part of women who have learned, usually the hard way, that they can take care of themselves has probably had an even greater impact on the self-concepts of men today than any law. With the phenomenal increase of wives working outside the home, women's lives are coming more and more to resemble those of men's. And that blurring of the sex roles is naturally accelerated as men and women approach the Age of Mastery in the postindustrial Information Era, where communication skills and endurance count for much more than brute physical strength.

Given this new set of conditions, men at middle life probably face the roughest patch of all in mapping the new adult life across time. Generally, it is a much harder passage for men than for women. When women in midlife go back to college and then find jobs that give them some dignity and paychecks that give them some authority, they are exhilarated. The psychic compensation is greater for women because they started with so much less. Men already had the good jobs and the greater authority in the family. To make a passage to the Age of Mastery often means for men giving up being the master.

What do they get for it?

The chance to create a new self. Men are going to live much longer than they expected, whether they like it or not. If they keep speeding along the old track, refusing to give up their Samson identity, they will miss the turnoff to Second Adulthood. They will age anyway, but it won't be fun. The question is, How to prepare to enjoy a Second Adulthood? How to pay for it? The competitive struggle alone will not satisfy a man's new appetites in Second Adulthood, which have to do with making closer human connections and releasing creativity.

But instead of taking the risk of change, many men in middle life keep hanging on to every vestige of power and pursue every opportunity for one-upmanship, even with their children, even when it makes them look ridiculous. In the title story of his collection of meditations on life after middle age, *The Afterlife*, John Updike memorably describes the dozey existence of a man in his fifties who resists fresh beginnings:

> At the office now—he was a lawyer—he was conscious of a curious lag, like the lag built into radio talk shows so that obscenities wouldn't get on the air. Just two or three seconds, between challenge and response, between achievement and gratification, but enough to tell him that something was out of sync. He was going through the motions, and all the younger people around him knew it.[1]

In Detroit a group of middle-American males came together in a modest suburban living room to discuss these issues further. Among them were an executive, an auto worker, a music teacher, a college dean, a hospital administrator. Within the first half hour these total strangers were baring their souls and self-doubts to one another. That's how pained they are. That's how deep is their need for vindication and validation that what they are feeling is not just something wrong with them.

THE EXCESSED VP, AGE 47

"I'm not going down the tubes. I resist that!"

Don Parrot has been stripped of his executive status at the age of 47, a casualty of corporate restructuring. He feels invisible in the workplace.

"You sure don't look invisible," the other men tease him.

Right. The Excessed VP is wearing a bold turquoise madras shirt and serious black cross-training shoes. There isn't a pinch of extra weight on him. And Don is proud of his hair, still thick as grass in midsummer. Yet for all his youthful appearance, he was made recently and painfully aware of being no longer a kid. He was mountain biking with his 16-year-old son and 18-year-old daughter. As they pumped up and down the rolling hills of a state park on a humid summer's day, his kids kept waving and shouting from up ahead, "Dad, Dad, aren't you coming?" His quads were on fire; his lungs felt like used birthday balloons.

"I was dying," he admits. "That was the first time it hit me. You can't take it for granted anymore. I resolved to do whatever conditioning I needed to put it back the way it was." Don's temples dot up with perspiration just remembering that day. "And I'll probably kill myself trying."

It is striking the lengths to which some men will go, including seriously injuring themselves, to deny that their bodies are not the same spring-loaded mechanisms at 50 that they were at 30. Given our culture's emphasis on killer competition in sports, it is understandable that many men equate their value with their Samson-like physical abilities. They cannot give up trying to prove themselves athletically because once they give it up, they cannot see anything else to replace that identity.

"Hell, I played football, baseball, and basketball when I was a kid, but I've moved on to other things now," says a 48-year-old hospital administrator with a barrel of a belly protruding under his big sweatshirt. "Why not take up sailing? You just sit there and move the tiller." Others talk about golf, softball, bowling.

But the Excessed VP shakes his head. "The idea that you can't physically perform the way you did when you were sixteen, so you take up sailing instead of jogging ten miles a day—no way! I have a lot of trouble admitting that."

Dr. Joseph Macri, a community college dean who is a little bit older, has already admitted this limitation and as a result has a much brighter perspective. His tennis game is obviously different from the game he played at 25, he says. He had to admit it when he played singles with a son of 25. "So at this age I *place* my shots rather than rely on running and a second wind."

Indeed, strategy based on experience—placing our shots in life—is perhaps the greatest advantage we have in Second Adulthood over younger greenhorns. The metaphor is lost on Parrot.

"I'm not going down the tubes. I resist that!" the Excessed VP shoots back. "I mean, I know enough about psychology and medicine that I ought to be able to reverse all this," he insists. He has been looking into cryogenics. "I thought I might consider having myself frozen at some point, while I'm still alive."

"Great," cracks another group member. "The only problem with that is, they have to chop your head off."

The end of physical dominance, of course, is not the end of life. On the contrary, letting go of some of the outer strengths that defined their masculinity in First Adulthood is exactly what allows men to discover and nourish the inner strengths that will sustain them through Second Adulthood. There is a way out. Men who accept change find it releases them to move on and find a new life.

Alan Alhadeff, a Seattle lawyer of 45, described his Aha! moment on a basketball court.

"This twenty-year-old kid was checking me real hard in the backcourt. I'm then about twenty pounds heavier than people my height should be. So I pushed him away, somewhat aggressively. I said, 'C'mon, I'm old enough to be your dad.'"

The young man looked the older man straight in the eye. "Then get off the court."

The lawyer had felt fairly invincible before that incident, he said. "There wasn't anything I felt I couldn't do. Skiing, climbing, whatever—I didn't mind putting myself in dangerous circumstances. But after that day on the basketball court I mellowed. I realized *I don't have to* prove myself in physical contests anymore. I don't see that as a negative at all." On the contrary, it frees him to try other forms of expression he had never entertained before: art, music, gardening, gourmet cooking. "And they're all a lot easier on the knees!"

Several of the men in the Louisville group, having already moved well into middle life, were scoring themselves differently now. From a rough, aggressive approach to the game of life, where only conquering and winning counted, their whole value system had shifted to one that prized human interactions. Even one of the athletes had found a new way to enjoy ballplaying.

THE SOCIABLE ATHLETE, AGE 59

"Now you're really friends playing against friends."

"I've graduated to senior softball, and I play now in senior tournaments all over the country," Bill Newkirk told us. He is now 59.

Did that give him a new burst?

"Absolutely. Felt like a kid again. You're playing with your peers, rather than competing against people you just can't compete against anymore."

"Or pretending that you're still twenty-five," added someone else.

"Hey, everybody playing is just glad to be still alive and competing," said Newkirk. Everyone chuckled. "And there's a real social situation. You find that before the ball game, during the game, after the game, the men are *talking* to each other. Now you're really *friends* playing against *friends*." Once in a while Newkirk still plays against kids, but now he sees them differently: "They're very aggressive, very competitive, and sometimes a little bit rough.

It is just two totally different cultures," he said, unconsciously making a profound comment on younger versus older men through the metaphor of sports.

He also felt a need to connect with a woman. "I went through divorce a year ago. I realized I could *not* stay alone. My sense is the conquering drive is not a quest by the time you hit forty-five. Even the sexual fantasy of conquering loses a lot of appeal. You think about the social consequences of catting around."

In shopping around for a wife, he had looked specifically for "a smile and communication." By now he was engaged to be married and anticipated the added pleasure of having a loving partner to share the later years.

Certain sports lend themselves to greater affinity with other men or with nature. A New York real estate developer told me he had taken up golf a few years ago and added somewhat sheepishly, "It's probably because it's a middle-aged sport." He confessed that he had become a fanatic.

"What is it that really draws you?" I asked.

"Well, it's the companionship. I use it to get close to other men."

He contrasted it with tennis, which he had loved at 40. "On a tennis court you show up, take your rackets out, you grunt 'Hello,' each gets on either side of the net, you rally, play a few sets, maybe you exchange a few words when you change sides, and you're gone. There's no real depth of exchange or friendship."

He described the many different opportunities for closeness on a golf course. You might be walking down the fairway with one of your party, having a deep personal conversation about your dreams or disappointments and offering each other a lot of support. Then you rejoin the foursome and tell silly jokes. On the way to another hole you might have a spirited political discussion or trade tips on your health problems. "By the time you stop for a bite to eat together, and you do this week after week, you have reached a level of depth and meaning in your friendship with these other men that you can't do in any other way. It's a huge commitment of time to one another."

This same man, however, is no slouch when it comes to competitiveness. He runs one of the more successful real estate development operations in Greater New York. I asked him if golf afforded him release from competitiveness.

"Golf isn't like any other sport in that regard, and that also appeals to me," he said. "When you're playing basketball, baseball, tennis, squash, you're always trying to beat the other guy to the ball. With golf, you're not playing against the other guys; you're playing against the course—this inanimate thing." The level of intimacy fostered by the game was best expressed by this man's golf partner: "When Dave makes a good shot, it thrills me, because I love Dave. I know he's enjoying himself, and that gives me pleasure." That is worlds apart from what a man at 30 would feel if he watched his racquetball partner hit a great three-wall shot or his tennis buddy aced him with a smashing serve. There is clear evidence here of the shift in satisfaction from competing to the pleasure in companionship.

But there was another, metaphysical level of the game that the developer wanted to convey. He sent me a little book written by the founder of Esalen, Michael Murphy, that describes golf as "yoga for the supermind" and interprets why people love to hit their drives so far. "The flight of the ball, the sight of it hanging there in space, anticipates our desire for transcendence."[2]

Howell Raines, the author and *New York Times* editorial-page editor, described another sport that can move the spirit to self-transcendence in his book *Fly Fishing Through the Midlife Crisis*.[3] Unlike Ernest Hemingway, who used fly-fishing scenes to illustrate the impotence of faith and who gave up fighting for life in his forties, Raines describes being alone in the natural sanctuary of red rock canyons where he can lose the boundaries of time and space and body and be open to truth.

> . . . many men come to fly fishing after they have been through other kinds of fishing, usually forms that involve powerful boats, heavy rods and brutally strong fish . . . perhaps it is that as men get older, some of them develop holes in their souls, and they think this disciplined, beautiful and unessential activity might close those holes.[4]
>
> Fly-fishing is also the most feminine form of the sport,
>
> relying as it does on touch, intuition and a more relaxed, nurturing and uncompetitive feeling for the quarry and its home. Perhaps that is why men discover fly fishing when they age past the point where, as Tom McGuane puts it, they are simply "running on testosterone."[5]

MACHO MEN HOLDING THE LINE

There is an important class distinction to be made here. The *Family Circle* Life History Survey drew responses from 394 men, the largest and most diverse group of men I have studied. They are largely skilled workers and technicians or administrators/managers who do not have college degrees and who earn an average of $45,000 a year. They average 47 in age. Almost all are married with children, and two thirds of them are still with their first wives, demonstrating a much more traditional family orientation than the more highly educated Professional Men. Indeed, the *Family Circle* men derive their greatest pleasure from their children and being fathers and from their marriages. What does 50 look like to them?

Most appear to be more resigned to accepting life as it is: Two thirds are not anticipating any major change, and one third feel more concerned about just getting by. Half these men feel tired and as if they are "running out of gas."

Like their wives, they sense they have little power in the outside world, although they do have more power at work than the women do. There is little altruism here; very few are devoted to any cause outside themselves. These men are not introspective, they have very few close friends, and they seem averse to admitting problems that might stigmatize them as being less of a man. In fact, 78 percent of them find it difficult to express their worries and almost impossible to ask for help. As explained by the Berkeley longitudinal study of personality patterns from adolescence to middle age, "From early adolescence on, traditional men are overcontrolled and value thinking rather than feeling."[6]

The overall picture of the traditional men from the *Family Circle* survey, by their late forties and fifties, is an extreme need for control in the one arena where they *do* have power: over their wives and children. There are hints that exploitative and condescending macho behavior is used to mask their inchoate insecurities. Their anger and frustration at aging they tend to project outward, through punitive actions or blame games.

Their greatest worry is that they can no longer take their health for granted. Longevity is not as alluring to them. Of those over 45, *half* have fathers who are already deceased.

BUT MY BODY IS BULLETPROOF!

At the turn of the century women lived, on average, only a year longer than their husbands.[7] Although both men and women live much longer today, men do die, on average, seven years earlier than their wives. Men are more likely to be depressed in old age,[8] and they are at four times greater risk for suicide.[9] While the number of women over 45 who take their own lives has gone down in every age-group over the last decade and a half, the suicide rate for men aged 45 to 49 is up significantly.[10]

Why should a man die sooner than his wife?

"Just what I've been wondering!" exclaimed historian Robert Caro. For one thing, men are usually in more of a hurry in First Adulthood and may suffer more stress along with less emotional support. "My father told me straight out, you've got to make it by the time you're forty," admitted writer Peter Prescott.

But the greater handicap, I submit, is the life-and-death chances men choose to take with their second half by pretending their bodies remain bulletproof.

Most men take better care of their cars than their own bodies. At least they take their cars in for regular inspections and tune-ups. I routinely threw out this question to the men's interview groups: "If you suspected you had a physical problem—say, you've felt some chest pains or discomfort in urinating—would you be most likely to check it out with a doctor and change your habits? Or go pedal to the metal and wait until you flame out?"

The replies always shocked me.

"I'm going to keep going until I crash and burn." The 55-year-old Dallas man, John Bredehoft, had been prematurely retired by his company. He felt very insecure about age discrimination and was remarried to a younger woman. Having chosen to deny any evidence of aging, he refused to go to a doctor or pay attention to his own health.

An extremely overweight 57-year-old Florida man boasted, "I just enjoy eating all the wrong things. As long as I'm not faced with a health crisis, I'd rather enjoy life to the fullest. I like to feel I have control over my life and I decide when I die." Of course, by ignoring the need to change his diet and get enough exercise to accommodate aging, he is doing just the opposite: forfeiting control over his life. Jim Bullard, a 52-year-old professional writer, was sharply perceptive about the delusions he noticed among other men in the Orlando group interview, but while he noted his own increasingly sedentary lifestyle and the poundage that has accumulated along with it, he was characteristically nonchalant.

"I'm consciously aware that I haven't changed my lifestyle in twenty years," he said. "Maybe this is immature or lazy, but I'm operating on the assumption that my first heart attack isn't going to be fatal, and that's going to be the alert. I'm just playin' the percentages. I think a lot of men do that."

This is Bullard's way of demonstrating that he is the same man he was at 32, a dangerous invitation to serious health consequences. "Do you resist going to the doctor?" I asked him.

"Yeah," he grumbled. "He's going to scold me. I hate to be scolded. It goes back to how my mother used to scold me." The writer takes pleasure in being the Peck's bad boy who resists his wife's prodding. Many married men I have interviewed harbor this same attitude.

The traditional working-class men in the *Family Circle* survey also worry about their health and bulging bellies. But few of them exercise or play sports anymore. They admit to being far less physically active than their wives.

Traditional men often become so stressed by intense emotional states they barely comprehend that they experience their feelings only as *physical* sensations: headaches or indigestion, low back pain or tingling in the extremities, or just "feeling blah." Even if the man is able to recognize the feeling underneath, he seldom has the vocabulary to express it, as, say, a fight-or-flight reaction, or shame, or the desperate need for a tender touch. Feelings so undiscovered are seldom able to be conveyed in appropriate ways. Instead many men allow their defensive beliefs about masculinity to lock them into behaviors that deprive them of fully enjoying their Flaming Fifties. This is especially true when it comes to taking care of their bodies. If they deny or resist the necessity of change, men in their fifties may be inviting psychological or physical problems.

The high school music teacher who joined the Detroit group is a good example. At first Ray Kudzia appeared to be somewhat sensitive and open. A compact man with a decent head of brown hair, he wore a crew-neck sweater and an open shirt. But Ray's extreme reticence to allow himself to know what he really feels has already cost him physiologically. In his thirties, he admits, he had a couple of small strokes. The platelets in his blood, he says, just, well, stuck together. It left him partially blind.

"Then I totally withdrew," he tells the group. "If I were my wife, I would have divorced me." But it's hard to change, he says. "This is the way my dad was, and he's my idol."

Ray's wife, to whom he has been married for twenty-three years, told me before the meeting, "Ray has been acting very weird. Blowing up at the kids, at me—and he never did that before." As a nurse she is especially worried about his holding everything in. Theirs is a grand extended Polish family, and family always takes top priority with Ray. He is highly responsible. He even cooks family meals now and then. But there are no *close-in* feelings allowed.

"I take after my dad," Ray says proudly. "He never expressed any feelings. I never tell anyone my problems."

Others ask, "Can you keep going that way?"

"Yup." The mouth clamps shut. "Well, every once in a while I'll explode at my wife. She's good. She'll listen."

Ray is like most men of the Silent Generation in this regard. He has no truly close men friends. While women have on the average four or five close confidantes to whom they can reveal their insecurities, men of this generation usually have only one source of emotional support: their wives. They rely on their wives to decode their own feelings.[11]

Ray doesn't connect his physical problems with the psychological hammerlock he keeps on his inner life. On his questionnaire he revealed that he has no close friends, and no source of intimacy, and his sex life is abysmal; hence he thinks about sex now twenty-four hours a day. "I guess I'm just pushing everything deeper and deeper," Ray tells the group.

What bugs you the most at this stage? I ask. Long silence.

"All these things are back here irritating me." He rubs the back of his head, as if to keep the currents moving. "I just keep pushing anything that's bothering me out of my mind. Maybe when I'm fifty, I'll become a serial killer."

Men's bodies, just like women's, naturally undergo changes in shape and stamina in middle life. After age 45, men who are sedentary rapidly lose lean muscle mass and, consequently, strength. For every pound of muscle lost, for instance, a man's resting metabolic rate drops by nearly fifty calories a day. And as his metabolism slows down, his endurance and energy will ebb, and his well-being and self-confidence will be compromised. Unless—and this is a solid promise—he compensates by being disciplined about maintaining his body as rigorously as he does his car.

Studies show that older men who do strength training (lifting weights or working out against resistance on machines) as well as aerobics can rebuild their muscle power, make it much easier to lose unwanted pounds and inches, and actually improve their physical and sexual prowess in defiance of their biological clocks.[12]

As men get older, their immune systems also need support. We now know that untreated depression is correlated with the onset of cancer. The risk of heart disease can be diminished by taking aspirin daily and going for regular cardiovascular exams, but millions of men refuse these simple precautions because they think they're unmanly.[13] Prostate cancer is a hush-

hush disease that now strikes one in ten American men,[14] a figure as daunting as the number of women who will get breast cancer. The difference is
that if it is caught early, prostate cancer is 80 percent curable.[15] Yet thirty-
five thousand men a year are literally dying from embarrassment, most of
them because they were humiliated by the very thought of having the
anal/digital exam that, together with a blood test, might have detected a
malignancy while it was still contained in the prostate gland.[16]

An increasing number of men, however, are beginning to make major life
changes to promote and take pleasure in their new longevity. A heart attack
or some other physical scare may be what gets their attention at first. For a
few weeks they will do whatever the doctor tells them—give up drinking,
buy a treadmill, get religion, almost anything—but fear is not enough to
sustain major life changes. The Samson Complex reasserts itself, and denial
comes back. It is too frightening to face the possibility of dying, so most
men forget the incident and return to their old ways.

"Changes need to be based not of fear of dying but on joy of living,"
says Dr. Dean Ornish, the pioneer of nonmedical reversal of heart disease.[17] His nonprofit research institute in Sausalito, California, tries to teach
people that illness or suffering can be a doorway for transforming one's life
in ways that go well beyond just prolonging life. And this isn't just a prescription for high-income professionals. In fact, says Dr. Ornish, people in
lower socioeconomic groups can benefit *more* from making decisive changes
in their habits to regain their health. Why? Because upper-income men take
it for granted that the decisions they make can create a big difference in
their lives. As we know from the *Family Circle* survey, fewer working-class
men feel anything like that kind of personal power. Further, about 90 percent of the cardiac bypass surgery is performed on white upper-middle-
class men despite the fact that heart disease affects all income groups.

An ordinary man, once exposed to the right tools and techniques for
reclaiming his health without surgery, feels a thrill of empowerment, perhaps for the first time. That experience often spills over into other areas of
his life, says Dr. Ornish, and becomes a driving force that sustains him in
making lasting changes.

Crises are doorways. Even Samson can benefit by stepping through and
enjoying the transformation.

12

FALL GUYS OF THE
ECONOMIC REVOLUTION

"I don't want to retire at sixty-five. I want to work until I'm shot by a jealous spouse."

That remark, which came up in almost every one of the men's discussion groups, sums up two sources of male power that men in middle life worry most about preserving: They want to continue to be valued in work and in bed.

Sexual confidence is inescapably linked with financial security for most men. In fact, one of the most important elements that contribute to a sense of mastery overall is financial security. Already close to half of America's discretionary income (spending money beyond necessities) nestles in the sixty million wallets of those grown-up individuals in their fifties, sixties, seventies, and beyond.[1]

> Households headed by someone over 55 control 56 percent of all the net worth in the nation's homes.[2]

The fact that mature households control such a money lake comes as a pleasant surprise to many of those in Second Adulthood. And that money lake will only overflow with riches in the next ten years, as the 50 to 64 age-group swells by 25 percent.[3] By the year 2000, with Baby Boomers crossing the Great Divide by the legions, the number of Americans over 50 is expected to hit the staggering figure of seventy-six million. These wealthiest members of a hot new market are not only living longer but thinking younger. Market research has revealed that members of the 50-plus set consider themselves ten to fifteen years younger than society perceives them to be.[4]

The other surprise is not so pleasant. Men who are in their fifties probably expected fallen arches, a bad hair stage, maybe a divorce, or one rotten kid in the barrel, but not unemployment, never unemployment, or even underemployment. The old 50 usually found a man in a safe corporate environment, with a planned retirement, able to count out almost to the penny what he would be worth when he was given the gold watch at 65. Not today. Something new and contradictory is happening. Here are some sobering figures pulled from the PUMS file:

> For the first time since the World War II Generation, men in their late forties and early fifties are suffering a steep decline in wages.

This phenomenon affects primarily the two million American men, aged 46 to 55 in 1995, who have four years of college but no graduate school.[5] They belong to the younger half of the Silent Generation who finished college in the prosperous late 1950s or 1960s and entered corporate jobs confident of steady promotions and rising incomes well into their middle age. Instead, when they were between 45 and 54, at the tail end of the go-go years, their median incomes plunged by 16 percent—from more than $50,000 in 1987 to $41,898 by 1992.[6]

In the recent past corporations didn't even think of cutting off their managers before 60. Lee Iacocca, when he was still president of the Ford Motor Company in the late 1970s, admitted to me that he felt guilty about nudging his mid- to top managers toward early retirement at 55. And for good reason; no matter what they had achieved up to that point, those men felt worthless, depressed, and often joined the walking dead.

Today men in their fifties in corporate life are in a precarious position. They are a high-ticket item in an era of downsizing. Boards of directors are impressed when downsizing is done as a "clean sweep"—usually by slashing senior managers who command the highest salaries and ominous retirement benefits. In a matter of months a restructured company's fiftyish management appears to have been "morphed" into a fortyish management. Since the mid-Eighties, layers of middle management have also been stripped away in company after company. And many men who are not fired are downsized in rank and income, with the clear implication that their jobs may be the next to go.

What do these prematurely obsolescent men do? They are too young to retire for good but usually too old to shift gears and work in an aggressive, growing, restructured company. Most of them have been conditioned to be good corporate citizens, to go with the flow, be chameleons, and to choose their wives and build their lives around external values and material accomplishments.[7] Suddenly they are expected to fall back on inner resources and to lower their expectations financially and socially. Senior executives who are likely to be computer-phobic must learn how to deal with a new digital culture.[8] Acculturated under the old corporate paternalism of the 1950s and 1960s, they harbor such loyalty to the company-as-father that even after the Gordian knot has been hacked in two, many of them are left numb and disbelieving.

This chapter will explore variations on the predicament and the most promising new adaptations men are making to this passage.

CORPORATE REFUGEES

Everybody tells you it's a great deal, you'd be crazy to pass up "the package." The company is desperate to downsize, and the offer of premature retirement is tempting. Your wife insists you've been miserable for years as a corporate cog and starts planning a monthlong sojourn of golf or skiing to celebrate your freedom. But freedom can be a terrifying burden.

"It felt like a mass burial" was how one robust-looking former Kodak executive described the day he and hundreds of others took the package. "You expected to reach a top job level, say, from fifty to sixty-two, where you'd make a significant contribution to the company," he ruminated. "Instead the best thing they think we can contribute at fifty is to get out— so they can hire younger people and pay them less."

Bill belonged to a group of corporate refugees. Six men, all of whom were high-level managers in different departments of the big yellow-brick Kodak tower that dominates their city of Rochester, they have been meeting for fifteen years to discuss the stresses of working in a large corporation. Rochester is a little big town in upstate New York, a complacent, conservative, insiders' town, dominated by several world-class corporations. For the upper middle class it's a country club town, very social and cliquey. There isn't much elasticity for accepting men in their fifties—corporate used-to-bes—who are trying to find more creative, self-generated lives, and work.

This private men's group was designed as a safe refuge, outside marriage, where these company men could relax their false fronts, spill their truths, and *not* get advice. Here they get listening. In April 1993, and again in November 1993, they allowed me to sit in on their group. Four had been prematurely retired. These were not tired old men. They were the lean and handsome, craggy-browed, button-down model organization men of their era—Joe College types thirty years later. As they gathered, greeting one another with big bear hugs, it was clear that their fellowship is what keeps them going.

THE LIFER, AGE 53

"It's like being alone in the woods without a flashlight."

Like most senior managers, Bill came to Kodak right out of college. "We're lifers," he admitted. "A lot of our identity is tied up with the company. We didn't prepare for this transition. Who's Bill and who's Kodak? I have a lot of trouble sorting that out." Little wonder. There was even an expression to honor the consanguinity of company and company man. Good loyal Kodak employees were said to have "yellow blood" because Kodak had become part of their bloodstreams. After thirty-two years and a day working for Kodak, Bill and thousands of others were given a couple of days to make the decision to accept the early-retirement package. The bitter pill was sugarcoated: Either take double your pension or lose thousands of dollars a year. But what seemed to make sense on paper registered differently in the gut. "I expected to be at Kodak until I was sixty-five," Bill said, "and they change the rules on you at fifty. It's a betrayal. It's like being alone in the woods without a flashlight."

These golden prisoners of the paternalistic corporate culture, after twenty or thirty years of being stripped of their individuality in exchange for security and status, were suddenly released like domesticated animals with their natural competitive instincts blunted and their fighting claws clipped. This wasn't how their fifties were supposed to be for these men. The usual plan was that all the children would be out of the house, the corporation man would be at peak income, and after all the years of sacrificing for the kids, he and his wife would be able to live life to the fullest. Instead many corporate couples are back to scrimping and saving like newlyweds. Or rather, they should be. It doesn't help matters to sit around bemoaning a betrayal. But the psychological impact of such a reversal in expectations is as stunning as a knockout punch. It is a life accident. And as with most life accidents, it takes at least two years to internalize the new reality and move ahead.

THE MEANT-TO-BE-PRESIDENT, AGE 55

"Now, if I run into a former colleague's wife in the grocery store, I want to talk to her."

A former senior staff man who harbored plausible notions of becoming president of Kodak, Bert (a pseudonym) makes a painful confession. "I used to be mortified going to the grocery store in the middle of the day. Inevitably I'd run into one of my former colleagues' wives." But things changed since this son of a rigid military man left the company three years before.

"I couldn't have left if my father hadn't died," he realizes now. As he has lived an unstructured existence for the first time in his life, all sorts of vivid, unexplored feelings have broken through his defenses. For a while after he left Kodak Bert had felt compelled to drop into the office and give advice to his friends. But whenever he drove up within a hundred yards of that yellow-brick tower, and walked through a parking lot that today is filled with beat-up Toyotas and Mazdas and budget cars, and went "back inside," through the executive entrance past the brass plaque that boasts: KODAK: IMAGINATION FOR THE WORLD, his chest would start heaving with incoherent emotions.

"It's disappointment, anger, um, something like love that you feel wasn't returned." He gropes for the key. "It's a parental thing. Maybe I'm disappointing my father. I'm not fully in touch with all of it yet, but I feel like I've lived a very fearful life, trying to realize somebody else's expectations. I went through all that pain, and it didn't work out. I'm really pissed off about that."

Bert is still in passage. He plays a lot of golf and has involved himself in some community work, but he doesn't pretend that it fills the void. The most important thing going on is that beneath the layers of false self he composed to please the corporate parent, he is uncovering the outlines of a real self.

"One of the markers of progress that causes me to feel better is that now, if I run into a former colleague's wife in the grocery store, I want to *talk to her!* It's a good feeling. A significant change. I don't have the same trepidations. That may have taken three years."

PSYCHIC CONSEQUENCES

There is another way to look at these dislocations. First, it is not your fault. You are simply caught up in a huge historical turn of the wheel. Understanding that reality, and facing it squarely, is the best defense. The human organism knows how to heal itself, once it has validation that its symptoms are normal.

As more and more men topple from the middle or upper rungs of their corporate ladders, or are laid off in middle age from white- and blue-collar jobs, they should know they are not the only ones. They belong to an endangered species. A great developmental splat can be heard from East Coast to West. "Men over forty-five are becoming the new at-risk population for significant problems with anxiety and depression," says a national expert on depression, Ellen McGrath, the psychologist and author of *When Feeling Bad Is Good.* "And for the first time ever, some of them are acknowledging it and reaching out for help. This is a brand-new trend."[9]

Experts say the men most likely to be affected are accustomed to being successful. Now past their mid-forties, they find themselves either unemployed or underemployed, or they hate their jobs. Many are in long-term marriages that have become vacuous, but so long as the men gained sufficient self-esteem from their work, it was tolerable to have empty but functional marriages. Once they lose the ego boost of a decent job, the vacuousness of the marriage is revealed. On the surface they may still look fat and happy, but the flashy car is leased, the luxury lifestyle is probably being financed by a home equity loan, and the family's assets and savings are being inexorably stripped in order to maintain the good life. Will the savings flow be there to get the kids through college? Hell, will there even be enough cash flow to get themselves through to Social Security?

Some men start falling apart within months after losing a job or being induced to retire, particularly those shaped by the Silent Generation who are unaccustomed to dealing with feelings. Here are some danger signs: Feeling betrayed, perhaps with good cause, the unemployed man runs in circles around his anger, concentrating on how to sue the company or sabotage it in some way. He begins using alcohol to buffer the pain. But since alcohol is a depressant, the more he pours the scotch, the worse he feels, and the less effective he becomes in dealing with the reality of his situation. With no one left to prove himself to, no office to go to, he starts picking on his wife and family as a way of registering some power in a domain where the wife rules. Trying to work from home reminds him of being a helpless little boy dominated by Mother. He vacillates between feeling helpless and withdrawing into mute and phony self-sufficiency. His wife is damned if she does help him and damned if she doesn't. Gradually he waits later and later to get dressed, vegetates in front of the TV, watching sports rather than doing them, while refusing to take responsibility for maintaining his health and improving his fitness—all signs of male depression.

"These men, whose psychological and emotional issues are least examined, find themselves much farther along on the decline curve in sexual function as well as physical aging," says Ken Goldberg, a Texas urologist who sees hundreds of such men a month at his Male Health Center in Dallas.[10]

This is the truth of the passage into late middle life for a significant number of men today. If they try to relive First Adulthood without the same physical and economic resources that went with it, they are almost certain to feel lost in the woods without a flashlight. They are going to have to change, to accommodate the fact that we all are living longer with fewer dependable resources. They will need reeducation and retraining. It is not easy. This is a passage that our society has not yet recognized. There are no ground rules for it, and not much impetus to attempt it. Most people don't even know it exists.

ANGRY AND ANXIOUS WHITE MALES

The voices of these angry and anxious men are the staple of hate-talk radio today. Research has found the audiences of most political talk radio shows to be 97 percent white and 60 percent male and middle-aged.[11] These men are often at home, with too much time on their hands, and vent their personal frustrations through interlocuters who encourage open racism and homophobia and personal slander.

"Men like this never developed the inner resources they need to make this transition," observes Jungian analyst Aryeh Maidenbaum from his years of clinical practice. "They start reverting to childlike behavior and turn the wife into mother. They demand constant companionship and attention."

But instead of shutting down for good, at least some of them are reaching out to men's groups, spiritual guides, and psychotherapists for guidance through this perilous transition. Dr. McGrath, who maintains a clinical practice in New York and in an affluent beach community in Southern California, sees herself as part of the cleanup crew for this great developmental splat. "These men are literally dragging in their bag of body and mind parts and saying, 'Help!'" She starts by giving them new communication and behavioral tools so they can regain a feeling of control. Once they feel some of their power restored, they can begin to put the pieces of their lives back together in a new way.

On Wall Street the high fliers have even farther to fall. A clinical psychologist in private practice and formerly on staff at Citibank, Marilyn Puder-York specializes in coaching the executive casualties from the powerhouse investment banks, brokerage houses, legal and accounting firms. Even though they still work at the high end of the income spectrum, they have been downsized in status and income. She finds they tend to waste a lot of very valuable time wallowing in their anger and in self-blame. Dr. Puder-York tries to supply the reality testing: "Read the headlines. You are part of a phenomenon." She pushes them to *feel* their real feelings, then to move along in the painful transition through acceptance, resignation, and on to practical career replanning and a new approach to life, looking for meaning and purpose based on values that are more inner-directed, rather than allow their worth to be determined by institutions and material possessions.

Marital conflict is almost inevitable. "I hate to say this," a securities analyst confessed to Dr. Puder-York, "but since downsizing I'm only making a hundred fifty thousand dollars a year." The psychologist asked, "What's wrong with that?" "Well, my wife's a schoolteacher," he said guiltily. "She really wants a bigger house, and she wants to have more than two kids. She says I'm just not making enough."

Many wives also need reality testing. A spouse who doesn't understand the limitations of the new marketplace may blame her husband and compound his problems. She may simply be naïve. But even wives who are earning good incomes themselves are often negative about their husband's efforts to accept change because they can't bear to give up the fantasy of the high-status husband earning big money in corporate America.

Children can also be unwittingly cruel. When a man is in precarious financial and psychological straits at the same time, he needs reassurance to make the transition, but instead he may sense an erosion of respect from his children. A heartbreaking scene was described in a *Wall Street Journal* article about midlife victims of corporate downsizing who find themselves stranded in the suburbs, hiding in their makeshift bedroom "offices." Husband, wife, and 12-year-old son were having a discussion of family finances. Suddenly the son told his father to butt out.

"You don't work, Dad," the boy said. "It's not *your* money."[12]

The tasks are multiplied for a man trying to move into the Age of Mastery during a period of unprecedented social dislocation. It's not just dealing with the threat of job loss. He may not be able to recover his income or lifestyle; he may have to move and give up some of his country club friends and put up with his family's resistance to these changes.

"These men need courage to look at this transition as something positive that will change their life, as well as the courage to handle the negative reactions of others," says Dr. Puder-York. "*Simultaneously* they need to learn new skills to make themselves more marketable. That is a tremendous amount to ask of one human being who is fifty years old and has spent maybe thirty years being rewarded for accepting the status quo."

THE NEW (HOSTILE) DEPENDENCE ON WIVES

Men in middle or late-middle life today may become increasingly dependent on their wives for financial help. This can be looked upon as a blessing or a curse.

Leonard Lyons, another Kodak early retiree at age 51, can't face changing his lifestyle. His wife is working full-time now, but they are still spending as if they had two incomes. They keep saying, "We've *got* to sit down and make out a budget," but they don't. "Where's the money going to come from?" Leonard asks rhetorically. Many other corporate refugees are in the same boat, sitting with fattened retirement accounts they can't touch without severe tax penalties until they are much older. In the meantime they're living off their charge cards and leaning on their wives.

"The biggest change I'm seeing is role reversal," Leonard says. "My wife goes off in the morning now, and *I* make *her* breakfast." He stretches out one cleanly creased pant leg. "I ironed these pants myself. My wife showed me how." His face twitches as he speaks. The other men in the group shift uncomfortably. The tension of this rapid role reversal often disrupts a couple's sex life. At a stage when Leonard was expecting to enjoy being closer to his wife, he feels too threatened to let down his guard.

Given the lack of interpersonal skills with which men of the Silent Generation were raised, if they feel their careers in descent, they may become envious of their wives, who at 50 are often just taking off in their careers.

This envy cuts across class lines. "It's always been the man who came riding in on a white horse to save the princess from the dragon." A salesman was describing the humiliation of accepting a loan from his working wife to bail himself out of near bankruptcy. "Now it's the princess riding in on her own horse. She owns the farm. And she's saying 'Is there anything I can do to help you out?' "

While men continue to drop out of the work force at earlier ages—fewer than 40 percent of all American men age 55 and over are still salaried job-holders—their wives (and former wives) are toiling longer and later.[13]

In 1993, almost half of all American women age 55 to 64 were still in the work force, compared to 41 percent fifteen years before.[14]

And as they take up the slack in household income, women are exerting greater control over the purse strings. Amazingly in 1992 almost a third of American women who worked full-time earned more than their working spouses, according to the Bureau of Labor Statistics.[15] The percentage is even higher among professional women, 42 percent of whom earned more than their male partners in a survey of forty-five hundred readers by *Working Woman* magazine.

A man who will not take responsibility for managing his own fears of obsolescence is likely to punish his wife for the fact that he cannot hold on to everything he had. Once this neurotic pattern develops, a man becomes stuck in hostile dependency. His working wife may become increasingly intolerant of his refusal to change to adapt to their new reality. And the couple is doomed to fight about every little thing.

But again, there is an opportunity here to see these realities for what they are and make the most of them. If a man can be secure enough in his intrinsic worth, and if he has a solid working partnership in his marriage, he may be able to relax and enjoy being partially subsidized by his wife's income while he indulges himself in a full-scale passage. After all, he has earned a period of reflection and redirection. It is no more an evidence of failure than is a working wife who takes an extended leave to give birth and early nurturing to a new baby. Claiming his earned reward could make the difference between enjoying his Flaming Fifties or flaming out.

When *USA Today* asked readers to share their experiences in households in which the woman outearns the man, most of those who replied said women's added economic clout is *not* creating conflicts or being used to trample on the egos of their partners.[16] The happiest couples who wrote back are those who take an egalitarian view of family finances, decision making, and housework. Chores are divided according to which tasks a spouse prefers or is better at doing. And their combined earnings go into one pot, or three pots—his, hers, and theirs—so that no one has to ask permission before spending money.

Class differences in expectations are important here. Within traditional working-class families, most wives are completely unprepared for these new middle-life role reversals. Their cultural instructions never called for the wife to be "stuck" with the breadwinner role. Such wives may have left the work force prematurely, expecting to settle into a pleasant existence as grandmothers and garden keepers. But as their husband's jobs begin to look shakier, and the pension plan slimmer, they may have to return to work in a serious way, training for more skilled jobs or starting their own small businesses.

Therapists and career counselors usually try to convert a resistant wife into becoming an ally to a husband who is trying to shape a new life beyond the economic revolution. Some of the more desperate among corporate refugees are the men whose marriages crumble while they are out of work. Not only does the man lose his only confidante, who has turned adversary, but he is likely to lose custody of his children. That leaves an enormous vacuum. However, admits one therapist, "There have been times when I have wanted to say to the husband, 'Cut your losses.' If the spouse is just resistant, let her go look elsewhere for the prince on the white horse."

REALITY TESTING FOR THE FUTURE

Is this just a temporarily painful but passing phase for certain corporation men now in middle life? No one knows for sure. But it seems that business and society are only at the beginning of a Digital Revolution comparable in scale to the Industrial Revolution, and the cost in human displacement will be enormous. As we know, the Fortune 500 have lost 24 percent of their work force since 1980. And the rate of turbulence in births and deaths of companies continues to increase in velocity exponentially. In the 1950s and 1960s, one third of the Fortune 500 turned over in a twenty-year period. In the 1970s it took eleven years for the names to change. In the 1980s it took only five years.[17] Companies must transform themselves radically to survive global competition, and this means that the downsizing of a stable labor force and greater reliance on robotics and computerization will continue even through periods of economic recovery.

"Of the seven million presently unemployed in the United States, about one third who were in middle management will never, ever work again at those jobs or even comparable positions in work or pay," says corporate-restructuring specialist Robert Sind.[18]

And it's not only America. More people are competing for fewer full-time jobs all over Western Europe, where an alienated army of tens of millions of idle workers contributes to social unrest. Eight of ten Britons call unemployment the most serious issue facing their country. France's government tries schemes to help companies avoid huge layoffs. Even Japanese workers, the ultimate company men, see their companies quietly pushing hundreds of thousands of white-collar workers into "voluntary" retirement. They join the "window tribe" of unneeded men who collect paychecks to sit and look out the window.[19]

And so, even as we are living longer and healthier, the economic cycle is rendering many corporate citizens obsolete earlier and earlier. Just as the forward guard of America's Boomers is entering the Flaming Fifties, wedged between responsibilities for still-young children (who will continue to need support through longer periods of education) and custodianship for their superannuated parents (who seem to be living indefinitely), the companies they work for are cutting many of them loose from the conventional work force with twenty or thirty years left to give.

The bottom line is, we are living longer, but most Americans are using up their assets faster. Is this any way for modern postindustrial societies to utilize their human resources? In 1994 I put the question to a top Clinton administration economic adviser.

"We haven't gotten to that problem yet" was the reply.

It is a problem that government, corporations, and private-sector institutions all are going to have to address sooner rather than later. "Economic insecurity can be totally debilitating, emotionally and physically, for these men who have been terminated," says Sind, the corporate restructuring expert, who moves around the country talking to displaced men. But *only* if an individual allows himself to be defined and limited by the life accident of termination. "In that case he begins to fill his time by moving the ashtray a little bit to the left and a little bit to the right," says Sind about some of the corporate casualties he sees. "Sooner or later he will find himself wallowing in self-pity and his family will feel the strain. Mild depression is a very good cover for anything we don't want to confront. After a while it becomes chronic."[20]

Management experts have observed that when people no longer believe they are working successfully at being good and becoming better, they will become frustrated and depressed and feel worthless, *no matter what they have achieved up to that point.*[21] This is particularly true for an individual in passage to the Age of Mastery. To feel alive and hopeful, he has to be able to master something!

Sind's prescription: Find something you can learn and master so you will feel good about yourself. For example, a man might draft his kids to teach him how to use a computer. As he becomes more proficient, he can use the computer to replace the secretary he once had, even program it to remind him when to pay bills and eventually to master the family finances and investments. Men who have always hankered to work with their hands can get serious about building bookcases or making over the garage into a workroom. Learning new skills can allow a man, even while unemployed, to contribute to his family in other ways.

THE REHABILITATION OF
THE CORPORATE REFUGEE

If men are going to remap their lives for exciting and fruitful Second Adulthoods, they should not wait until something blows—in the body, on the job, or in bed. They need to begin laying the groundwork early, at least in their forties, so they have the flexibility to make major occupational changes in their fifties and sixties as conditions call for them.

And there's a silver lining.

In terms of adult development a man has a much better chance of reviving his zest for life if he is shaken out of the complacency of coasting along in corporate life. Change will awaken his survival instincts, stimulate his brain, and renovate the very habits of thinking and behavior that may be contributing to his premature obsolescence.

As it becomes harder to achieve material success as a result of one's efforts, and being a good corporate citizen no longer carries the same sense of mission, people are looking elsewhere for meaning and purpose—often to the spiritual realm. "I have seen spiritualism increase in direct relation to the trauma of the marketplace," confirms Dr. Puder-York. She used to have a Wall Street trader as a patient. A million-and-a-half-dollar man, he lost his job in 1991. He had been very narrow and rigid. This life accident coincided with his entry into Second Adulthood in his mid-forties. Forced to become more entrepreneurial, he found a marketable health care product and started his own business. In the process he realized how totally he had surrendered power to the corporation. Raised to cauterize his emotions, he was also persuaded to become introspective for the first time. He found himself volunteering to help the homeless and from there became interested in working with foster children. That opened up for him a whole spiritual dimension and an interest in the cosmos.

Today, in his late forties, the Wall Street survivor is lucky if he can gross $200,000 from his business. But he is excited by the much greater balance in his life. Had he not lost the all-consuming job, he could never have become the well-rounded, spiritually nourished person he is today.

In a later meeting with the Kodak refugees, one of the "lifers" spoke honestly in our group interview about how fearful he had been while making the same kind of passage but how exhilarated he feels now as he finds himself becoming a new man.

THE COMPANY MAN AS FREE AGENT, AGE 48

"Freedom is the scariest freakin' thing in the world."

Gary Whelpley had come to Kodak straight from school. A photographer, he viewed his existence as the picture-perfect layout of successful adulthood—candids of him shooting pictures for the company all over the world, a blowup of his solid suburban home, the dynamic businesswoman wife, and himself, tanned and rugged and totally secure—until the day he caught the last train out and watched, helpless, while his whole life crashed.

"Once I took the package and left, I realized what an incredible part of my life that company was," lamented Whelpley. "It was my friends, my support system. I knew that every day I was going to get up and go to the same place. I was set. I loved the company; it gave me everything that I ever dreamed of. These last two years"—he throttled back the swill of regret—"they've been like a death for me."

But the Gary Whelpley who now occupies a tiny matchbox of a house, while he is in the transition of divorce, is far more provocative and alive-looking than any Bachrach company man portrait. Beneath dark brows, Gary's dreamy blue eyes roam the listener's face for reactions. Having weaned himself from the company's "yellow blood," he now wears a bold flowered shirt and a big silver ring and keeps his pewtered hair youthfully scissored. But the hardest part of the "little death" of his First Adulthood has been to realize that he almost killed his creativity in exchange for making it into management status. "Looking for total security was making me sick with frustration." Once he left, he looked beneath his picture-book life and said, "Where's the meaning?" Where was the artist and dreamer he had left behind?

"I get up now and think, *I can do anything I want. My God, how can this be?* That freedom is the scariest freakin' thing in the world!" It is not easy to transform oneself from an institutionalized team player into a self-promoting entrepreneur. *Jesus*, he thought, *here I am, about to turn fifty!* But Gary refused to be in a hurry to produce. He decided to give himself a couple of years to seek serenity and balance and to look for a way to give a little something back. He has found a church that truly reaches the community. "I walk in there, and I feel there's a place for me to contribute, something I've never felt before." Gary's thoughts turned more and more toward the children of his first marriage, the scattered seed; he hadn't seen them more than once or twice a year since his first divorce. His daughter was eight then. He could rationalize and say it was his second wife's fault; like many second wives, she was reluctant to share him with children from a former marriage. But the reconstruction work was his to initiate.

"To have meaning in my relationships with my three kids is now my major drive. You don't know how many years you'll have left. My father died when I was very small, and I never got to say good-bye." Gary had recently spent two weeks with his 29-year-old daughter. "Just intimate sharing—it's a good thing to do. I feel it helps me to do the work of this transition."

Intuitively Gary is working on exactly the task that will benefit him most. The divorced men in my surveys who rarely see the grown children from their first marriages, now having passed 50, usually turn out in interviews to be suffering from a sense of personal failure or to feel they are running out of gas. They stand in strong contrast with the more satisfied divorced men who usually say they have become *more* attentive parents in middle life.[22]

Men in their forties, as we have seen, still have time on their side. Men who reach 50 realize there isn't a lot of time. But it is a seminal purpose of this book to persuade them that there is a lot more time left than they think. Eventually they may look back upon the Samson Complex, or even the life accident of termination, as the catalyst that forced them to give up their false selves and to see the absolute necessity of shaping a "new self" to take advantage of Second Adulthood.

13

THE OPTIMISM SURGE

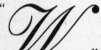e are all hungry for connection," said James Sniechowski, a 51-year-old men's group leader in Santa Monica, California. It was a word that came up again and again in the midlife men's groups: *connection.*

Another word often repeated was *optimism.* A healthy majority of the Professional Men over 45 I have surveyed and interviewed are enjoying a surge in optimism and a sense of serenity that are a recent development in their outlook.[1] The conflicted values of their thirties and forties are sorting themselves out around core beliefs affirmed by their life experiences. Most say the best thing about being in middle life is feeling "clearer about what is personally right."[2] They register a stronger self-awareness and increasing inner peace.

What's the secret?

The most strikingly consistent result to come out of my surveys and focus groups with men is the evidence of a clear and finite change in the poles of the battery sometime between ages 45 and 55. The happiest men move from devoting most of their energy to competing and sexual conquest to devoting more and more of their energy to finding emotional intimacy, trust, and companionship and community with others. I see this as the essential task for men in middle life: to move from competing to connecting.

Robert Bly, the poet-author of *Iron John* and Pied Piper of the new masculinity, drawing on the confessions of men at his workshops, told me he had arrived at the same formulation. The young man is determined to dominate: nature, women, younger men, everything. His force field is directed straight ahead, and he ignores most community and family obligations. "As that arc of intensity reaches a peak, at about age fifty, he feels it faltering."[3] Bly extended the metaphor. "As the poles on the battery change, a man finds himself more in receiver mode. He doesn't feel like firing his vice-president anymore. He's liable to stop at a pay phone and call his wife. He suddenly develops a sense of community. He feels warmth toward younger men that he never felt before. His sexuality also becomes more receptive. He's on the way to becoming a human being, but he doesn't know it. He thinks he's on the way to becoming a failure. The problem with the capitalist life is they don't tell any of the men about this."

A Park Avenue dermatologist who graduated from an all-male Princeton University in 1961 noted the dramatic shift in the way his classmates related to one another during their twenty-fifth reunion. "At the fifth reunion we were still all Joe College. At the tenth and fifteenth, we were horribly competitive and full of ourselves. At our twentieth, we were a little nicer to each other. By the time we gathered for our twenty-fifth, we were all in our mid-forties, and almost nobody reaches his mid-forties without some pain in his life. It was as though we'd been through some kind of metamorphosis."

Instead of breaking off into little cliques, with the jocks at one table and the bookworms at another and an invisible quarantine around the less-than-successes, guys who had never spoken a word during college were talking to one another. They were much more open.

"This time we all were looking for friendship, for what we can share rather than how we compare," noted the dermatologist in relief. "Everybody seemed to want to connect."

From very early in their lives most men bend their efforts toward proving themselves unique. Being "best boy" or star athlete or "baddest dude" on the block means defining themselves in terms of how they differ from others. And having made every effort to shuck any dependency on parents, bosses, wives, or friends, they now discover they feel somewhat isolated from others. It is no wonder that once they are older and more aware of their human vulnerabilities, men find themselves looking for opportunities for human closeness rather than differentiation.

FROM COMPETING TO CONNECTING

The real winners among men in middle life do make this shift. The 110 Professional Men I've studied have reached an average age of 52. Most at this age feel closer than ever before to their wives.[4] They are also hungry for closer contacts with their children and a different level of friendship with other men and women. The edge of competitiveness has softened.

If these men were ranked on mental health, most of them would get an A at this stage. Nearly all have developed passions or hobbies that happily occupy and challenge them *outside their workaday routines.* This is crucial in offsetting the disenchantment in their profession that polls show is now felt by large numbers of doctors, or the boredom of the accountant defending yet another tax audit of a rich client, or the dentist who cannot expect to be wildly stimulated by drilling his billionth bicuspid. Almost half of the 110 Professional Men are "delighted" or "pleased" with their lives as a whole at this stage. This was not true in their mid-forties, when *almost half* went through a depressive period. Now they are more open to discovering the emotional parts of themselves that didn't fit with the posture of the tough, combative, straight-ahead, rational men they were supposed to be in First Adulthood. The healthy ones recognize the presence of an inner life and start paying attention to its muffled messages.

As their power orientation subsides in their fifties, the happiest men grow noticeably more expressive and sensuous, more gregarious and likable. Once they are able to satisfy the heightened need for human closeness they formerly suppressed, they are able to be more perceptive in their reactions to other people. That makes them more valuable as managers, husbands, fathers, and friends. And they show a corresponding rise in psychological health. According to the Berkeley studies, *non*traditional men often repossess by age 50 the opposite-sex characteristics they suppressed in early adulthood. "They are now able to move toward intimacy with others and a sense of personal meaning in life."[5]

This was exactly the transition described by Dr. Harold Wahking, a toweringly tall, ruggedly handsome man who is a licensed marriage and family therapist in St. Petersburg, Florida. Dr. Wahking was among those in the last chapter who expressed the high cost of adhering to the masculine code of his generation. As he told the men's group in Tampa, Florida, "Becoming a naval officer was a very important symbol of manhood to me. Another was to allow myself to feel only two feelings—either anger or sexual desire—because all other emotions were 'feminine' and therefore weak and to be abhorred. That caused me a lot of stress, especially in my forties, because it meant denying a big chunk of who I was in order to try to prove I really was a man."

Studies have by now tracked the ways in which nontraditional men, like Wahking, often suffer in their forties from adhering to the overcontrolled, power-oriented, exploitative behavior expected of high-achieving men.[6] "Until I graduated into my fifties, I used to belittle my wife's 'intuitive hunches,'" Dr. Wahking conceded. "I felt it gave her an unfair edge over me. Since then I've spent a lot of time learning how to feel and tune into other people's feelings, meanings, hidden motives. I'm in a substantially different place by now." He is almost 62 and much more contented with himself today. "I've cultivated the feminine side of myself, and integrated that with the masculine side, so now I'm intuitive too!"

Of the many observable contrasts between these Professional Men and the working-class men in the *Family Circle* survey, the most important one concerns their readiness to make this shift from competing to connecting. Fewer than one third of the traditional *Family Circle* men over 45 are more interested in close relationships at this stage. They don't understand what they need or how to go about getting it. The exception proves the point: When we look at the top hundred *Family Circle* men with the highest scores on overall well-being, almost all seem to have achieved an enviable degree of intimacy in their marriages. They spend significantly more time with their wives than do men of low well-being—an average of six hours a day—and they have sex more often than their peers. These men *do* recognize that competition is less important, and they say that close relationships are now a higher priority.

Lorn Bown, a retired trucker in Webster, Wisconsin, who was part of the *Family Circle* study, has been the partner of Jeanette Tull for the last ten years. In his fifties, when he worked as a garbage hauler, Jeanette would work alongside him. That meant they spent about ten hours a day together, shouldering the same workload. Now that he's retired, Lorn says, "We spend sixteen to eighteen hours a day together. She takes awful damn good care of me, and I take good care of her." Lorn has also honed a tight network of male friends he's met through the years. "In my mind, a lot of good friendships is better than a lot of money."[7]

MEN'S ANGUISH OVER EMPTY NEST

It is a paradox that this very movement toward a hunger for closeness usually brings with it an unanticipated pang of regret. Men at this stage also yearn for connection with their children. It is not so easily satisfied as one might think. Surprisingly the subject of the empty nest came up in almost all my men's groups, even among the hypertraditional males in Detroit.

Don Parrot, the Excessed VP in Detroit, describes a common ambivalence: "We've worked very hard to teach our kids to be independent, but now we're saying, 'Whoa, don't get *that* independent.' You know, first they get their driver's license, so they're not dependent on you to be mobile. Then they get a part-time job, so they're not entirely dependent on you for money. Finally they move out." It was yet another measure of aging for him. "The dog's getting on in life too."

All the men laugh, but it has an undercurrent of rue. Don thrusts his arms outward as if giving up. "I can just see our family going to the wind."

Does his wife feel the same way about the empty nest? I ask.

"No. She says she's looking forward to it." Typical.

Ray, the high school music teacher in Detroit, is prompted to show a glimpse of his own regrets. "I'm surprised at how important my kids are becoming in my life," he says. "I didn't have much time for them before."

"And now they don't have any time for you, right?" guesses another man.

"Right." A wistful expression settles on Ray's face as he describes waiting up for his 16-year-old daughter to come in after an evening with her boyfriend. Ray just wants to sit and talk to her. "She might give me an hour before she goes to bed," he says, but he is aware all the while that the nature of the transaction is very different from when she was Daddy's little girl. "It's like I'm being appeased."

It's only a matter of time before his teenage daughter will start making excuses for why she can't eat meals with the family. His son is busy with his own activities. And when Ray suggests to his wife that they go off for a romantic weekend, she looks at him as if he's an addled teenager. She probably has an exam for her specialized nursing degree. She's just coming into her own.

We don't hear much about the sadness and longing men feel as they see their children slipping out of reach or resisting the love and guidance they long to give. Yet this is a systemic problem for men in middle life. By the time Dad is ready to clear his calendar to make room for his children, because he needs *them*, they've usually "left home" in spirit. For men who were socialized to the old dominance-and-control model by their own fathers, it is difficult to acknowledge the regret, even the sorrow, that comes with losing the chance for closeness with their children.

And there is likely to be a greater sorrow, hidden underneath, that is not even made conscious. Letting their children slip out of their arms, silently, stoically, often reopens the wound of losing touch with their own fathers. The repetition of this dark cycle is depicted as inevitable by no less a writer than Thomas Wolfe:

> We are the sons of our father,
> Whose life like ours
> Was lived in solitude and in the wilderness,
> We are the sons of our father,
> To whom only we can speak out
> The strange, dark burden of our heart and spirit,
> We are the sons of our father,
> And we shall follow the print of his foot forever.[8]

But does a man have to follow his father in working harder and holding back on his tender needs, so that his children, too, will carry the dark burden of the heart, while he continues on through Second Adulthood as only half a man? No. The melancholy a man may feel as he anticipates the emancipation of his children should be read as a signal, another door, an opportunity to explore a deeper wound that may have been hidden from him.

FATHER, I HARDLY KNEW YE

The lack of loving, respectful relationships with their fathers is one of the greatest tragedies males suffer. Remember the forcibly retired photographer in the last chapter, whose father had died when he was very young and who looked to Kodak as a surrogate, almost as a blood father? Even when fathers are physically living in the home, they are often absent emotionally. Bernie Zilbergeld writes movingly of the father-son divide in his book *The New Male Sexuality.*

> Physical affection, emotional sharing, expressions of approval and love—these are the human experiences that very few boys get from their dads. . . . Consider what it must be like to be a boy child and never know if your father loves or even likes you or, worse, but quite common, to believe in your guts that he does not.[9]

When we met, Zilbergeld urged me, "If you want to see grown men cry, give them a safe setting and get them to talk about their fathers."

This was one of the dominant themes in the men's groups: their search for the missing father. Only a handful out of the 110 men who attended one of my group sessions described their boyhood relationships with their fathers as close. No more than two or three of them answered yes to the question, Was your father emotionally close to you?

❧ "No, I can't ever remember him saying, 'I love you.'"

❧ "I never had a dad. Men in my life were brutal."

❧ "The concept of Father in our home was 'Leave him alone. He's working.'"

❧ "My father was tough, a wounded World War Two veteran. You got an allowance and discipline, period."

❧ "I'm eerily like my father. He never thought about *Am I showing enough love to my children?* I think about it a lot. But then the old tapes will go on, and I'll hear my father speaking through me: *Did I really think that? Or is that just something my father would have said?*"

Ray Bunch, a 53-year-old Chrysler service manager, was one of the walking wounded who attended the men's session in Santa Monica. "What we're doing in men's groups like this is looking for the fathering we didn't have," he acknowledged.

World War II Generation fathers adhered to a rigid code of masculinity; they were supposed to be breadwinners and disciplinarians while all the emotional support was supposed to come from mothers. And parents of that generation had to be stalwart through the Depression. Their sons from the Silent Generation recalled doing only sports or mechanical projects with their fathers, activities that were almost entirely nonverbal and involved no touching. Many of the men recalled vividly being afraid of their fathers.

Now, in middle life, the men are conscious of suffering from "father hunger," as Bly calls it. Quite a number have been attempting to break the cycle and warm up to their own sons and daughters. "I'm very conscious of it, but I never spent much time with my own father, so it just doesn't come naturally," said Ken Piel of Dallas about attempts to reconnect with the children of his first marriage. "The hugging part . . . I have to work real hard at it, and I think it shows." Others mentioned they have an easier time bridging the awkwardness with their youngest children. Almost all seemed to sense that reconnecting with their children could be a way to repossess emotional lives that had been largely shut down for most of their adult years.

But such men also fear releasing the tenderness buried in their souls that would foster those intimate connections. "It's fear of our own femininity in ourselves," said Jordan Good, a Santa Monica construction engineer who, at 50, is now daring to act on his dream of becoming a psychologist. "The tension for men is in the ambivalence between wanting to keep our aggression and wanting to give up retaliation when it's not necessary or appropriate. To function in the world without attack is a hard task for a man to learn."

Men in the Santa Monica group also talked about learning to trust enough to be "fertilized by another man's soul." These strong, virile men found ways to touch one another. They butted heads, poked sides, and came at one another frontally to grip elbows or give hugs. But they also respected men's boundaries. Having been expected to be "success objects," they now yearned to revive the kids in themselves. Meeting in groups like this gave them a chance to rediscover their playful sides.

"Feel this room." James Sniechowski interrupted us at one point. "There's raucousness; there's gibing; there's emotional arm wrestling. There's an erection allowed that is honored."

"Yes!" chorused the men. (It was California, after all.)

REINVENTING FATHERHOOD

Contrary to conventional wisdom, fatherhood has just as significant an impact on the mental and physical health of many men as career achievement.[10] New parenting research shows that fathers who are highly invested in their work, but who also care about their children and spend significant time with them, can still have an important effect on the emotional well-being of their sons and daughters—and, by extension, on their own emotional well-being.

These are among the research findings of William S. Pollack, Ph.D., assistant clinical professor of psychology in the Department of Psychiatry at Harvard Medical School and coeditor of *Toward a New Psychology of Men.*[11] Along with Ronald Levant, Ed.D., Pollack is beginning an effort toward redefining a new, postfeminist masculinity and freeing the John Waynes and Iron Johns still snared in the myth of the fully autonomous man. The most promising direction for redefining masculinity, they believe, is in reinventing fatherhood.

The new-model father is on display at any airport today. One spots his toddler first, grandly portaged high above the crowds, his little legs clasped around Daddy's neck while he makes reins of his father's hair. Daddy's stride is sure, proud, infallible; he moves like some glorious new animal form, bonded with his own image—a Manboy. (Well, at least until he sets down his charge on the changing table in the men's room.) These daddies are different. They are discovering a secret that women have always known: The easiest way to feel loved and needed and ten feet tall is to be an involved parent.

Most of these reinvented fathers are in their twenties and thirties. But not all. Many are Start-Over Dads in their late forties and fifties, raising second families.

In my group interviews with men all over the country, the same sentiment was repeated: "I don't want to have the relationship with my children that I had with my father." These men want to be seen by their children not as remote disciplinarians but as friendly, trustworthy, and kind. "Over the course of the past 200 years, fatherhood has lost, in full or in large part, each of its four traditional roles: primary caregiver, moral educator, head of family and family breadwinner," as tracked by David Blankenhorn, president and founder of the Institute for American Values.[12] But rather than be retired to the bench as pinch hitters, American men are becoming more expressive as fathers. According to a 1992 Roper poll, nearly five times as many men would rather be viewed today as sensitive and caring than as rugged and masculine.[13] But that wasn't the way most men were brought up.

Pollack proposes that boys are put at risk by the premature separation from both their mothers and fathers. Mothers are supposed to push their sons toward a clear-cut separation. Already hurt, boys are doubly wounded when their fathers are unable to assume the nurturing role. The reason so many men feel emotionally frozen, even though they want desperately to connect with their own children, Pollack contends, is fear of reexperiencing the repressed pain or sadness or depression that they buried in their hearts when their own parents pulled away.

Pollack and Levant's research in fatherhood workshops is borne out in my interviews. Men can come to recognize that the way to find the father they lost is to find him in themselves and then give him to the next generation. As this yearning for wholeness is revealed, "men's anger will be turned into a sense of grief, which is the harbinger of transformation."[14]

"Fathering is one of men's greatest opportunities for personal transformation," says Dr. Pollack. How do men already in their middle years or older accomplish this transformation?

They have to be willing to suspend decades of cultural conditioning and learn how to be nurturers as well as providers. They learn the language of the heart; they try to feel what a child is feeling, and to acknowledge the truth of those feelings, before doling out correction or punishment. Divorced fathers who have been estranged from the children of their first families can also become Start-Over Dads. Again, recall the Kodak photographer Gary Whelpley, whose painful forced retirement freed him to recognize a much more fundamental need: "To have meaning in my relationships with my three kids is now my major drive." The great opportunity is to offer their children much of what they failed to receive from their own fathers, and in the bargain they are likely to salve that old wound and boost their own self-esteem.

Younger fathers are making tremendous strides in focusing attention on their children and deriving the benefits therefrom. But even a man from an older generation can be transformed by a late-life baby.

THE START-OVER DAD, AGE 59

"I knew my son and he knew me before he was born."

Frank Gifford, a fabled halfback for the New York Giants four decades ago, was a traditional 1950s absent father the first time around. He went straight from football into television. His three kids were asleep when he left the house to do the morning news, and they were asleep when he came home from doing the evening news. But he got a second chance. In 1986 he married Kathie Lee Johnson. He was secure in being a star sports commentator and already a grandfather. His new wife was more than a quarter century his junior. But after some initial reluctance, Gifford became a Start-Over Dad at the age of 59. He told Aaron Latham in an interview how it had changed his life.[15]

> I thought, "To hell with it, I'm just going to take the time to get to know him." I went to every doctor's appointment. I went to every Lamaze class. . . . The birth itself was a really wonderful experience for me. I just had no idea how it worked. . . . It offers a bonding not only with the baby but also with your wife.

Kathie Lee Gifford endured a long labor, determined to have natural childbirth, but the baby was too big and a cesarean had to be performed. But even a cesarean can be a transformative experience for a new father, as Gifford describes it:

> I watched the surgery. I was looking at her face. I watched them make the incision. I watched them take him out. I was scared because he was blue. Then, WAAAA! I'll never forget it. They wiped him off a little bit and handed him to me. And he stopped crying. The doctor said that was perfectly understandable. He had been through this trauma and then he heard a familiar voice. My voice. So I knew my son and he knew me before he was born.

As famous as they are, Frank and Kathie Lee Gifford found themselves switching roles in a mode very familiar for Start-Over Dads. The arc of success is so much earlier and steeper for most men. Gifford was already leveling off at a high plateau while his much younger wife was just coming into her own. The enormous popularity of the *Live with Regis & Kathie Lee* TV talk show and her best-selling book all erupted after motherhood. So it's the older father who makes breakfast for his son every morning: "If I'm late for work, screw it." It is often humbling for fathers to realize the second time around how vital they are to a growing child's grounding in security. "For the child to know that Daddy will be there . . . it's much more important that I ever realized," says Gifford. "We *are* somebody."

Today close to 90 percent of fathers are present in the delivery rooms when their children are born—a huge increase over the last twenty years.[16] And since more and more fathers want to stay at home for a few days or a few months with their newborns, by popular demand a third of American companies now offer paternity leaves.[17] With so many wives necessarily working for pay outside the home, or part-time inside the home, older fathers have little choice but to pitch in.

Once they stumble upon the tender delights of sharing in the delivery and day-to-day nurturing of a baby, Start-Over Dads often become besotted by the offspring of their middle lives. It feels good to make up for the "lost opportunity time" when the children of their first families were young. You see older dads now constantly kissing the heads of their newborns or beaming from the stands at soccer games, as they assume more of the responsibility for teaching their kids the ropes. You see gay men forming stable households around the gift of an adopted child. Their own "father hunger" is assuaged as they learn how to give and receive with a growing child the full range of emotions: anxiety, joy, pride, dependence, and unconditional love.

All these elements combine to give fatherhood a new power: not that of the distant disciplinarian and salary drone but the power of the fully nurturant co-parent. Children have always thrived best when they have had both a father and a mother, who allow them to turn to the appropriate model at the right time to mimic the behavior they need to learn. Dads are finding out how good it feels to be depended upon not just instrumentally but *emotionally.*

And now we learn that being a success as a nurturing father is actually good for a man's mental and physical health. Studies on fatherhood at Wellesley College Center for Women find that fathers who get along well with their children are better insulated from the emotional ups and downs of work and careers. Moreover, says research director Rosalind Barnett, "the better the quality of your relationship with your children, the fewer physical health problems you experience."[18]

But not every man has children or necessarily wants them. Is it possible to move from competing to connecting without being a parent?

THE MEDIATOR, AGE 48

"I'm not so worried about what life didn't bring to me."

Alan Alhadeff married late. He and his wife waited too long to have children. He told our Seattle men's group that the preoccupation with childlessness became acute in his early forties. Every time he'd step off an airplane and pass families greeting one another at the exit, seeing children lifted toward their fathers and lights going on in the faces, one after another, he would feel more than ever shut out of these bright little globes of happiness. Waves of sadness engulfed him.

"During the early stages of my life I had vague unrequited desires. There was always something out there that I didn't have. I couldn't figure out why, and it would be very frustrating. But when I was forty-four or forty-five, I sensed the angst and dissatisfaction leaving me. Then, in the last year, my whole attitude seems to have shifted."

At 48, as he feels himself coming through the passage to the Age of Mastery, Alhadeff now sees his work, his marriage, and his relationship to others in a very different light. He describes consciously cultivating a greater connectedness with others, which offsets his regret at having no children. As a mediator he has chosen a profession that calls upon him to connect emotionally with two sides. "I try to create a rapport. It's a good feeling. My work also gives me a chance to be creative and introspective and . . . even get some recognition."

This surge of optimism came as a complete surprise to him. His wife of twenty years has been changing dramatically over the last five years as well. Although she has often seemed to him self-absorbed with her own menopausal problems, it was she who would catch him brooding in a midlife funk and remind him that life is not a bowl of cherries for anybody. "She taught me how to focus on the good things going on in life."

Approaching the half-century mark, this nontraditional man looks sexy and alive. He is tall and trim with dark, glossy hair, and a salt-and-pepper beard and mustache, and his eyes flash with curiosity and intelligence. He chooses not to wear jeans but dresses distinctively in an unusual green and red plaid shirt, well-tailored slacks, and suede loafers.

"I still have everything I could do at thirty—well, almost everything— but I bring more to it because I'm less distracted and a lot more focused," Alhadeff says without vanity. "It's certainly related to this phase of life. I'm not so worried about what life didn't bring to me. I can look back on every stage and say, 'What I have now is better than what I had yesterday.'"

Finally he laughs at himself. "Fifty always seemed real old to me. Now it's two years away, and I'm amazed at how *young* fifty sounds!"

14

THE UNSPEAKABLE PASSAGE: MALE MENOPAUSE

"*I* had a permanent erection from the age of eighteen to thirty-five," a dashing bicontinental publisher boasted to me during a dinner party. "Never gave it a thought. At forty-five I had a sexual failure for the first time." It was a moment he will never forget. He leaned closer to confide the rest: "Here was this naked girl beneath me, ready to surrender herself—and I couldn't perform. I looked down at myself. What I saw paralyzed me. What a devastating reality!"

Now in his early sixties, with a demonstrably fertile young wife across the table to remind him of his burning youth, the publisher still felt the sting of that moment two decades before, that harbinger of sexual death. "It was a cruel hormonal backfire. Now I can see it as the beginning of male menopause, probably the exact equivalent of the female menopause."

This story is probably one that every man can relate to, although it's hardly the sort of light banter one expects while passing the macadamia nuts at a party. But the publisher knew I was researching the murky subject of male menopause, and his revelation was the first of many surprises.

"My wife and I are both going through menopause, and I'm not sure whose is worse," the college professor confessed to the group of strangers sitting around a large conference table, intent as if they were negotiating a treaty between Babylonia and Abyssinia. Florida Hospital in Orlando had been flooded with calls: "I've heard you're having a men's breakfast to talk about male menopause. Can I come?" Others phoned to say, "I sent in my Life History Survey and attached a letter so Ms. Sheehy will know who I *really* am."

At eight o'clock on a workaday morning twenty-four men turned up. It was that rarest of American social gatherings: A group of open, communicative men had come together to talk frankly about the doubts and demons that affect them. Among them were a "bad boy" adman, a New Age electrician, and an African American prison counselor, all of whom seemed eager to compare notes with the Baptist geologist who had lost his libido in Indonesia and the 70-year-old engineer who had found his in Palm Beach.

The professor who broke the ice was southern, 50, deeply tanned, and feeling ashamed and alone. "The sexual area is where I feel the most vulnerable. It's not that *she's* keeping score. *I* am."

A tall, rangy 55-year-old business consultant I'll call Walt jumped in to describe the severe physical and emotional changes that he had seen in his wife.

"We were just sitting there at dinner, and *her glasses steamed up,*" he said. "I could have fried an egg on her forehead. She became standoffish. Here I was, only fifty-two, and she'd stay up real late, watching TV in the den, so she wouldn't have to go to bed with me. She developed all her own interests. She goes off on horrendous shopping sprees and spends money. Her menopause destroyed the intimacy. We used to be thick as thieves."

Did you divorce? I asked.

"No, we're still married, we still live under the same roof, but separately."

You really have an "internal divorce," I suggested.

"Something like that." Normally an upbeat guy, according to his friends, Walt wore a hangdog expression. His wife had refused to see a doctor or to consider hormones. Walt leaned back and folded his hands over the top of his still-thick hair. "But what can you do if your woman won't admit she's having a hot flash even when her glasses steam up?"

This telling vignette launched a spirited debate during which each man tried to decide for himself: *Is it her, or is it me?* Several other men talked about how helpful hormone medication had been to their wives.

Jim Bracewell, a big man in a blue work shirt and chinos with a full head of blow-dried gray hair, had been sexually involved with only two women in his 52 years. One was his wife, from whom he had been divorced for a dozen years. He had been in recovery programs and therapy and had become active in a local men's group. Now, he said, he was in a relationship with a younger woman, an "empowered" woman.

How much younger is she? he was asked.

"Twenty-four years younger." They had had some sexual difficulties. He hastened to add, "I don't feel driven about sex with her." His priorities had changed, he said, because he now saw women as human beings and not as objects. "Sure, I'm aware of my body changing. It takes longer to get an erection, and it doesn't last as long. But we've talked about it, and we've arrived at a cognitive understanding."

The 51-year-old "bad boy" adman, a man I'll call Deke, leaned over and needled Jim. "Yeah, now. Wait until she reaches her sexual peak and you can't reach your toes. Let's hear about your *cognitive understanding* then."

Everyone in the room heard the wisecrack. It confirmed Jim's concern that people would discount anything he had to say, on the basis of their prejudgment of men who marry much younger women. Privately he had two greater fears. One was that he would never be in a healthy relationship with a woman. The other was that he would. Both were dangerous. What he didn't feel comfortable enough to tell the group was that after struggling alone for so long, he had met this young woman at a seminar for Adult Children of Alcoholics. Because of their age difference, they initially rejected any possibility of a romantic entanglement. They came to know each other as friends. And that friendship turned into the sanctum allowing them both to explore a love more tender than anything they had known.

Walt, the man with an internal divorce, then showed a glimpse of his own fears. "You don't know how it's gonna feel in six or eight years. I have a buddy my age who was laid off, and his potency went to zip. His wife was in tears. She's only fifty-six, and she can't stand losing it. She told me she just longs to be touched." He sighed in exasperation, "I just can't buy the idea that fifty-six is old. The thing that angers me is my sexual drive is still strong."

The next speaker was a geologist who had been raised a Southern Baptist in a small town where the natural inclinations of any young person—partying, dancing, sexual feelings—were considered sinful and wrong. Not surprisingly, a normal lustiness fermented under pressure into a heady preoccupation with sexual fantasies. His friends once gave him a T-shirt that spelled out his dual nature: REVEREND RICHARD up front and MR. HORNY MAN on the back. He had tried developing a uranium mine in the Southwest, retrieving gold in Africa, brokering real estate, even mining in Borneo, but each ship he'd captained had gone under to sea changes in the economy. At age 56, while deep in the interior of Borneo, he developed a deadly fever that led to the discovery of a condition requiring prostate surgery. In the past few years this formerly trim, ambitious man had accumulated fifty or sixty extra pounds and stopped fantasizing.

"My sex problems I'm pretty sure are related to my heart medication," he told the group. "The lust part of it left me a few years ago. But I choose to see the lessening of sexual drive as spiritual progress, instead of just getting old."

The guffaws were only barely muffled. Deke, the bad boy adman, rolled his eyes. Being a brilliant copywriter, he couldn't resist whispering a sound bite: "The reverend overthrows the Hornyman in midlife. Maybe male menopause is a slap from God himself—enough already!"

Deke had told us he based his masculinity as a young man solely on sexual conquest. He loved relating stories of how he and eight other airborne radar crewmen would hook up on an intercom, while flying long missions over Southeast Asia, and try to outbrag one another about their contortions with the likes of "Crabby Abby" and "Mona the Hummer," prostitutes most had shared. Now 51, and fiercely resistant to self-reflection, Deke admitted having to make a major shift. "Now my masculine identity is totally career-based." Given the shrinkage of corporate ad budgets and companies in general, his narrow base was obviously precarious.

But I was curious about the geologist's way of adapting to a physical condition that curtailed his sexual activities. Was it a release for him, I asked, not to have the monkey of sexual horniness on his back all the time?

"Yes, that expresses it exactly," he said. "My sexual fixation in youth was driven by whaddyacallit—test—" The other men supplied the name of the hormone typically thought of as the male sex steroid: testosterone. "Yes, testosterone. But as the lust loses its hold on you, it opens up avenues for spiritual development."

The next speaker brought another level of complexity to this problem with no proper name. A tall, attractive, mustached man of mixed blood, he looked the picture of an uptight professional in his precisely tailored pink shirt and wine-colored suspenders. Art (a pseudonym) squinted nervously behind thick glasses as he told his story. He had been married three times. When he was in his mid-forties, having sex with his wife became more and more of a chore, and he often failed.

"My doctor gave me testosterone supplements—little black and white pills," he relayed. "For the next two years I went around with a full erection. I felt crazy for sex all the time. I couldn't tell if I was horny or a hat rack."

The raucous laughter was interrupted by one man who shouted, "What color were those pills?"

But Art was wincing. He then put himself at some risk by revealing to the group that he had recently come out. "I got divorced because I could no longer live the lie. I'm a gay male."

The others wanted to know if being gay made it easier or harder to overcome male menopause. "It's much harder to be a middle-aged gay male dealing with the changes in sexual potency," Art acknowledged. "The flip side is, at fifty, I'm in a second adolescence, by virtue of getting divorced and coming out. But what I need at this stage is different. I'm not so much looking for pure sex as for intimacy and support."

The professor who had started the discussion chimed in. "I'm so relieved to hear from some of the men here that you can relax and get away from performance. I feel I have moved on in all other areas in my life but this one."

Before the group broke up, everyone looked to the oldest man there for reassurance. Herb Harrington was 70, with abundant silvery hair, flaring brows, gentle features, and a physique that showed the beneficial effects of continued vigorous activities, both indoor and outdoor. He had divorced in his mid-fifties, joined Al-Anon, and, when he retired as an engineer at 60, begun adventuring in Palm Beach. "At sixty, with a prostate in great shape, Palm Beach is a great place to be!"

"I'll bet," said some of the other men enviously.

Herb had initially had no intention of becoming attached. But having met an artist who opened up another whole side of life to him, he had happily acquiesced to marriage. He was willing to admit that remarriage had probably prolonged and certainly vastly enhanced his later life. At 70 he was starting a new business venture and enjoying a still-robust libido.

We adjourned feeling good. The gathering had introduced the men to other men who were potentially an ongoing source of real information, support, and friendship. They were all as cheered as I was at the willingness of two dozen strangers to have a conversation that only a few years ago would have been unimaginable.

The prevalence of this unexplored phenomenon is beginning to force such conversations. Since my report "The Unspeakable Passage: Is There a Male Menopause?" was published in *Vanity Fair* in April 1993, men and women have been opening up to me and talking candidly about this problem without a proper name. Having by now done seventy interviews in the United States and Britain—both anonymous in-depth interviews with males from 40 to 70, and with the top experts in the United States and Europe who study or treat men over 40 having impotence problems—I can report a broad consensus that there is a middle-life male potency crisis. This chapter will present many witnesses to the phenomenon, the cutting-edge research, and the good news.

A man need not panic. Male menopause is often just that: a pause in virility and vitality that is most alarming at the start. It need not become permanent.

I'D RATHER HAVE A TALKING FROG

It soon became apparent to me that if menopause is the silent passage, male menopause is the unspeakable passage. It is fraught with secrecy, shame, and denial. Everyone has some anxiety about aging, of course. Men of a certain age simply stop bragging about their sexual conquests. Or they may make jokes. What's the difference between anxiety and panic? Anxiety is the first time a man can't get it up the second time. Panic is the second time he can't get it up the first time.

Groucho Marx, leaving a poker game with his friends one night, said, "So long, fellas. I guess I'll go upstairs now and see if I can bend one in."

The frog joke has been repeated to me by at least four different men in their fifties or sixties. "An older man is walking down the street when he hears a frog talking. The frog says, 'If you pick me up and kiss me, I'll turn into a beautiful woman.' The man picks up the frog and puts it in his pocket. The frog complains. 'Aren't you going to kiss me? I'll turn into a ravishing woman, and you can have me all you want.'

"The man replies: 'I'd rather have a talking frog in my pocket.' "

"How old is this man?" I asked one middle-aged joke teller. He fell silent.

One of the most advanced researchers in the field, Dr. Fran Kaiser, a professor of medicine at St. Louis University School of Medicine, is not bothered by the popular term; asked if there is a male menopause, she says, flatly, "Yes, there is."[1]

Dr. Isadore Rosenfeld, one of the top cardiologists in New York City and a best-selling author, could boast of a patient list that includes some of the most fearsome rogue elephants in the business world. I asked him if he thought there was a male menopause.

"Yes, I think there is," he replied without hesitation.[2] He hears evidence of it all the time in his practice, but he has to drag out the admission. "I think the majority of men—that is, greater than fifty percent—have sexual problems after age fifty. They don't discuss it, but they do." He bases his observation not on measuring their hormones but on calibrating how drastically men's values and needs and behavior change between 50 and 60.

Women probably think they are the only ones who begin to feel invisible over 50. It was surprising to find out how vulnerable men are to the evaporation of admiring looks. Men who have relied on being handsome and strong to pave the way for sexual conquest are especially stung by the sudden indifference of younger women. A well-known entertainer in his fifties confided to me that unless he is clearly identified by the prestige of his TV and movie credits, he is now invisible to young women.

"When you go through the supermarket line, the checkout girl doesn't meet your eyes anymore." Many women would imagine that his graduation into middle age would only enhance his powers of attraction. Instead, describing how he and many of his male friends in their fifties see themselves, the entertainer said, "You feel separated from youth at the same time you're feeling diminished in physical strength and stamina; you start being passed over by younger men; the sex isn't as great as it was; an incredible desire to be young again comes over you."

Would you believe that one of the most ravishing leading men in movieland history—Cary Grant—was insecure about his physical charms in middle life? At 59 he refused to make *Charade* until the producers guaranteed he wouldn't have to attempt to seduce Audrey Hepburn, who was then more than twenty-five years his junior. "He wouldn't do love scenes per se, no kisses," the actress revealed in 1991, "because he was so much older."[3]

A male potency crisis may flare abruptly when a man faces the loss of his job, unleashing a vicious circle. In the movie *Glengarry Glen Ross*, the sagging egos and precarious potency among middle-aged salesmen lead to blind boasting and balls kicking and, finally, utter self-debasement. One of the older salesmen struggles against the younger men to keep his ego and his world from collapsing. He keeps saying about his attempts at deal making, "I just can't close anymore. I try, I really try, but I just can't *push through*." The sexual metaphors are vivid.

"Men go off the boil for a couple of years" was the colorful description of this mysterious slump in élan offered by one of Britain's most successful industrialists, Sir John Harvey-Jones.[4] He has seen male menopause in so many of his employees that he thinks it may be inescapable. Can they regain the boil? "Some of them do," he says, "but corporate life is very punishing, and many seem to lose their drive, their push, their will."

"You can tell with men, by the time they're in their early forties, which ones are going to succeed. If that effort to succeed fails in the forties and a man can't come to terms with it, it's devastating!" related a wife with first-hand experience. Margaret was part of a group of middle-life women who met with me on the West Coast to share sightings of male menopause. A highly articulate woman just over 50, Margaret was married to a prominent endocrinologist. "When my husband heard I was coming today, he gave me a lecture about testosterone." She rattled off all the safe, clinical terms her husband uses. Her personal experience was far more telling.

"At age fifty-six my husband got a call from the NIH. He didn't get his grant. He's been impotent ever since." She hastened to add, protectively, that he remains an extremely affectionate and loving husband.

No less an expert than the dean of the Gerontology Center at the University of California at Los Angeles, Dr. Edward Schneider, gave me his personal, nonscientific opinion: "All my male friends between forty and fifty-five have gone through a major life readjustment. Probably the vast majority of people do not achieve their goals. We don't know what biochemical changes accompany it, but there are so many analogies between men and women and their reproductive systems, I really do believe there is a male hormonal counterpart [to menopause]."[5]

THE PROBLEM WITHOUT A PROPER NAME

In fact, it is a misnomer to call it male menopause, although the term has achieved widespread popular acceptance. What happens to men is more gradual than female menopause. Their reproductive glands do not all shut down around the same age, the way women's ovaries do. It also has little to do with fertility; a healthy proportion of men continue to have sufficient sperm to sire children well into older age. But although it is not strictly a menopause, many men in middle or later life do experience a lapse in virility and vitality and a decline in well-being. This decline can definitely be delayed. It can even be corrected. In the near future it may even become preventable. But first a man must understand it and be prepared to master it.

In Britain the problem is sometimes called viropause, and on the Continent andropause. *Viropause* refers to a suspension of virility in middle and later life that may be correctable in some men by hormone replacement therapy.[6] The term *andropause* has been used in France since 1952, but the conventional definition is very narrow: the natural cessation of sexual function in old males.[7] Serious clinical trials under way all over Europe are now viewing andropause not just as the lack of potency but as a fully developed syndrome. At medical conferences on the subject, one tends to get narrow definitions from highly skilled scientific researchers with tunnel vision. I heard one of Europe's top experts, Dr. Georges Debled, define andropause as that whole roster of "physical and psychological pathologies going on with the progressive decrease of sexuality in men."[8] But the famous urologist focused almost entirely on the hormone testosterone as the main problem behind andropause. To facilitate understanding of this complex mind-body syndrome, I have chosen to stay with the popularly accepted term *male menopause.*

An artist of the human heart, like novelist John Cheever, doesn't need any numbers to render painfully recognizable this mental and spiritual breakdown. In *The Journals of John Cheever* he starts out showing the usual ambivalence toward such a painful subject—"The male menopause is, as we know, an old wives' tale"—but he goes on to dissect the symptoms with devastating accuracy:

> Their friends, if they are left with any, say that X seems to be going through some sort of psychological crisis. It usually begins with sharp discontents about their business life. They have been treated shabbily and cheated out of the promotions and raises they deserved, but their position at this time of life, their security, is too precarious to allow them to express any grievance. They are sick of ball bearings and bedsheets or whatever it is they sell. Sexually their wives have come to seem unattractive, but they have not been able to find mistresses. Their friends bore them. Their children seem, oftener than not, strange and ungrateful. The financial burdens they have been forced to assume are backbreaking.
>
> All of this is true, but none of this would account for the wanton disappointment that engorges them. Something of more magnitude, something much more mysterious than these bare facts would show, has taken place. Valor, lustiness, hope—all these good things seem to have been misplaced.... Was he growing old? Was this the rumored falling off?[9]

Cheever then describes the conversion of one man's psychological panic into excruciating physical symptoms which afflict him whenever he drives his car over a bridge. He would feel his member shrink, his blood pressure drop, and at the summit the seizure would overwhelm him with dizziness, weakness, a darkening of his vision. He could not admit his symptoms to his wife. One might say X did not dare cross the bridge—

or make the passage—into Second Adulthood. Thus he lived in a state of suspended panic.

> He is lost . . . tyrannized by a fable of herculean sexual prowess . . . yet the way in which he reached this tragic wilderness is hidden from him and from the rest of us. . . .[10]

HARD STATISTICS AND HOPEFUL SCIENCE

What really excites andrologists—scientists who study hormones—is their speculation that hormone research will eventually uncover a biological basis for the male middle-life potency crisis, much the way research into brain chemistry has turned up a biological basis for depression. Even the National Institute on Aging is supporting three different studies to investigate whether testosterone supplements might benefit older men by preventing bone loss, depression, and other symptoms.[11]

Hard statistical evidence has been piling up for the first time to reveal how widespread this phenomenon really is, and the figures projected for the next two decades are sobering. In the largest study of impotence since the Kinsey Report it was found in 1993:

> About half of American men over 40 have experienced middle-life impotence to varying degrees.[12]

The federally financed Massachusetts Male Aging Study took a cross-sectional random sample of 1,709 men between 40 and 70 years of age from eleven different communities in Massachusetts and asked them a variety of questions about their sexual potency during the previous six months. The men's self-reports showed the steepest of changes was in the onset of moderate impotence, meaning a problem with attaining and maintaining an erection half the time.[13] If those numbers are extrapolated to the national male population of the same age-group (more than thirty-seven million men in 1994), the current estimate that ten million men are suffering from impotence would have to be doubled.

> Problems of declining sexual potency may already affect nineteen million men in the United States.[14]

Like the attention now being paid to perimenopause in women for the first time, we can expect a demographically driven interest in male menopause as a serious public health problem. As the first battalions of Baby Boom men march toward 50, the number of males between 40 and 70 is projected by the Census Bureau to grow to fifty-four million by 2010.[15] That means:

> America's male menopause population will increase by almost 60 percent during the next twenty years.

In Britain current estimates are just as startling, according to a 1993 study of 802 older men conducted by the respected market research organization, MORI.[16] Even among the men who were still sexually active, almost half complained of poor erections since they had turned 50. The study estimated:

> Nearly a third of all British men over the age of 50 do not have sexual intercourse.

In Germany the subject made a splash in the summer of '94, when a psychologist reported results of a medical study that suggested men might suffer the effects of midlife hormonal changes the way women do. The study at Frankfurt's Goethe University of 240 healthy men between 35 and 64 found "an astonishing number" of participants complaining of ailments commonly associated with menopause, including increased irritability, depression, and even hot flashes![17]

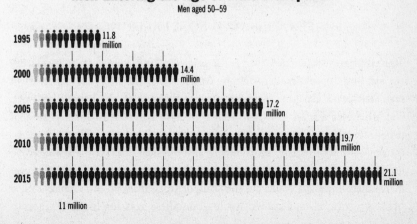

Men Entering the Age of Male Menopause
Men aged 50–59

1995 — 11.8 million

2000 — 14.4 million

2005 — 17.2 million

2010 — 19.7 million

2015 — 21.1 million

11 million

Physically a man notices a gradual decrease in muscle mass and strength and an increase in body fat. Hormonal changes can bring on symptoms ranging from broken sleep, lethargy, and depression to the cerebral signs of irritability, nervousness, trouble concentrating, memory lapses, and mood swings. In addition, there may be circulatory signs such as numbness and tingling, headaches, dizzy spells, and even night sweats. The most upsetting symptoms, however, are significant changes in virility that become noticeable as men move into their fifties. Along with intermittent problems of gaining and sustaining erections, men may start to notice a soft-pedaling of sexual desire. Unless a man is in a good relationship with a knowing partner, that psychological shock can bring on a full-fledged sexual shutdown.

A quite amazing response came back from the nationally representative sample of more than a thousand middle- and working-class American husbands and wives in my *Family Circle* survey:

> Fully 82 percent of these traditional women said they believe that men experience a menopause.[18] More than half these traditional working-class men over 45 are ready to acknowledge that a male menopause exists.

But they are sure it's going to happen to some other poor sap. Almost two thirds of the same four hundred men insist that they won't personally go through a menopause. Fewer than a third say they are now experiencing or have already been through a male menopause.[19]

SEX, LIES, AND SCOREKEEPING

The emphasis on performance is the single greatest enemy of a satisfactory sex life. "Intercourse is identified by Americans as the true religious heart of sexuality," says Dr. June Reinisch, former director of the Kinsey Institute. "So whenever a man loses the ability to have an erection for a period of time—whether it's because he's anxious or it's related to an illness or medications—he will usually stop having any physical contact."[20] I wanted to learn more about the tyranny of herculean sexual prowess that Cheever mentioned. I knew I could get the straight story from an old friend, a New York art critic always known for his boundless zest for life and vigorous appetite for the pleasures of Eros. I'll call him Fitzgerald, since like F. Scott, he likes to think, *I always had the top girl.*

When Fitzgerald was in his thirties and splitting from his first wife, a lay analyst asked him, "Now, what do you think about when your mind is completely free?"

"Sex," Fitzgerald said.

The analyst dismissed this frivolous reply. "No, no, no. What do you think of when there's nothing on your mind?"

"Sex," Fitzgerald said. "That's all I ever thought about," he recalled recently. "I think most men are like me. I thought of sex day and night. Is that unusual?"

Hardly. I told him about my surveys of men, most of whom were helplessly led around by their phallic urges as young men in their twenties:

> Fully half the middle-class *Family Circle* men thought about, pursued, or engaged in sex from twelve to twenty-four hours a day during their salad days.[21]

Among the Professional Men surveyed, other interests or necessities took up at least some of their twenties: Only one in three men studying to be professionals spent most of his days and nights thinking about or enjoying sex![22] It gives some idea how omnipotent is the issue of sexual potency for young men. What was striking was how sharply sexual fantasizing dropped off after the age of 45. Half the men over 45 now focus on sex for only an hour a day or less.

Fitzgerald, when he's candid, admits that he was a little scared of women in his younger years. But by the time he was 40 and divorced, his appetite was voracious. "Finally I had all the girlfriends and all the sex I could ask for." He chuckled. "It was like having all the lobster you could want, for once— instead of just picking away at the little legs." At 42 Fitzgerald found the woman of his dreams, the beautiful, gentle, considerably younger soul mate to whom he was married for the next twenty-three years. She had made only one demand: "You've got to promise me fifty years." He did a quick calculation. His father and mother both were still alive. So he said sure.

Fitzgerald is 65 now. He lost his beloved wife in the last year. During her years of illness their sexual life had languished and stopped. When I first saw him after the funeral, the armor against his tragedy was anger. "You know why I'm angry?" he said. "She didn't give *me* the fifty years. It never occurred to me . . ." The emotion rattled in his throat. "I mean, I held to my end of the bargain. I really feel sad for her, and of course, as time goes on, I feel sadder for me. It never occurred to me—you mean, I might have to start all over again?"

Fitzgerald still transmits an infectious enthusiasm, still cuts a dapper figure in his blue blazer and jeans, and before a year of mourning was out, he had a very desirable new lady friend. We met to talk about male menopause. As he ran a hand over the top of his head, to finger-comb the last threads of his once-grand thatch, he began confessing the most amazingly painful changes.

"This is a very hard age. I turn the key, but I don't hear the hum of the motor anymore. You wonder, *Has the motor shut down for good?*"

Ironically every now-single woman with whom Fitzgerald had enjoyed a passionate love affair prior to his fifties sought him out over the past year. Flattering, yes. The redheaded virgin, the blonde, the married woman— their memories of him were still strong! He too remembered how delightful they had been, "but obviously they no longer had the same physical attraction for me."

Except one. Fitzgerald tells the story of his desperate infatuation with one woman—his last grand affair, while he was in his forties and between marriages. He describes her ravishing body and how it so overwhelmed him on their first encounter that he failed. But one night, after he had made love to her three times within a few hours and was savoring this irrefutable evidence of his potency, she rolled over with her back to him without a word of affection and said, "You're angry with me, aren't you?" Though he protested up and down, they both knew she would never return a single endearment. She didn't love him; she was simply allowing herself to be loved.

"I left this, this"—his hands all but conjured her up in front of us— "this honeypot and walked away from her and never went back. It was too humiliating."

She was 55 and still a stunning woman when she looked him up this year. She admitted being very afraid of losing her looks, her lifelong trump card. She wanted to be desired again in the old manic way. Fitzgerald pulled back. The bitter irony of it: Suppose the divine woman of his fantasies suddenly surrendered to him, to his 65-year-old carcass, and it died on him?

"I don't want to be challenged on that level," he said forcefully. "At forty-five I was on top of the world. At sixty-five I am a very vulnerable creature!

I don't want to take the chance of being impotent with them. That would destroy their memory of me." He didn't take any of his old loves to bed.

"When you were young you could say, 'Look what I have to offer you, baby: I'm gonna give you love. I'm gonna give you children. I'm gonna give you a great time in bed.' But when you're sixty-five, there's no use pretending. You're not thirty-five." Older women—although he has deep suspicions about this—at least act as if they're more understanding. "If *I* were they"— Fitzgerald sneered—"I wouldn't put up with me. To be fooling around with some woman to arouse her and then not be able to really, you know, carry through. When she says, 'Never mind, it's great,' I think, *If this is great, she's an idiot.* I know better. I was a young man, after all."

But your new lady friend doesn't seem to be keeping score, I suggested. Why are you so hard on yourself?

"Any man who tells you nobody's keeping score anymore is lying. Somebody is always keeping score—and it's *him*."

AM I JUST GETTING OLD?

It is a universal phenomenon that male sexual function ebbs with age. And the frequency of impotence did steadily increase with age in the Massachusetts Male Aging Study. Given that about half of American men over 40 have already experienced the problem to varying degrees, does this mean a man should expect the decline and fall of the phallus as a natural insult brought on by aging?

No, the decline is gradual, and in a man without major physical problems there is enough of a threshold of male sex hormone to allow him to have satisfactory sexual functioning well into his seventies, and for some men well beyond.

In younger men psychological stress is the primary cause of impotence, says Dr. Tom Lue of the University of California, San Francisco, one of the top urologists in the United States. Stress constricts the blood vessels that allow the penis to become engorged. In men over 55, he finds, the root cause of impotence is usually physical—anything that interferes with the blood and oxygen supply to the penis. "Even at the age of 40, nearly two thirds of those men reporting a diagnosis of heart disease exhibit at least moderate impotence," says the Massachusetts study. Men aged 45 to 55— in passage to the Age of Mastery—fall somewhere in between. "They don't have any obvious disease, but they're not as good as when they were twenty, says Dr. Lue. "It's a matter of expectations."[23]

In *City Slickers*, the movie about Boomer men's midlife crisis, Billy Cryst. and his buddies hunger for vicarious youth and bemoan the staleness c monogamous marriage. "Have you noticed the older you get, the younge your girlfriends get? Soon you'll be dating sperm!"

One of his pals is remarried to a 24-year-old underwear model, but eve he complains it's like having eaten all his life from the Kellogg's Variety Pal and now it's the same cereal every day. "And then you wake up one mornin and you're just not hungry anymore."

Another buddy spells it out: "You can't get an erection."

But instead of dumping his own wife, Crystal's character has his Wil Man experience on a cattle drive, delivers a calf, feels a new pride in h maleness as a protector of the young, and goes home eager to enjoy this ne role with his original wife and kids.

When does this male potency crisis begin? I asked Fitzgerald. "It start going in your fifties, there's no question about it," he grumbled. "Men ofte will run after other women at that age because there's no doubt that new lo is invigorating. But the point is that the same cycle starts all over again."

One of my sources, a driven entrepreneur who cashed in and found him self retired and restless in his mid-fifties, says, "Renting a porno movie isn enough, or reading *Playboy*, or even having a naked woman in your bed. It a depends on what she *does* to you—her sexual skills." His married friend titans of finance, law, and medicine, say the only way they can feel excite now is with the novelty of someone new—not necessarily younger, but ne and different, exotic in some way. The first time with a novelty woman a ma often regains the athletic performance level of his youth. It's thrilling. In sub sequent encounters it's hard work. "After that," the entrepreneur report "most of them say, 'I'd rather play golf.'"

Dr. Richard Spark, a Harvard Medical School urologist, describes a "stut tering effect" in men who come to him in their forties or fifties complainin of impotence problems.[24] This early phase of stuttering potency might b termed *periviropause*, corresponding to *perimenopause* in women—a baffling, gradual, change in sexual responsiveness that is often psychologically toxic.

"Even men whose testosterone level is perfectly normal experience a de inite slowdown," says Dr. Helen Singer Kaplan, the psychiatrist and se researcher who first identified the syndrome of low sexual desire back i 1979. In her two decades of clinical work Dr. Kaplan has observed that "a a man gets older, the critical difference is he becomes much more dependent on the physical stimulation and emotional support of his partner."[25]

Two major studies of the incidence of impotence show that the big jump occurs around age 60.[26] By age 70, among men in the Massachusetts Male Aging Study, the prevalence of complete impotence tripled to 15 percent.[27] But it's important to underscore that there is a robust population of gray-templed men who survive this potential crisis with their egos and erectile tissues intact.

> The Massachusetts study found that 40 percent of these normal, healthy males remained completely potent at age 70.[28]

Another academic study, *The 1993 Janus Report on Sexual Behavior*, confirms that almost 40 percent of men age 65 and over are functioning just fine, thank you, having sex a few times a week.[29] Until very recently our National Institutes of Health had no statement on the subject. After the very first NIH conference on impotence, held in December 1992, a consensus statement was drafted: "The likelihood of erectile dysfunction increases with age but is not an inevitable consequence of aging."[30] Thus, although impotence is definitely age-related, much is not explained by aging alone.

THE MIND-BODY LINK

The American medical profession has basically ignored the syndrome of male menopause up until now. It has been shunted, first to psychiatrists and then to urologists, who among themselves refer to the problem as "just putting some lead back in the pencil." They've gone from surgical implants in the penis to promoting vacuum erection devices and now penile injections. Let's reframe the problem.

Male menopause may not be a medical problem at all, but a mind-body syndrome with many factors that interact reciprocally: A man's age, hormonal activity, and general health level are mediated by the psychological confrontation he has in middle life over what it means to be "manly," as his physical strength ebbs and his occupational status changes and he finds he cannot depend on being aroused at the drop of a bra. Technological male medicine refuses to acknowledge a mind-body connection, however, and that is probably the main reason so many men cannot get help before they panic and render themselves psychologically impotent.

Attitudes that are precursors to male menopausal impotence are:

- It's not going to happen to me.
- My body is bulletproof.
- It's too late to make any big changes in my life.
- The state of my sexual potency is nobody's business but mine. I don't want to talk about it to anybody else.
- If I can't perform up to my old standards, forget the whole thing.

Dr. Herbert Benson, who holds a chair in the Mind/Body Medical Institute at the Harvard Medical School, suggests that "men do not recognize the worth of mind/body work as intuitively as women. But once a man gets initiated, we can deal with male menopause." Even in its watered-down consensus statement, the NIH acknowledges the impact of the mind over the matter of male potency: "In reality, while patients with erectile dysfunction are thought to demonstrate an organic component, psychological aspects of self-confidence, anxiety, and partner communication and conflict are often important contributing factors."[31]

Although the most obvious and threatening aspect of male menopause concerns a diminishing sexual performance, there is a larger cultural context: the challenge a man faces in maintaining his potency in the world as he ages in a society that does not value older people. Currently, American society presents many added toxins to the middle-aged male: a downward economic spiral, a postfeminist consciousness that has pulled the rug out from under the white male's assumption of dominance, and the increasing terror of joblessness.

Dr. Spark reports from his practice, "Losing a job has been a major issue with the current economy. For an awful lot of people, sexual dysfunction seems to correspond with their loss of sense of self-worth."

But it has been ever thus. Going back to the Bible, the lusty story of King David's adventures with Bathsheba has a cautionary postscript. Despite his ten wives and countless concubines, there came a time when the king grew weaker and his advisers feared he was losing his potency. They brought in the young virgin Abishag, the Shunammite, to rekindle his desires. She cherished the king, the Bible says, "but the king was not intimate with her." So what did his subjects do? They deposed him as a weak, impotent ruler.

The first dictionary definition of *impotent* does not refer to a loss of sexual function, but to a loss of power. Synonyms are "powerless, helpless, ineffectual, feeble, weak"—a murderous indictment of masculinity.[32]

People have always equated sexual potency with power and continue to do the same thing to men today. As a result, the slightest hint of diminishing sexual performance can create performance anxiety. After the first few times a man has problems, he becomes anxious, and from then on there is a "spectator" in bed with him and his partner, as veteran sexologist Dr. William Masters has described the phenomenon.[33] With a spectator watching, if a man fails to come up to his own standards of performance, he is flooded with shame, and shame almost certainly will bring on the dreaded sexual deflation.

Men who are afraid to perform pull away from intimacy. They stop hugging and even holding hands. They become socially isolated. After a while they develop *the habit of impotence.* And once a man develops the habit of impotence, it is extremely hard to break.

This was my friend Fitzgerald's problem, exacerbated by his loss of a wife whom he loved very much and who he fully expected would outlast and take care of *him*. He had developed the habit of *widower's impotence.* For companionship he smoked a pipe, smoked it all day long, lit up at four in the morning when he couldn't sleep, puffed while he paced up and down "talking" to the ghost of his wife, smoked until his blood vessels blued like a road map tracing up and down his empty arms. He refused to see a doctor or to consider giving up smoking. I was worried about him.

"Promise me one thing," he implored. "If you stumble upon an easy surefire way to overcome this problem, you will tip me off."

"You'll be the first to know," I assured my miserable friend, and gave him the name of an excellent sex therapist. We'll come back to Fitzgerald at a later stage, in Chapter 16, "The Serene Sixties."

HIGH-TECH SOLUTIONS

Following the publication of my male menopause article, I had a call from the Texas doctor Kenneth Goldberg, a urologist dedicated to doing preventive health care with men. That's when I learned about his Male Health Clinic, the first in the United States to specialize in men's medical concerns. Dr. Goldberg, who later wrote the book *How Men Can Live as Long as Women*, has treated thousands of men since opening up in Dallas in 1988.[34]

He now sees sixty impotent men a month. Typical profile: He's middle-aged, out of shape, overstressed, still smoking, and hung up with sexist attitudes; his cholesterol is high, and he sees himself going straight downhill, but he's reluctant to talk to anyone about it. All these men want the problem to be physical so they can find a quick fix: a pill, a shot, a sure cure. "It's wrong to blame male menopause on lowered testosterone," Dr. Goldberg has concluded. "For years all doctors had to give to men who complained about declining potency was testosterone injections. The problems are still with us, so we know testosterone isn't the answer."

Dr. Goldberg invited me down to Dallas to sit in on his men's groups where patients fighting male menopause compare their progress. "I assure you, some of them will talk about your unspeakable passage because they're getting help." I did go down, and he was right. These were men forged in the macho Texas tradition "to talk rough and swing a big dick," as one of them summed it up. But moving into Second Adulthood without an ethos to replace their performance as young studs, they were as helpless as beached whales.

Bill Howie had been fishing off the Florida Keys when he hooked a big kingfish. Only 44, he fought it in the Hemingwayesque spirit but with flesh that was heir to mean genes and bad habits. Afterward, with his heart leaping like a frog trapped in a jar, he smoked a pack of Marlboros "to calm down." Howie believed he was bulletproof, better than bulletproof; he didn't need doctors or diets or stress tests. Four days later he went under the surgeon's knife for a quadruple bypass; a majority of the vessels that carried life's blood to his heart were blocked.

It was five years and several other surgeries later when we met. "And after all the surgeries *that thang* doesn't work anymore," said Howie. He was eager to share with the other men in the group what they were learning about the road back from impotence. "In my mind the problem had to be entirely physical," he said. "It's all the macho crap that my dad put on me until I was eighteen years old." After a sexually prolific period of running single, Howie had remarried in 1987 at the age of 40. She was younger. *This is it, Lord,* he told himself. "I had all that I wanted, the intimacy and the trust. Our problems began less than a year later. She thought it was *her* fault."

Grunts and murmurs around the room confirmed this was a typical story. The next speaker was a jolly-looking, red-faced man with fuzzy dyed strawberry hair and several bushelsful of flesh into which his double chins spread whenever he laughed.

"My name is Roy Bielich," he said. "I started in the airline business thirty-five years ago, and I stayed in it until June of this year, when I took a nice little early retirement which I was really looking forward to." Roy had patterned himself after his father, his idol. "Dad was a good old Serbian carpenter who played horses, loved women, drank, and indulged his violent temper. We were buddies. I wanted to live the same way." His father died of cancer of the prostate at the age of 57—exactly the age that Roy faced his own mortality crisis. He casually slipped in that fact.

"I had the cancer last year. It will be a year and six days since they took it out."

"You had a prostatectomy?"

"Yeah. But I've always been in good shape, no problems."

I asked if he had noticed any changes since the operation.

"Well, the sex life changed quite a bit because I'm impotent. But my friends here at the health center have fixed that up for me." He laughed heartily.

Both men fitted the profile sketched by Dr. Goldberg and by novelist Cheever. They earned between $50,000 and $75,000 a year but were not stimulated by their jobs, didn't exercise, wouldn't give up smoking, and had gained a dangerous amount of weight. They believed all their problems would be solved when they found a *Playboy* centerfold wife, and both of them did just that. They had each married knockout women, younger women, and then set about to do everything in their power to please them. At a second session they told what had happened.

"I had remarried in 1974 to a very beautiful lady who was sixteen years younger than me," Bielich boasted.

"Did you think she'd do it for you?" I asked.

"Oh, she did it for me. She really did it. We had a very passionate love affair. In fact, number two was the reason I left number one."

But in his early fifties Bielich began failing to please his beautiful young second wife. His desire flagged as his erections faltered. "I wanted to have more sex, but I'd say to myself, *It ain't gonna work tonight; don't start something you can't finish.*"

"Fear of rejection—is that the worst part?" I asked.

Bill Howie interrupted and, clutching his insides, confessed, "Let me tell you something. When you're laying there at night, okay?, and you're trying to make love and it does not work, and you hear your wife sigh, like she's saying, 'Not again,' it'll rip your guts out."

Roy Bielich nodded. "Snuggle and sleep, that's all you're good for. I thought it was all over—until my friends at the clinic here gave me the needle!" He began chortling. "Funniest damn thing that ever happened to me."

Every man in the room leaned forward and hung on Roy's description of the "magic" injection that made him feel like a lion again. After Bielich had recovered from prostate surgery, Dr. Goldberg told him he could now help him with his erection problems. Bielich admitted that he had been impotent for some time. A technician said, "Okay, we're going to try the needle."

"You're gonna put a needle in my *what!*" Bielich bellowed.

"You won't even feel it," the technician promised. They laid him out on an examining table. He felt a little pinprick in the base of his penis. It didn't hurt as much as Roy expected. "Okay, in about ten minutes we'll see what kind of reaction you get," the technician said.

"I'm laying there, and I just can't fathom what's happening," Roy continued. "It's like a button was pushed. The tech comes back and tells me, 'Fondle it a little bit.' He says, 'Good, you're up to about an eight on a scale of ten.' I says, '*Eight!* Hell, that's a forty-two!' The doc comes in and says, 'All right, Roy, you can go.' Here you are with this enormous hard-on. Where the hell are you going to go?"

The room began to rock with horse laughs.

"I told the doc he oughta at least have a whorehouse next door," Bielich continued. "They'd be payin' *me!* So now I gotta go to the Galleria for a sales meeting with one of my clients. I can't even do up my pants. Course, in Texas you never wear a suit coat. Alls I had was my briefcase. And you know travel agencies—they're ninety-nine percent women."

By now the men were doubled over in hilarity. Bielich stood up to demonstrate his moment of macho ignominy. "So I walk in with this briefcase in front of me—boom, ba boom, ba boom. The secretary looks up, shoulda seen her eyes. She says, 'Is there something wrong?' "

Roy Bielich's future dream, the funny man told the group, is to find a woman "with big knockers and a little money," preferably a registered nurse who could give him his penile injections. "I'm lookin' forward to dyin' in the saddle with the needle goin'."

The sad part of his story was this: He didn't admit his problem and get help until two years after his young wife had walked out on him. Did a wall grow up between the two of you? I asked the beefy Bielich.

"I guess so," he said. "To this day I still don't understand why she left. I talk to her once a week, and I always say, 'You want to explain it to me now?' "

Perhaps his wife feared that raising the subject of his impotence would be devastating to him, I suggested.

"Probably." He reflected. "Her and I did not talk about it. We talked about her female problems."

Married men who haven't been able to perform in the bedroom for months or years, once they do disclose their problem to a doctor, almost always reveal the same jarring truth. All the time this eight-hundred-pound gorilla (impotence) has been in their bedroom, *the couple has never talked about it.* Just breaking through the silence and shame by admitting they have the problem is the hardest part, say experts. But talking about it, and taking the pressure of performance off the man, can be the most effective medicine of all.

Bill Howie, by contrast, did keep his marriage together and broke through to a much deeper level of communication. But it took a few years. "My wife would just pitch a fit," Howie remembered. "She wanted to know, 'Why, am I not attractive anymore?' I mean, we were practically newlyweds." After a year of problems she confronted him. "Do you have a girlfriend?" Howie shot back, "What the hell would I be doing with a girlfriend? I can't get it up with you. Get real, lady."

One day, after two years of sexual freeze, Howie's wife stood in his face, holding up a newspaper ad with this headline: ƎꙄЯƎVƎЯ IMPOTENCE! *COME TO THE MALE HEALTH CLINIC.*

"What the hell is that?"

"It's where you're fixin' to go," his wife said.

So the first step is honesty with yourself and your partner, I suggested.

"Oh, yeah," Howie agreed. "I had to convince her that it was not her problem." Once he could empathize with his partner's frustration, Howie found the courage to ask for help. But he brought his East Texas macho bias to the first visit. "I don't want to hear that 'It's all in your head' bullshit," he protested. The wife is often the one who calls to make the first appointment, as in Howie's case. When men shuffle in to the first of Dr. Goldberg's seminars on impotence, they make no eye contact. A patient-lecturer says, "I know you can't look at me. I know you're having trouble with your sexual performance. How many of you are blaming your wife or your girlfriend?" The men's eyes remain pasted to the floor as their hands inch upward. At the same time the wives' arms slip around their mates' shoulders to give them support. Tears of relief dampen cheeks with the flush of honesty.

"It's amazing what's happened to our marriage since then," says Howie. "I don't feel numb anymore. I feel a lot more love and emotion along with my wife, instead of pretending to be some phony cowboy."

Over the last five years of treating middle-life impotence, Dr. Goldberg has developed a humble respect for the power of the mind. "We can get most of these men erections," with the needle, drugs, or other devices, "but too often it doesn't make a difference in restoring their confidence so they can function sexually on their own. This is where the medical profession fails when it refuses to look at the whole man." This unusual, visionary urologist firmly believes that a physician must check out a man's physical plant—his blood pressure and cholesterol and smoking and exercise habits—yes, but also look at social, hormonal, and especially psychological causes.

"If these guys are so concerned about their sexual performance that they're keeping score, they're not going to be able to perform independently no matter how many hormones we give them," says Dr. Goldberg. "Thinking about their sexual problem consumes their life. Every minute of the day they are telling themselves: *What kind of man are you? You can't even get it up.*"

In keeping with America's obsession with high technology, for treatment of total impotence our urologists rely on devices that are aesthetically daunting. They used to prescribe surgical implants in the penis, which were found to *decrease* sexual activity. Injections with vasoactive drugs—the needle used by Bielich—are the latest advance in the technological treatment of impotence. In less than a minute the tiny blood vessels in the penis dilate and an erection begins to occur. The correct dose will last about an hour. A man can learn to give himself the injection with a minute needle just before intercourse.[35] (The latest version of the needle works like a Mont Blanc pen.) Increasingly popular is a natural herb called yohimbine, made from the bark of an African tree, which is taken in tablet form. Dr. Goldberg finds this remedy to be effective in up to 30 percent of his patients with middle-life erection problems, but these are not the men with major physical problems.

It is a lot easier to prevent male menopausal impotence than to correct it, however. The portion of fully impotent men who can be successfully restored to independent functioning is only about 15 to 20 percent, acknowledges Dr. Goldberg. "The vast majority of these guys just can't accept that it's their mind-set that's doing this to them."

Prevention calls for a change of mind-set about where a man is in his sexual life cycle. How does a man tap into the strengths particular to Second Adulthood? The solution is to become the master of his sexual energy—a major task for men that is part of executing a successful passage into the Age of Mastery.

HIGH-TECHNIQUE SOLUTION

Young men often approach sex as if they were racing a Porsche—*See how I can accelerate from zero to a hundred miles an hour in thirty seconds!*—whereupon they screech to a halt, roll over, fully spent, and fall asleep. They miss savoring the tenderness and affection their partners are probably longing to share with them to seal the act of love. Let's call this "racing-car sex." It's instant gratification and fast crash. It's stud power. It can be very exciting for a man, but often unsatisfying for his partner. It is also often unavoidable for young men, because they haven't learned yet how to control or prolong their sexual responses. But it's an adolescent pattern and appropriate only to First Adulthood.

The high point of a man's sexual life cycle is in his forties. By then his sexual responses have usually slowed just enough for him to control and choreograph, prolong, and savor each erotic encounter, taking pride in his virtuoso performance. But as a man moves into Second Adulthood, the amount of time he must wait after ejaculation before he can become fully aroused again noticeably lengthens. If he remains committed to the "cock as performer," it will eventually fail him, and the source of his power will turn into the instrument of his disempowerment. If he minimizes sexual tension and maximizes the time he enjoys intimacy before he has an orgasm, he will be able to master his sexuality so that it contributes to his personal power rather than depletes it. How?

The mature man is ready to graduate from adolescent "racing-car sex" to "body-surfing sex." Imagine riding the waves of love, moving up with the swells of pleasure when sexual energy is high and down with ebbs of intensity, when love and stroking can be enjoyed, then up on the next pleasure wave, and down in the rest cycle, when partners just lie there breathing and holding each other and whispering love, until they feel the next wave of sexual energy starting to rise again.

In her best-seller *How to Make Love All the Time*, psychologist Barbara De Angelis describes this method as the "Continuing Pleasure Wave."[36] Lovemaking is like a spiral, without a sense of beginning, middle, and end. The couple doesn't try to control or force the waves of sexual energy, and nobody asks tensely, "Did you come yet?" She contrasts this with traditional lovemaking, which is a goal-oriented, frenetic effort to reach orgasm. She says the longer one allows sexual energy to circulate in the body, the more powerful will be its effect. Each new wave increases rather than depletes the sexual energy and *builds the trust of the man in his partner and himself* so he is able to prolong the act well beyond traditional lovemaking, until he and his partner's bodies are so saturated with sexual energy they experience a flood of orgasm and afterward feel refreshed and renewed.

Dr. Harry K. Wexler, a widely respected clinical and research psychologist, slips into youthful vernacular to describe the hope for sustained male potency that is shared by many middle-aged men. "Young men see their cocks as a solution to life," he says. "As they get older, their cocks become the problem. Don't worry about the cock; discover the tongue. The tongue will work until ninety. Men really have to let go of their flashy boy cock to gain the stronger sense of potency that will rejuvenate them."[37]

The pioneering sex therapist Dr. Helen Singer Kaplan has found that a change in sexual technique, together with a closer, more intimate relationship with a partner, will compensate for the age-related slowdown in most older men. Many men in their sixties report back to the Kinsey Institute that they find they don't need to have an orgasm every time they have sex. This allows the next encounter to be more robust. "In fact, if they have a reasonable level of self-esteem and a woman who supports them," says Dr. Reinisch, "they often see this as an enhancement of their sexuality. It doesn't control them; now they start to control *it*."[38]

But a man who has known the thrill of sexual conquests—those moments when he felt he was controlling the world—does not forget that feeling. "It's like a warrior who remembers his great victories," Fitzgerald explains. "The memory of those sexual triumphs is poignant."

Isn't this another form of competition? When a man loses out in job competition, he can always blame the company or the person who stole his job. With male potency, it's self-competition, you competing with your younger self. The resolution is the same. A man has to let go of the old scoring system in order to enjoy learning and playing a whole new game.

"Sexual drive, desire, and orgasm definitely have something to do with male hormone versus female hormone in the male body," confirms Dr. Samuel Yen, a gynecologist and endocrinologist at the University of California at San Diego, who is on the cutting edge of research into hormones relevant to aging. "But the level maintained in the aging population is definitely sufficient to conduct satisfactory and enjoyable sexual activity." In fact, he told me anecdotally from observing many of his patients—mostly educated Professional Men—those *who understand the process* enjoy their sexual intimacies even more. "They're retired, free of stress, they have security and a lot of time for exercise. Those are the best medicines of all."[39]

The men of high well-being among the Professionals I have studied *have shifted* to a preference for intimacy over sex per se *and have not lost their erections*. Once men come through this passage and accept that they are free of the burden of sexual predatoriness, they can open up to receive and express love in its many shadings.

The Safe Woman or Man—the partner a man can trust—becomes the most desirable partner at this stage. Then a man can relax and be himself. "Particularly as a man becomes more vulnerable, he's going to need somebody who is not going to use his weaknesses and frailties against him," observes Dr. Stuart Fischoff, a professor of psychology at California State University in Los Angeles. "Trust becomes a pivotal issue."[40]

HOW TO RESTORE VITALITY AND VIRILITY

There are many safe, natural steps a man can take to make himself potent again. Smoking is devastating to male potency, since it damages the tiny blood vessels in the penis that must enlarge to allow the substantial rush of blood during an erection. Diet matters; high cholesterol levels can clog arteries. Alcohol abuse over ten to fifteen years actually kills the nerves in the penis. Taking medication for hypertension *doubles* the risk of impotence. A man may have to try four or five different medications before he finds the drug that will control his blood pressure without affecting his capacity to have erections. And stress may be the final straw.[41]

"We now believe that some of the symptoms we call aging are really due to hormone deficiencies," says S. Mitchell Harman of the NIH.[42] Indeed, researchers have discovered that just as estrogen production drops during female menopause, so testosterone production in men diminishes markedly in many men over 50.

About a third of men over 50 have a testosterone deficiency, estimates Dr. John Morely, a professor of geriatrics at St. Louis University School of Medicine and one of the leading researchers in the field. By age 65, according to his colleague endocrinologist Fran Kaiser, at least 40 percent of men produce such low amounts of testosterone that their health may be compromised.[43] "Males have been unwilling to recognize that they lose their sexual hormones and the sexual prowess that goes with it," says Dr. Morely. "They are much readier to study female sex hormones than to look at themselves."

Having recently reviewed the charts of five thousand of the patients she has seen over twenty years, Dr. Helen Kaplan insists that without clinical hormone tests "no physician can tell if the lack of desire is due to psychological inhibition or a hormonal deficit." Some hormone researchers claim that the most common cause of low sex drive for midlifers is not low testosterone but low moods prompted by chronic low-level depression.[44] Indeed, both depression and repressed anger were strongly associated with men's potency problems in the Massachusetts study.[45] But it's a chicken-and-egg argument. Testosterone definitely alters men's moods. We know that in male competition, whether it's tennis or chess, testosterone levels rise with victory and fall with defeat. For the loser the drop in testosterone may blunt his sex drive along with his self-esteem, and as he continues to lose confidence, he is likely to perform poorly both in future sports competitions and in bed, until it becomes a vicious circle.

What surprised me most in researching the effects of testosterone is that the primary action is not on our sexual drive. Testosterone is the leading hormone for metabolism in both males and females—the very fuel that burns the proteins that keep us going day to day. There are testosterone receptors in the brain, the bone marrow, the kidneys, just about everywhere in the body.[46]

"If a man has a low testosterone level," Dr. Kaplan says, "you can do all the psychotherapy in the world, but you are much better off replacing his hormones. Then it's magic. But if there's no deficiency, it is dangerous quackery to give it."[47] Dr. Kaplan encourages men to make the same sort of risk/benefit calculation that women must make in considering whether or not to replace estrogen.

Other hormones under study may prove to be even more relevant to the aging process and, as they ebb with age, to contribute to male menopause. Dr. Daniel Rudman, the late pioneering hormone investigator at the Medical College of Wisconsin, demonstrated that about a third of men between 60 and 70 are deficient in *human growth hormone* (GH). And in the age-group between 70 and 80 more than half of all men have no detectible growth hormone.[48] When Dr. Rudman gave injections of growth hormone to twelve men, aged 61 to 81, their excess body fat dissolved and muscle mass returned, their bones firmed up, their skin thickened, and their sex drive came back full force.[49] The landmark medical study published in 1990 reported these changes were equivalent in magnitude to reversing aging by ten to twenty years.[50] An antiaging panacea?

Not quite. These good effects occur only if a person is genuinely deficient in growth hormone. That decline is probably inconsequential in most people until age 60. Supplements given before then in small studies have caused some carpal tunnel syndrome, gynecomastia (breast enlargement in men), or diabetes-like symptoms.[51] Most of these problems seem to be related to dose and have since been minimized by low-dose regimens. A review of current scientific literature turned up guarded optimism that GH may increase quality of life both physically and psychologically in people over 50.[52] But treatment at present is only experimental and very expensive.

The good news is, men and women can stimulate this elixir on their own. Numerous studies have now demonstrated that growth hormone is acutely elevated by vigorous exercise and remains elevated for up to a half hour after an aerobic workout.[53]

Yet it is a measure of the viropausal panic that a Houston businessman has been able to set up a "clinic" in Mexico, appropriately named El Dorado, where he has supplied more than a hundred clients with self-injectable growth hormone and on-ice shipments every three months at a cost of about $12,000 a year.[54] "Men here want sexual potency," says client Sandy Highland, a Seattle nurse. "That's what every man here talked about; it's on the top of their list." Dr. Rudman himself warned that taking growth hormone on one's own was a bad idea. "We know it can produce negative side effects and damage health," he said.[55] Very few doctors are experts in measuring or administering growth hormone in adults (although it has been used safely and effectively for years with growth-deficient children).[56]

But many scientific and commercial investigations are now devising strategies to augment the body's natural secretion of growth hormone, as an alternative to replacing it.[57] The National Institutes of Health have funded no fewer than four major clinical trials of growth hormone in older adults.[58] Now along comes a promising new study which raises the likelihood that men over 50 may soon be offered a custom-made "hormonal cocktail" to keep themselves virile and vital and to protect against other assaults of aging.

Dr. Samuel Yen, the endocrinologist at the University of California at San Diego, has been studying the hormones most relevant to aging. He has also been noticing the phenomenon I'm describing. "Men between fifty and sixty, when they refer to male menopause, suddenly realize well-being is not there," he told me.[59] The most important group of hormones related to aging are growth hormones, one of which (IGFI) declines quite rapidly in that decade of life. Metabolism slumps, and the sense of well-being slumps along with it. Dr. Yen and his team propose that a sex hormone known as DHEA (dehydroepiandrosterone) may have a central effect on restoring the élan, sexual and otherwise, as well as the physical stamina and the immune response of both men and women in the menopausal years.[60] It accomplishes this by reviving growth hormone.

In the first study of DHEA on humans, men and women were given replacement doses. A remarkable increase in both physical and psychological well-being was reported by both genders: an 84 percent increase in the women and 67 percent in the men. Subjects in this reliable double-blind study said they felt increased energy and improved mood, slept more deeply, and felt more relaxed and better able to handle stressful events. Within the first two weeks they were back at the level of growth hormone normally enjoyed by 30-year-olds. "We're finding in our latest study that DHEA also activates the immune system," says Dr. Yen.

BEYOND MALE MENOPAUSE

The real relief for men in making the passage into the second half of adult life is that they no longer have to keep proving themselves as young studs. On the contrary, nature provides relief for a man who is patient enough to take his place in the cycle of generations. He becomes the Great Father. The famous entertainer I interviewed was overcome in his mid-fifties with a craving for youth, until the experience of holding his first grandchild in his arms.

"It all came in a flash," he says. "This tiny girl, I was young again with her, but when she grows up, I'll be gone. So it was the experience of rebirth and death all in the same overpowering moment."

He began to think about being descended from primates. "There comes a time when you can't fight off younger males much longer, and you don't have to beat your chest anymore. Chasing young girls offers only temporary relief. If you stay with your wife (which is hard) and stay close to your children (which is also hard, because they're pulling away), when it's time for the next generation to be born, you can enjoy being part of the whole evolutionary process. What having grandchildren does is put you in touch with youth again. If you try to rush it, by dumping your wife and kids and trying to re-create the young family, sooner or later you're going to be the old fart in the picture."

Men who continue to try to drown their stress in sexual hedonism will predictably have the rockiest passage into the sixties, just as the women most miserable upon reaching menopause are those who were always heavily invested in their looks. But the man who has cultivated new roles—replacing his retired mentor, becoming a "father" to his community and a grandfather to his family—who savors the freedom to explore the world with his Safe Woman or Man, and who perhaps finds a deeper spiritual companionship, may be able to relinquish the status of his professional role, when the time inevitably comes, without feeling extinct. If he has prepared himself with an image appropriate to his sixties and found a passion he's eager to pursue, even being brutally forced out of a job can occasion not impotence, but an opening up of creative potency.

I asked the still-reigning authority Dr. William Masters what was the best advice he could give to an older man who is worried he's losing his potency. The 77-year-old pioneer's reedy voice suddenly filled with tenderness: "Talk to your partner. Tell her you have these concerns. She's probably concerned and afraid to tell you. Then talk to a competent sexologist about how to reactivate your bedroom scene."

After almost fifty years of treating sexual dysfunction, Masters has a humble definition of good communication in a relationship: "It's the privilege of exchanging vulnerabilities."

15

MEN AND WOMEN:
THE NEW GEOMETRY OF
THE SEXUAL DIAMOND

*M*ales and females are very much alike for the first ten years of life. We become radically differentiated at puberty and arrive at the farthest reaches of our oppositeness in our late thirties, the most distant poles of the Sexual Diamond. But in our fifties men and women begin moving closer together again and take on many characteristics of our gender opposite, and by our sixties each becomes something of what the other used to be. Injunctions about what it is to be a man or a woman lose force as we age. Rigid role divisions melt away. Changes in life tasks and the dramatic shift in our time perspective in middle life shake up old patterns and allow new ones to form. At last we have permission to become more accepting of all that we are.

The solitary, disciplined, emotionally detached stance that allows men in First Adulthood to master a skill or conquer an adversary or solve a political problem, while essential to survival, taps only part of their personality potential. By learning early how to shut off their feelings, they also develop weaker attachments to people and even have weaker bridges between the emotional and the intellectual hemispheres of their brains than women do.[1]

Women's hypersensitivity to their own and others' feelings in First Adulthood guarantees the survival of their young and helps them weave a dense fabric of human ties and family rituals to keep the males around during the long parental emergency. But this diffuse attention to human connections often translates as "fuzzy thinking" in the larger sphere where rational, objective analysis is required and rules and abstract principles must also be respected.

Voilà! A massive shift takes place across gender lines as we grow older. What is observable empirically is that women begin to be more focused, more interested in tasks and accomplishments than in nurturing, whereas men start to show greater interest in nurturing and being nurtured, in expressing themselves artistically and appreciating their surroundings. Each sex adds some of the characteristics that distinguished its opposite in First Adulthood, women becoming more independent and assertive, men more expressive and emotionally responsive. These changes in middle and later life are developmental, not circumstantial, and they occur in predictable sequence across widely disparate cultures.

Anthropological studies tell us, however, that men remain identified with being male, rather than become femininized or androgynous. It is their need to prove themselves through sexual and aggressive conquest that diminishes to a great degree.[2] Women across cultures age psychologically in the reverse direction, becoming more aggressive and managerial and political. While they remain identified with being female, their focus is no longer diffused by caring for young children or the conflict between seduction/childbearing and career achievement.[3]

There is mounting evidence that the sexual aggression of younger men can later be recruited in the service of a mature heroism, in which passion is harnessed into a compassionate, community-building cause rather than a violent Rambo rampage. Think of some of the former terrorists turned peacemakers in later life: Anwar Sadat, Menachem Begin, Yasir Arafat, and, more recently, the IRA's Gerry Adams. At the same time the dependence of younger fertile women congeals in middle life. Given an open society with sexist barriers that are not insurmountable, a woman's full political potential can at last be tapped. Consider recently famous female leaders who were postmenopausal: Golda Meir, Indira Gandhi, Margaret Thatcher.

A POINT OF HARMONY

Couples should expect a switch of polarities in marriage. But rather than the sexes' simply trading roles in middle life, men and women become freer to express both the masculine and feminine sides of their personalities. We have the chance to reach a point of harmony—the upper point of the Sexual Diamond—where the tension of male-female differences relaxes at last. This is one more stage-linked transition that makes Second Adulthood so exciting. (See the diagram visualizing this dynamic on the next page.)

The Sexual Diamond

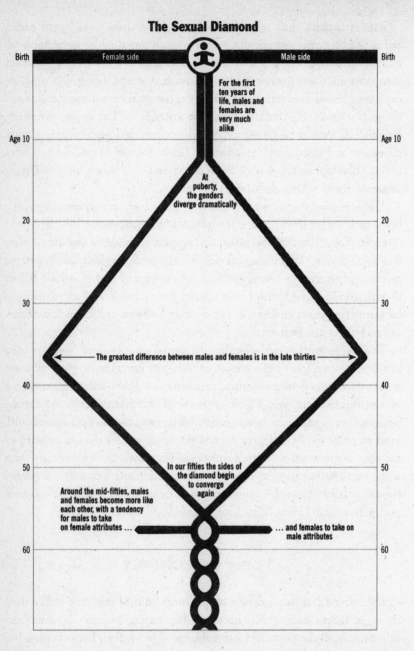

Birth — Female side — Male side — Birth

For the first ten years of life, males and females are very much alike

Age 10 — Age 10

At puberty, the genders diverge dramatically

20 — 20

30 — 30

The greatest difference between males and females is in the late thirties

40 — 40

50 — 50

In our fifties the sides of the diamond begin to converge again

Around the mid-fifties, males and females become more like each other, with a tendency for males to take on female attributes ...

... and females to take on male attributes

60 — 60

One very public couple that exhibits this dynamic in a middle-life marriage is the former treasurer of the state of California and her husband. Kathleen Brown's story traces the classical outlines of the Sexual Diamond.

Just past seven on almost any morning the odds are that Kathleen Brown will just be winding up her daily hike. A great yolk of sun will be breaking over the hills at the top of Doheny Drive and running down the sides of her canyon into the basin of Los Angeles. This lean, fit 49-year-old grandmother takes the same fast walk alone every day, as if pacing herself to run a marathon in her Second Adulthood.

Indeed, she ran a two-year race from 1992 to 1994 for the governorship of the largest state in the Union. She lost that contest. But her political drive is still strong. On the brink of her fifties Brown is driven by a redirected maternal instinct to help save the state her father governed through its Great Arc of Prosperity.[4] The expectations she carries on her shoulders are gargantuan. Certain advisers to the highest circles of the White House size her up and say, "Because she's young, attractive, bright, the odds are that she could be on the ticket as a vice presidential candidate with a Gore in the year 2000."

This amalgam of male and female strengths has been a long time in developing.

Kathleen is the daughter of California's First Couple of politics, Bernice and former Governor Edmund ("Pat") Brown. "Kathy" was the only one of Pat Brown's children to grow up in the governor's mansion in Sacramento, where she absorbed the cultural and political message of California in its ascendancy. She was a natural politician, charming and pragmatic. But her brother, Jerry, prince of the family, was the one charged with perpetuating a new California dynasty.

"I was pretty convinced that I would never run for public office in the adult world," Kathleen told me.[5] "It was just too hard." And so, during most of her young adulthood, Kathleen Brown tried to fit the traditional female mold she had watched her mother carry off with style and self-sacrifice. "Kathleen came up thinking that her lot in life was to be a good Catholic mother and wife," says family friend Karl Fleming, "to raise her children and belong to the PTA, get on the school board, and do all those wifely and motherly things."

She eloped at 20 and dropped out of Stanford University in 1966 to have her first child. Young women today might see this as a shrewd move:

the "early option" it's called now. But the concept of "options" did not enter the vocabulary of the female life cycle until maybe ten years later. "It all just happened," Kathleen told me. "There was no great plan or design." She followed her husband to Cambridge, Massachusetts, where George Rice entered Harvard Law School, and his wife settled into the comfortable anonymity of being Kathy Brown Rice.

"It was the Sixties. I made his ties," Kathleen recalls.

It was also her twenties, a period when the natural female tendency is to want to feel cherished and to be responsive to others, expressive and empathetic. Toward the end of her twenties, typically, she felt hemmed in by domesticity. Her frustration was expressed in exasperation with the school board of Los Angeles, where she now lived. She toppled a veteran conservative to gain her own seat, but she saw her first political post merely as an extension of the altruistic works of a caregiver. Her husband saw it differently, as a threat.

In their early thirties the couple began to diverge more dramatically. She had performed the role assigned to her—good Catholic wife and mother—but after fourteen years of marriage and three children it blew up in her face. On Memorial Day 1979 her husband announced he was leaving her for another woman.

Stunned, she sat in the library staring at the wall for three weeks, neither sleeping nor eating, dropping seventeen pounds, and finally fled to the sanctuary of the old family house in San Francisco. "I felt totally adrift, totally terrified about how was I going to manage," Brown told me. "Most women don't have the half of what I had. My parents were there, and my settlement was very fair. But it gave me that sense of urgency: You've got to develop an awareness of finances and not expect to be taken care of your whole life."

Kathleen Brown was not on the remarriage market for long before an unlikely Tracy-and-Hepburn match was cooked up by friends. Van Gordon Sauter, an older, bow-tied conservative who ran a local CBS-TV station, used to watch the liberal Democrat Kathleen Brown on television and think: *How can a woman that beautiful be so stupid?* He let it be known he'd like to meet her. Kathleen intended to give this blowhard a piece of her mind.

Sauter took her breath away by announcing on that first date, "Hey, I want to marry you." He was in his early forties and presumably feeling the urgency of "time running out" that accompanies the early midlife transition. She held him off, but not for long. One April evening in 1980 she left a hysterical session of the school board to meet Sauter at a romantic Italian restaurant. "So when are we going to get married?" was his opener.

"I'm not even divorced yet," she said, stalling. "Maybe two years, something like that."

"That doesn't fit into my timetable," he towel-snapped, whereupon he got up and left the restaurant. Kathleen got in her car and followed him. Catching up, she motioned for him to roll down the window. "Can we talk?" She laughs uproariously at the memory. "Guys like ultimatums; I believe in keeping on talking."

"She decided it was time to close," says Sauter.

But for all the jollity of their courtship, the decision to throw together two families of divorce with a total of five children in various stages of adolescence set off emotional havoc. To complicate matters, Sauter was immediately summoned to New York to become president of CBS Sports. Kathleen, like her mother before her, again followed her husband unquestioningly, although it meant leaving behind a daughter in rebellion and giving up her own fledgling political career.

In New York she took easily to the role of Mrs. Van Gordon Sauter. She entertained network bigwigs and traveled with her husband to boring meetings with affiliates in the hinterlands. "She was a superb corporate wife," says a somewhat nostalgic Sauter, "without a doubt the *ultimate corporate wife*."

But reaching the crossroads of her mid-thirties, Kathleen hit upon the idea that she could become a late-blooming lawyer. She decided to apply to Fordham and had her course all planned before she broke the news to her husband.

"She nailed me on the law school idea when we were going eighty miles an hour on the Wilbur Cross Parkway," says Sauter.

Predictably he exploded. "A lawyer! I loathe lawyers! The last thing the world needs is another lawyer, particularly *my wife*." He wound up his fusillade by suggesting that anything short of streetwalking would be more constructive than becoming a lawyer. Kathleen held her ground.

"Since I can't talk without my hands," says Sauter, "there was nothing I could do except run off the road."

Kathleen's abrupt change in course was the result of an Age 35 Inventory. Like many women in their mid-thirties, she had an epiphany: She would have to be more assertive and independent to survive. Her children were grown and gone, and she wanted a new life. In private, however, she had grave doubts. As a woman formed in the prefeminist era, she had never been given permission to want something for herself. She had to fight off her inner fears. "I didn't think I could ever catch up."

When I asked Bernice Brown, "What dream did you have for your daughter, Kathleen?" her mother was surprised by the question. "Oh, I didn't think of that."

"Were you surprised when Kathleen decided to go to law school and did so well?" I asked Bernice Brown.

"Yes, I was."

Kathleen stuck to her guns. She threw herself into law school studies, but without giving up her friends, her family obligations, or the corporate dinner parties. Still, she managed by the age of 40 to finish in the top 15 percent of her class. Her decision to become a corporate bond lawyer was driven by the painful experiences of her young adulthood: She wasn't taking any chances on drowning again in her dependency on a man. "Whether I liked what I was doing or not," says Brown, "I knew I had to have an oxygen tank to support me."

An "oxygen tank" becomes vitally important to women as they begin traveling across the Sexual Diamond in their forties toward greater autonomy. It became even more urgent in Brown's case when her husband ran into a life accident. Sauter was suddenly and unceremoniously fired by CBS. The couple left New York to return home to L.A. But not in defeat. Kathleen was exhilarated. She loved the sprawling openness of the place, which demands an assertion of will against its void. And she felt ready. It was time for Governor Brown's daughter/Kathy Brown Rice/Mrs. Van Gordon Sauter to reinvent herself.

I asked if there was a point where she finally turned to embrace the political life. Yes. One night, slaving over a bond document to finance a state health facility, she finally permitted herself an individual ambition. *This is an all-right thing, going into politics through finance,* she remembers thinking. *And this is probably more fun than being a lawyer.*

Politics is a field women can enter without the lifetime of training and seniority that is expected in corporate life. Kathleen decided to run for state treasurer. From then on, according to Fleming, the family friend, "she was like a flower slowly opening. I watched her week by week by week just get stronger, more confident, more her own person, more sure of her own ideas. The way she wore her hair changed; the way she dressed changed. In the old times there were a lot of bows and scarves, like her mother. The clothes got simpler, the colors stronger. She became more sure of her own view of life."

Now what emerged in her was the rippling Irish political charm of her father. Sauter told me he recognized the zeal for public life that overtook his wife as coming "directly from her father. Not diluted. From the father." Ethnic particularities aside, it is a classic switch in identifications as a woman begins moving in the opposite direction along the Sexual Diamond. Brown built a staggering campaign chest and won the treasurer's race handily. When her party tapped her to challenge Pete Wilson, and vie for the highest-profile governorship in the land, she was ready. She ran hard right up to the end.

How does her husband react to this extreme switch in polarities on the Sexual Diamond? Quite contentedly, it appears. Once the fearsome president of CBS News, Sauter now works only three days a week as a consultant to Rupert Murdoch's Fox News. He is ten years older than his wife, just short of 60.

"I like the idea of being a semiretired kept man," he cracks. He cultivates a Hemingwayesque iconoclasm, walking his Border collie in khakis and Dock-Siders and sporting a long, snowy beard. When his wife is away campaigning, he'll jump into his Ford Bronco and drive north with a fishing buddy. When she's home, their life buzzes with entertaining friends, enjoying grandchildren, and staying on top of political trends.

Her second husband, at his mellowing stage of life, seems completely supportive of her political career, not threatened as her first husband was at a more distant pole on the Sexual Diamond. But he's no pushover. When the prickly conservative tangles with his liberal wife on an issue, friends attest that he will occasionally snap at her, "You're full of crap." He sees these contretemps as stimulating: "It's almost like two dogs fighting. There's a lot of noise but never any injury." Normally Sauter holds back on meddling in his wife's political life. But this was the media whiz who put the sweater on Dan Rather, after all; his stock-in-trade is making TV personalities connect emotionally with viewers. And so, when the moment calls for it, he will weigh in as his wife's senior producer and political manager.

This sort of integration and celebration of male-female strengths is probably not possible until we reach middle life. For couples who are conscious and confident enough to allow the Sexual Diamond to work for them, the reward is a richer, smarter, more attuned relationship in which each can come closer to being whole. But it must be said that whether we welcome them or not, these changes will take place anyway. They are not just social or psychological. There is a solid biological basis for men and women becoming more like their sexual opposites as they move beyond young parenthood. Now, to go back and fill in the story from birth.

BRAIN-SEX CHANGES

Biochemistry is at work long before society pigeonholes us into confining gender roles. Since I last wrote about this concept, in 1983, in *Pathfinders,*[6] strong evidence has emerged of brain-sex changes over the course of a lifetime that helps explain the biological basis of the Sexual Diamond. Just as puberty catapults us out of the simple polymorphic pleasures of childhood, so changes in hormones and brain chemistry in middle life return the two sexes closer to the neutrality they had as children.

It used to be thought, on the basis of animal studies, that neonatal factors, including perhaps hormones, fixed the brain at birth and that it was hard-wired forever. That whole notion has been changing over the last two decades. We now know that the brain is *physically* changed by experience. The work of neurobiologist Eric Kandel at Columbia Presbyterian Medical Center has clearly established that the brain has a "youthful plasticity" unmatched by any other organ of the body.[7] More pertinent to the Sexual Diamond is Dr. Kandel's finding that at certain stages of its development, the brain's very structure at a cellular level is dependent on its interaction with the environment.

The latest revelation by neurobiologists is that estrogen helps establish the brain's very architecture in the fetusus of both females and males and acts to maintain that intricate structure all through adulthood.[8] Roger Gorski, a neuroanatomist at UCLA known as the father of brain-sex research, along with his colleague Laura Allen, have proved beyond doubt that *hormones can change the very structure of our brains.*[9] In fact, throughout life our behavior is constantly modulated by the effect of hormones on our brains. But at certain periods in life their impact is greatly heightened.

During pubertal development, for instance, hormones have their greatest effect on body shape and size. But they also change the structure of the brain in significant ways. Androgens, primarily testosterone, are associated with a number of male traits that emerge vividly in males during puberty: assertive sexual behavior, status-related aggression, spatial reasoning, territoriality, pain tolerance, tenacity, transient bonding, sensation seeking, and predatory behavior. This list just about sums up the gripes females have about the opposite sex. Yet androgens make a boy out of a female fetus and a strong man out of a gentle boy; one cannot separate maleness from characteristic male traits.[10]

Similarly, before their ovaries begin to make estrogen, girls in prepuberty are exposed primarily to testosterone from their adrenal glands. That's why girls between nine and twelve sprout hair under their arms and around their genitals and suddenly shoot up in height. This relatively high-testosterone/low-estrogen phase is also a time of adventurousness and competitiveness for most girls, when they climb trees and play sports competitively and shout back at boys and aren't yet ashamed of their bodies.

But just wait. Both the male and female temperament will change in middle life, the result of an inexorable hormone decline in both sexes.

What is now known biochemically is that the ratio of "female" sex hormone (estrogen) to "male" sex hormone (testosterone) decreases markedly as women reach middle life. "In postmenopausal females, there is a shift toward the male sex hormone," confirms Dr. Pentti Siiteri, professor emeritus, University of California at San Francisco.[11] (Women continue to produce testosterone via their adrenal glands even after their ovaries have stopped making estrogen.) The ratio of testosterone to estrogen in a postmenopausal woman may be up to twenty times higher than in a woman who is still ovulating and making estrogen in her ovaries.[12] It is no accident that this second period of testosterone dominance coincides with a resurgence of adventurousness, independence, and assertiveness in women.[13]

In a man, as his testosterone levels decline, the ratio shifts in the opposite direction. In addition, more of his "male" sex hormone is converted into estrogen. "So his ratio of 'male to female' hormone is much lower than when he was a young man," says Siiteri. He points out, however, that with men it's not an abrupt change and males will always have at least ten times as much testosterone as females.

We know that the brain is a major target of both estrogen and testosterone. Given the fluidity of our brains and the hormonal volatility of the middle years for both men and women, it stands to reason that the brain would have to rebalance around the deprivation of hormones it was accustomed to having in full supply for thirty or forty years. I asked Professor Gorski if the brain structure could be changing markedly again for women in menopause and men in male menopause.

Gorski fully agreed this is plausible. Some of his studies show structural changes in the brains of older animals. Other scientists are beginning to appreciate the importance of estrogen to the health of the human brain of both sexes. As earlier described (in Chapter 9, "Wonder Woman Meets Menopause"), if estrogen levels drop sharply in early menopause and are not replaced, the connections between brain cells that are necessary for mastery of new facts and tasks can diminish. Such brain changes may even render women more susceptible to Alzheimer's disease.[14]

That our brains change structurally in middle life is a remarkable concept. Can this be part of the reason that men uncover more of their "feminine" side and women their "masculine" side in Second Adulthood? Maybe, as the ratio of hormones alters with age, men's and women's brains go through a passage and begin to approximate more of the brain structure of the opposite sex.

"It's a plausible and thought-provoking analysis," says Siiteri. "Postmenopausal women become more like men, in the endocrinological sense." In normal males, from their prime around age 25 to maturity at age 70, there is a 20 to 50 percent decline in testosterone available to the brain, Siiteri reaffirms. "Most scientists now ascribe not only functional but also mood and behavioral changes to that." As testosterone and DHEA decrease in men, and the female hormone estrogen increases, passivity and docility become characteristic of older males.[15]

TAKE BACK YOUR DIAMOND!

Wouldn't it be nice if human behavior played out as neatly as the drawing of the Sexual Diamond? It looks as though it automatically brings the sexes closer together. Actually, it creates a new dynamic. Today men and women in middle life don't just gently move back together; in fact, some couples may feel more out of sync than ever. Just as in all the other new stages and passages of Second Adulthood, the possibilities for men and women and couples are in flux. We cannot expect to live and love or be loved the way we were when men retired at the end of their fifties and stay-at-home wives were available to baby-sit the grandkids and keep their hubbies company while shelling peas.

A hip contemporary television director, for instance, recounted for me the moment of crisis in his trajectory as a sexual being, at 52. He insists that he was not the trigger, that it was his wife's entry into the Change of Life. The director was a boyish comic who went from stand-up acts in Greenwich Village clubs to Broadway and on to the *Tonight* show, while his wife of long standing played handmaiden to his success. But as she approached 50, he says, they hit a very rocky time together. He noticed his wife changing, dramatically. "As the woman finds her individuality and defines herself separately from you, it's at a time when you, the man, are *opening up* to the more tender, loving side. For the man at fifty, work is not so paramount. At the same time the woman is becoming more individualized, more assertive, less tolerant, just ... different. Harder, as opposed to softer. Not unloving, just not as involved with men who are still babies."

The director was describing a classical turnabout between married couples in their fifties. But displacing the whole change in dynamics on his wife's menopause did not sufficiently explain it. He was changing too. Fear about shifting gender characteristics can emerge on a deep emotional level. It may be another of the reasons we are so phobic about aging, because we feel ourselves changing in a Frankenstein-like way that is out of our control.

We are pretty familiar by now with the many ways in which males and females in the phase of young adulthood are out of sync. Although middle and later life does tend to bring both sexes back to a greater equilibrium between the self-assertive seeking drive and the merging and affiliative drive, men and women come to this point from opposing directions.[16] One member of a couple may be moving fast while the other is stuck in traditional role playing. A younger wife's career may be soaring while her older husband's is either static or in eclipse. Members of such couples seem to crisscross like trains in the night.

THE CROSSOVER CRISIS

Current historical trends are exaggerating the Sexual Diamond. Role reversals that would otherwise be more gradual and easily assimilated, even welcomed, are being accelerated. The gender crossover can throw husbands and wives out of sync. Yet the confusion of this Crossover Crisis has received little attention.

A typical role reversal situation was described to me by Dr. Judith Rosener, who was contentedly occupied into her forties as "just a corporate wife," tending children, doing volunteer work, and playing tennis. Like most women of her generation, she is still married to the same husband. She went back to school in midlife, part-time, with no career plans in mind. At least not until she was 52, when—watch out, world!—she found herself engrossed in a late-blooming career as a popular writer and lecturer. She locked up tenure as a full-time faculty member at the Graduate School of Management at the University of California at Irvine, but more amazing, even to her, she went on to write a best-selling book about male and female leadership styles.[17]

"I never made a dime in my life," marvels Rosener. "My husband was the provider. All of a sudden as a professor with all these lecture engagements and royalties, I find myself making big bucks. I'm writing thousand-dollar checks to political candidates and giving money to issues I care about. I have a new book coming out in '95, *America's Competitive Secret: How Organizations Can Gain the Advantage by Promoting Women into Top Management.* It is the most exciting time in my life!"

That is her perspective at age 65. Her husband, a former chief executive officer, is now 71. He just wants her physically there, sitting beside him, she says. He admits he preferred it when she was "just a wife," so she sometimes feels torn.

"The world is opening up to us women," she says, "while our husbands are slowing down professionally. My husband's an exception, because he's quite happy working out of our home in a relaxed manner and because he takes real pleasure in my success. But many of the men married to women like me are having a really tough time. Their husbands are very jealous of the time they spend working."

This is an increasingly common predicament. As more men over 50 are being induced to retract out of the work world earlier than they wished, their wives, freed from family duties, are being seduced at the same stage to expand fully into the world. Over the years, as former director of the Jung Institute, Aryeh Maidenbaum has observed the Sexual Diamond becoming more pronounced. "When women get to their fifties, they feel so much energy freed up. They're more likely to say, 'Hey, I've got thirty years ahead of me!' Men so often see this stage as a loss of power, a loss of potency. The sense of mortality really starts settling in for men about fifty. They become very threatened that they're less needed by women."

Most men and women in the Silent and World War II generations were not anticipating anything like this dramatic disruption in the power balance. For men who feel threatened or confused about letting go of stereotyped gender roles, the new geometry of the Sexual Diamond can register as pain, displacement, lost stamina, and a sense that time is running out. But who wants to be stuck in the rut of a First Adulthood role forever? A dentist in his fifties told me about his delightful epiphany. One day, all stiffly white-coated with his drill poised over a patient, he suddenly thought: *Who says some eighteen-year-old snot-nosed kid should decide you have to spend your whole life looking into people's mouths?*

When men begin to enjoy cooking, or landscaping their homes, or take up musical instruments they once loved, or start studying languages or exploring spiritual or philosophic realms, it is obvious that a major reorganization of their personalities is in progress. Instead of fighting a transition that allows them to be more, these men are tapping into new sources of energy and pleasure that are available to them naturally. The men of highest well-being in my current surveys, as well as pathfinders I have studied in the past, fit this model. They become much more open to new experiences in middle life and find it reinvigorates their senses and adds new flavor to life. They do not equate their expanding aesthetic interests with being "passive" or "femininized." By allowing themselves to stretch well beyond the narrow stereotype of "masculine," they turn the Sexual Diamond into a jewel that can make middle life sparkle.[18]

Dr. Rosener puts on her social scientist's hat to explain the female perspective. "A lot of the fulfillment we women used to get from our husbands, we are now getting at this stage from a sense of mastery. Traditional relationships aren't the be-all and end-all like they used to be. Women have found great excitement in being with other women. These relationships generate a different kind of intimacy than you get from a marriage. We're not talking about sex, which, by the way, continues to exist in long-married relationships, but a pleasure based on shared experiences as women."

The clash is most painfully evident between women in their fifties fired up by postmenopausal zest and men in their fifties slowed down by post-managerial slump—especially those "excessed" by the economic revolution.

A vivid display of this dyssynchrony took place halfway through a daylong interview with a group of male corporate refugees in a small community. The six wounded men were joined at lunch by a sales team of women, also mostly in their fifties, who work for an aggressive, all-female ad agency. The women's entrance had the effect of estrogen shock. They walked in, all sharply suited, almost swaggering with the novelty of competitiveness unleashed, quite full of themselves. They talked about how they work like an all-woman sports team, going up against the other area agencies. "Most of us women are all excited about being beginners again," said one. "And *all* of us are quite successful," asserted another.

The men literally began shrinking and folding their arms protectively around their bodies. One of them muttered, "They remind me of my first wife."

Therapists are seeing more couples distressed enough by this Crossover Crisis to seek help. The therapists tell me that the women tend to be snappish and judgmental with their husbands: "What's the matter with you? Get your act together." The men, they report, are usually in varying states of depression and denial. Some of the Type A men become hostile, acting out their humiliation and rage by blaming everybody else. Others retreat into overwork, diving into their computers from 7:00 A.M. to I:00 A.M., in order to deal with the anxiety of feeling worthless. One psychologist counsels her women clients in this predicament: "Be patient, or you won't *have* a husband at sixty."

Thus can sudden and severe role reversal take a toll, unless a couple understands how to use this exaggeration of the Sexual Diamond to their benefit.

SECRETS OF SERENE POTENCY

As we have seen, men over 45 feel *least* secure about their sexual prowess. Almost half of them admit that they no longer feel the same level of sexual desire.[19] But something else takes its place. There is a major shift in what they value in a relationship as they enter Second Adulthood and later stages. The need for intimacy and companionship eclipses the importance of sex.

The highly educated Professional Men I have surveyed and interviewed show a growing awareness and appreciation of this need for closeness. They now value "intimacy and trust" most in a loving relationship. What they mean by intimacy is closeness, emotional warmth, tenderness, private jokes, and a mutual acceptance of vulnerabilities. A new chemistry seems to come out of this admission of their need for closeness that binds their feelings into a more subtle sexual passion. Only a handful of the Professional Men over 45 say they most prize "revitalized sex." Yet most of them are fully enjoying their sex lives.

> All the Professional Men over 45 who are still in first marriages say that their spouses are now their primary source of intimacy and comfort, all of them—I00 percent.

This challenges the conventional excuse that it's the familiarity of the same old wife that deflates a man's desire and performance. And it's not about a much younger wife. None of these men is married to a woman under 35; they all are married to near peers. Quite a number of the remarried men lean on female friends outside their marriages for intimacy.

Men who make it through male menopause and do find intimacy and trust with one partner can enjoy an equivalent to postmenopausal zest (PMZ) for women; call it SP—Serene Potency. It helps if a man knows what to look for.

BUST-TO-BOOM BANKER, EARLY FIFTIES

"I still liked women's company very much, I liked to talk to them, but I didn't feel compelled to take them to bed. It was much more about affection."

An urbane investment banker described to me his bafflement at how the direction of his sexual energies changed dramatically in his fifties. He was divorced and constantly invited to parties as a highly eligible bachelor-around-town.

"I didn't feel like chasing women anymore. It wasn't a natural instinct, the way it was when I was younger (and then, although I loved the chase and the conquest, I don't remember much about the actual experiences of making love; I just remember the climax and release). I still liked women's company very much, I liked to talk to them, but I didn't feel compelled to take them to bed. It was much more about affection. And I had that from the woman I loved at the time. But I felt like I *should* chase women. They expected it. It went with being a man. So I'd do it. I'd go home with them and take them to bed. But it wasn't very successful, and sometimes it was just a bust. Because I didn't really *feel* it. I was just doing it because I thought I should. And after a while I felt like I was being false to myself, so I found ways to excuse myself from performing.

"This may sound sappy," the banker added. "What I discovered was, as I got older, sex for its own sake wasn't much fun. But sex as a way of expressing love, that is sublime."

In our secular culture sexuality often replaces religion as a means of pursuing the meaning of life. But as the late author Ernest Becker reminded us in *The Denial of Death*, "sex is of the body, and the body is of death."[20] Therefore, when relying upon the sex act as the bottomless well of continually renewed strength, a man sets himself an impossible standard: *perpetual virility.*

NEW-AGE ELECTRICIAN, AGE 52

"Another whole side of myself has been brought to life."

Robert White, an electrical contractor I interviewed in Florida, was conditioned to the standard of perpetual virility. But beneath the rigid behavior codes of his working-class upbringing were hidden the longings of a man both gentle and cerebral by nature.

As a young, broad-shouldered buck with an archetypal American cowboy face, Robert had grown up in an alcoholic household as his "mother's spear carrier," although he never bought into the John Wayne mystique. All the years he was working with his hands day by day as a self-taught multilicensed contractor, he hungered for some balance in his intellectual life. But it seemed he was valued only for his physical powers. He also believed it was his job to initiate any sexual advances.

Divorced in middle life, he met a woman who lectures on miracles. He was astonished at his own delight in being opened up to realms of the imagination and spiritual zones never mentioned inside the ritualized confessionals of organized religion. The woman lecturer also taught him how to enjoy being a receptor of sexual pleasure as well as an active partner in love. She represented *the radiant woman*, a female presence who so often awakens a midlife man to his own humanity. Robert readily acknowledges it was she who released the tenderness in his soul and freed him from his total preoccupation with technical performance on the job and in bed.

"Now it's not so much what's done *to*, as what's done *with*—sharing the experience—that makes sex in my middle life so much more satisfying," he told me. "I feel like another whole side of myself has been brought to life."

Men in Second Adulthood who still find meaning in their work or develop passionate interests or hobbies, who also expand the intimacy in their marriages, and who invest in their physical health and strength, seldom have potency problems. A successful New York surgeon, whose persona seemed all tied up in being the guru followed around on grand rounds by adoring pups in lab coats, retired in his seventies. "Just watch, he'll get depressed and dry up and die," fretted his family. But the man's inner vitality carried over into a passion for studying history, collecting coins, and playing chess until he became proficient enough to enter tournaments. He continued playing tennis twice a week to keep the body tuned up. "He never looked back and never missed a beat," says his admiring son-in-law.

You'll remember that most of the over-45 working-class men in the *Family Circle* survey did not have much intimacy in their marriages. They were more resistant than ever to admitting problems or troubles that might stigmatize them as less of a man. It was rare for them to have friends they could confide in, yet most still weren't interested in closer relationships. Their sex lives reflect this increasing distance from intimacy. The average *Family Circle* man over 45 has sex once a week. (This is less than the norm found in the recent large-scale government study of American sexual behavior: Forty-one percent of all married couples have sex twice a week or more.[21])

The contrast is striking when we look at the *Family Circle* men who scored highest in well-being. They spend a lot more time with their wives—an average of six hours a day—many of them presumably as partners in small businesses. They are more involved with friends and spiritual pursuits. These men seem to look upon the aging process as a second chance. And at the end of the day they enjoy sex with their wives much more often than the average *Family Circle* man.

THE SAVE-YOUR-LIFE WIFE

"I've come across a lot more women who can and do live alone in their fifties, sixties, and seventies," says Maidenbaum, the Jungian analyst. "Men, almost invariably, need a partner."

Men who do make the personality transformation from conquering to connecting may even learn how to create a friendship network or a men's group. These more extensive sources of intimacy become a lifeline—literally. But the biggest factor in protecting older men against depression and prolonging their lives may be the save-your-life wife.

> Men from the ages of 45 to 64 who live with wives are twice as likely to live ten years longer than their unmarried counterparts.

That was the stark conclusion of a large-scale study of survival factors in more than seven thousand American adults by the University of California, San Francisco.[22] Being married remains for men the strongest link with male survival, even after one accounts for differences in income and education and such risk factors as smoking, drinking, obesity, and inactivity. The greatest surprise to the researchers at the University of California, San Francisco, was to discover that it's not just *any* woman who is a lifesaver; the same benefit is not enjoyed by men who simply have live-in lady friends or who reside with their grown children, parents, or other relatives.[23] As other studies have confirmed, there is something special about wives that protects men from depression.[24]

Men often tell me in interviews, "My wife has helped me to discover aspects of myself I never knew were there." Wives are often able to put a man in touch with his repressed rage at having his talents or efforts ignored, or to help him bring to the surface corrosive emotions he didn't even know he had been feeling. Wives are the sensibility specialists.

First wives often get a bum rap. Many men I've interviewed describe their first wives the same way: "She's a nice lady, but . . ." What's surprising is how little they ever knew about this "nice lady." If they stick with the first wife until middle life, they may be as surprised as was John Updike when he wrote the Rabbit trilogy. In *Rabbit Is Rich*, Harry ("Rabbit") Angstrom is 46 and suddenly envious of the wisdom, energy, and "middle-aged friskiness" he sees in his wife, Janice, the "dumb mutt" of earlier books. Updike acknowledges: "The decade past has taught her more than it has taught him; often she has [the more] mature answers while he is the ignorant questioner."[25]

Of course, a husband and wife of roughly the same age may have such different needs and goals in Second Adulthood they simply cannot regenerate each other. To escape the sharper edges of the Sexual Diamond, a man may well marry a younger woman. All of a sudden there is another meaning in his life. He has someone new to protect. If she's a child-woman, he can teach her about the world. If she's a rising star in her field, he can become her promoter or her investor, if not her business partner. And if she wants a child, as she usually does, he becomes challenged to be the main provider all over again.

"Some of these men are attracted to a younger wife because they have the potential for remaining young themselves," says Maidenbaum. "In that case a man will learn from the marriage. But if he's really threatened by getting older, the contrast with his young wife will probably cause him to deteriorate faster. It can go either way."

THE DIVORCE SPRINGBOARD

One of the unmarked revolutions of the last twenty years is the resistance of women in middle life to remarriage. The ranks of divorcées between 40 and 54 have grown the most rapidly of any age-group since 1970, but these divorcées are radically different from the dumped middle-aged wives who were ubiquitous in an earlier generation.[26] Demographers say that increasingly these women are *choosing* to remain single, rather than sacrifice their independence. As long as they are able to support themselves in a reasonable style, once having tasted financial and sexual freedom, and now that they are beyond childbearing years, they view most offers of remarriage as a bad deal. They don't want to "knuckle under" ever again.[27]

While divorce is always painful, it is seen in retrospect as a springboard by many of the women I have interviewed in the Silent Generation. The forced assertion of self, plus the educational pursuits so many have resumed, open up a whole new range of possibilities for progress as women grow older. Only one of the divorced or widowed extraordinaries among the New Women over 50 whom I interviewed is losing sleep over finding a new husband. Having earned their self-confidence through crisis and turmoil, they guard it fiercely.[28] A recent study of several hundred "typical" white middle-class American women front-runners of the Baby Boom Generation, and their slightly older counterparts, confirmed that divorce spurs a woman's psychological growth: "Suddenly single—whether by choice or default—most felt unburdened for the first time in their lives. And they weren't risking remarriage if it meant being restricted. They were out to discover who they were."[29]

But what turns out to be a divorce springboard for many women represents a slippery slope for many men. Most middle-aged men are reluctant returnees to single life. In my interviews with divorced men of 40 to mid-fifties, the common theme is a sense of failure and downgraded self-worth. More often than not, these men will confess that their wives instigated the divorce.

VICTORIA'S REAL SECRET
—SEXUAL POWER SURGES

The best-kept secret about today's older woman is that once she has outgrown the proscriptions to be a good girl, she may allow herself a license for lust. Passion not only is possible after waists thicken but becomes a pursuit of women just as often as men. The *New Women* subscribers who responded to my survey are open about saying that part of their radical change was becoming sexually adventurous as they got older.[30] Half of all the women surveyed who are over 50, both married and single, admit to having taken younger lovers. And almost a quarter of them have made love with men who were *at least twenty years younger!*

Some of these women mention in interviews that their husbands are no longer as interested in sex as they themselves are. A substantial number of them—four in ten—have had extramarital affairs, a considerably higher infidelity rate than seen in most surveys of even younger married women. The reason often given is their husbands' impotency.

Mary Ann Goff rediscovered sexual passion in her Flaming Fifties. The small-town Ohio woman who attended the Flaming Fifties celebration brunch had endured years of sexual drought with a husband who refused to go for counseling before she left him and started over in a southern city. She had found an ardent younger lover, but her academic course work required them to live in different cities. A believer that being sexually active is the true fountain of youth, Mary Ann had proof during that semester-long near celibacy.

"I saw a great difference in my appearance and body," she says. "I think there's a particular sparkle in your eyes when you have constant touching and talking with a lover. And the actual intercourse keeps your sexual organs stimulated inside," she believes. "Without it, you're there but moving in slow motion, half depressed, half dead. When you're with someone, stimulated, being touched, you don't feel your age; you feel young!"

At present Mary Ann, who has turned 60, has a platonic relationship with a pleasant dinner partner, but she is confidently shopping for a new, healthy lover—a man not on heart medicine, not a smoker, and not an alcoholic. Her son-in-law told her, without a trace of irony, "Your standards are too high." Mary Ann finds her biggest critics are her prudish adult offspring. Her daughter keeps scolding, "Oh, *Mother.* What are we going to do with a mom who's sixty and wears string bikinis and sheer teddies?"

"Take heed!" Mary Ann tells her. "It might revive *your* marriage."

Women with younger lovers generally echo Mary Ann's view that lively lovers keep them youthful in body and spirit. Of course, older men have known this secret for years. For many women, however, the problem about sex over 50 is not their reluctance to follow Masters and Johnson's mantra—*Use it or lose it*—but rather, *Whom to use it with?* They often mark themselves down most cruelly as too old to be appealing when indeed, there is no reason a healthy, fit woman in her fifties shouldn't be sexually desirable.

FINDING YOUR PASSION WITHOUT A MAN

"The older I get, the less I find the men of my generation appealing," says Jeanette Fruen, then a vibrant divorcée in her fifties with a peripatetic career as a political consultant. She thought she should date only "age-appropriate men," meaning around her age. A male friend told her, "Oh, get off it. They'd never keep up with you. An age-appropriate man for you would be ten years younger."

Ann Stunden, the director of an academic computing center who pulled out of the pits of alcoholism in her late forties, found that once she was sober, 50, and more honest, direct, and charming than before, younger men seemed to get crushes on her. "Men of forty are so much more enlightened than the guys my age," she says, reflecting a common observation by older women. "And men in their thirties are even more so. They're not all hung up with the sexism and ownership that is ingrained in men over sixty. They're easier to connect to."

What does she get out of the relationship with a younger man?

Ann laughs heartily. "A bit of adoration. Tender loving care. Of course, I get love from my adult kids [who lived with her off and on until recently], but there's this little kicker that comes with it: *Did you go to the grocery store, Mom?* I've got one young man who floats in and out of my life. He doesn't ask for anything except my time. He's in another city."

Ann now places the greatest value on her long-term friendships with other women. "I find the women my age much more interesting than the men." When she visited her young lover's city for a recent weekend, she spent the whole time hanging out and howling at old stories with two of her soul sisters. The young man was hurt and curious. "Why did you prefer to be with them than with me?" Ann had to think about it. "My women friends feel like they're part of my life forever. You feel like you're part of my life just for now." He said he understood.

The great lure the older woman holds for the younger man seems to be sex and soul feeding without obligation. "I'm not looking to them to give up their life as they know it and marry me," says Ann. "I talk with them about their souls. And they enjoy the extra fifteen years of experience I bring to bear."

It would be nice to have a partner to share the in-between moments of life, but typical of formerly married women in the middle, Ann is not actively looking. "Living with a partner again would mean I'd have to give up some of the things I do, and run according to somebody else's schedule. Living alone or with adult kids means I can come and go at my pleasure."

Both men and women in the middle, if they're unattached, adopt the pattern of the early twenties. Half of all single American men between the ages of 45 and 64 live alone, but among the many who do share a household it is usually with women to whom they are not married. This is true for two thirds of men up to the age of 65, according to never-published data obtained from Census Bureau figures.[31] Women over 45 without husbands are very likely to be living with other relatives. But a great many unmarried, widowed, or divorced females between 45 and 65 are also living with men they have no plans to marry.[32] Others turn to celibacy, self-gratification, or recycling old boyfriends.

Still, many women in the middle, especially those who have lived with traditional men for most of their adult lives, are starving for intimacy. A growing issue for such women is opening up to the possibilities of same-sex intimacy. Clinical experience suggests that the number of women who were previously heterosexual and who are choosing or exploring gay lifestyles in middle life is growing and may well be above 50 percent. The psychological literature reports, "They describe finding intimacy with women at levels and depths they have never before imagined or experienced."[33]

Can a woman enjoy the new powers of the Sexual Diamond if she's on her own? You bet. Women don't have to apologize for wanting power after they're no longer sex objects. And once they hold postmenopausal high status, they find it easier to become peers with older men. The gender competition is noticeably diluted. It is observable in corridors of power—even in the United States Senate, as Barbara Mikulski discovered.

"I ran for the Senate *after* my midlife crisis," Senator Mikulski told me. She gave up her very safe seat in the House of Representatives to run for that more exclusive legislative body in her fiftieth year. "I didn't need to go for the Senate for life fulfillment," she emphasized, "and it was a *very* risky run. But I feel so much surer of myself and energetic after postmenopause. I just love my fifties!"

It shows. The diminutive Maryland activist was one of the nonconformists of the Silent Generation. The only aisle she has ever walked down is that of the U.S. Senate, where she was sworn in as the first Democratic woman to win a seat in her own right. She finds that the men in that chamber, who tend to be older than the men in the House, behave in a much more collegial manner toward her. At this stage in their lives, and hers, she is able to command their respect more than she arouses their competitive instincts. In 1994 Barbara Mikulski struck another first: She was elected by her Senate colleagues to be secretary of the Democratic caucus, the highest leadership position a Democratic woman has ever held in the U.S. legislature.

As people like Kathleen Brown and Dr. Judith Rosener and Barbara Mikulski break the old stereotypical molds in their respective fields, more women will be encouraged to expand their own managerial or political potentials. And as new men like the bachelor banker and the New Age electrician discover the subtler pleasures of sharing love over simply performing sex as they grow older, while other men demonstrate the possibilities for heroism in acts of conciliation and community building, the dimensions of the Sexual Diamond will be extended for everyone.

Part Six

PASSAGE
TO THE AGE OF
INTEGRITY

16

THE SERENE SIXTIES

*B*link. Even as he mixes bright colors, the zoo of animal-shaped clouds moving over his head metamorphoses into a dark and menacing mass. He changes brushes. His brush is still saturated with mauve when the dark clouds resorb and a sheet of white appears. Blink. Now sunlight rips a hole of blue through those opaque clouds, but as surely as he will dip a brush into the cerulean and a new glower will again fill the sky. How like his life. Was there no predictability?

After the widower had spent a month under the hood of Ireland's changeable clouds, his mood lifted of its own accord. He was bedding with nobody these nights, still alone and lonely, having buried his beloved wife two years before. But amazingly he seemed to have recovered his buoyancy. It wouldn't be going too far to say, as he later did to me, "I feel much younger. My whole time sense is rejiggered. I feel I have much more time now. Rationally I know that's ridiculous. Anything can happen, you can drop dead tomorrow, but I have something I love to do, a new dream."

You would never guess who was talking. It was Fitzgerald, the broody 65-year-old New York artist who had "retired" into male menopause in an earlier chapter. I promised we'd return to him. But where we find him, only a year later, is back with a burst of ebullience.

During the four long, involuntarily celibate years when his wife was too ill to want him, Fitzgerald had considered taking a mistress. "I didn't want my sex life to fade away," he admitted. But whenever he maneuvered a woman into position, he had to withdraw. "I would have felt terrible about betraying my wife." There was also the fear. His spouse had let him know that if he strayed, she would probably get a gun and blow him away. Even after her death the residual fear and guilt contributed to a classic Widower's Impotence. I had encouraged Fitzgerald to contact Dr. Helen Singer Kaplan and her brilliant team of sex therapists at New York Hospital. After some initial reluctance he made an appointment.

On the basis of his answers in the first interview, the therapist told Fitzgerald he was not impotent. What a reprieve! The man walked off sexual death row, but he wasn't dumb enough this time to resist professional help. He had gone back to the therapist once a month for the previous year. She gave him tricks and tips to encourage his erotic fantasies, cheering him on; she helped him rebuild his confidence chink by decayed chink. His lady friend fully cooperated. As his sex drive gradually returned, he began taking better care of himself, walking the forty blocks downtown to his studio and loving the freedom to notice his surroundings rather than crabbing up in the subway on the way to performing as an office slug. He cut down to one cocktail at dinner, or none. When Fitzgerald and I last met for dinner, he was in the final stage of his recovery from male menopause. He had thrown out his pipes and cigars.

"See how much whiter my teeth are?" He grinned. He did look and smell much fresher than the sourly sweet, tobacco-stained, timid and ghostly man who had just about given up on himself a year before. He had started breathing deeply again. He was even aware of the greater force of juices pumping into his phallus and supporting his sexual rehabilitation.

"Within three weeks of treatment I felt a surge of power," he enthused. "And my sexual revival has made a terrific difference. I'm back in my early forties again. Well, let's not go overboard, but the gap is rapidly narrowing. It's amazing I've come as far as I have."

Fitzgerald's revival cannot be ascribed simply to the change of mind-set that helped him cure his habit of impotence. Lust and hope are back, yes, but he also has an audacious new dream.

"Hell, I've been a breadwinner all my life," he recounted. "I've gone to the office and written jillions of inches of copy and enjoyed professional success [as an art critic]. But I'm no longer interested in being a shining success in the downtown world. Heading into my sixties, I wanted to do something different. Now I've found it. Painting."

The desire to paint had been there for years, maybe as far back as his high school days in Brooklyn, but the notion of making one's living in the arts was a fey and foreign concept among most men of the World War II Generation. Fine art was hardly something a Brooklyn boy could discuss with a father who spent himself as a foreman in a cap factory. The young Fitzgerald had no role models and furthermore didn't even know it. All he knew was he had to escape the highest aspiration his teachers had prepared for him: a Brooklyn high school principal.

Unknowingly in his late forties he had seeded the ground of being that would flourish for his third age. He had begun taking formal art classes. He studied portraiture and spent his Saturdays and certain designated evenings doing paintings of friends. After some years of this amateur dabbling, he had a gnawing thought that he might never have the chance to express himself fully in art. It wasn't enough anymore to be just a critic. He wanted to be the creator.

"At sixty-six, I can take the risk of being a professional painter," he said jauntily. "If it takes me twenty years to establish myself, that's little enough. It's a great challenge—more internal than external. I don't have to be scared the way I would have been as a younger man. I have nothing to lose. I've already proven myself in my first life."

He must earn an income from this painting business, of course. With a body of work to show, together with his enthusiasm as a huckster, he is attracting commissions to do portraits. A gallery showed his Irish paintings. A lifelong professional artist who saw the show addressed Fitzgerald with a new tone of respect and encouraged him to pitch his dream even higher— so high, it is guaranteed to outlast his lifetime. "I want to paint the kinds of paintings you see in museums."

More important than all the rest is this: Fitzgerald is in love again. With the clouds of Ireland, the landscapes of Europe, the faces of his friends just begging for portraiture—all of these ravish him now, the way his women used to do. And this expanding ardor gives him back his power. He can enter his subjects and explore their inner contradictions, even make love to them, all with his paintbrush.

When we last had dinner, an exquisite young Asian waitress asked us for our order. Fitzgerald was so intent upon studying her face, he forgot even food. As the waitress turned with a toss of her gleaming hair, he said, "Mmm, I'd *love* to paint her." He said it with devout desire, not with the desire for sexual conquest but for a full creative engagement with beauty and intimacy.

Still, the glint is back in his eye. Fitzgerald has begun thinking like a hunter again. *Hey, the sex isn't bad. Why not ask for love too?* "I have to face the fact I want a wife," he told me matter-of-factly. "I want the traditional marriage. Because the truth is, I'm scared of growing old alone."

Nothing wrong with Fitzgerald's survival instinct. The only problem is his lady friend, Elena, the same loving and sexually responsive woman he has been with since his wife's death. Elena too has endured the lingering death of a beloved spouse. She is allergic to remarriage. Her candid argument to Fitzgerald is simply "I don't want to go through that ever again. I'd be terrified you'd die on me."

"I'm not the one who goes!" he insisted. "It's my wives who go." But he hadn't had the courage to push her to an ultimatum; the nightmare was he'd sweep her off her feet and a few years later she'd be sorry: *Who is this tired old rooster sleeping in my bed?* Ah, but now he was crowing again. No more shying away from the M word. When Elena backed out of the apartment they were about to buy together, he confronted the issue: "My time line is this: Marry me next month, or forget it." It finally became clear that she was more terrified of taking the chance of commitment and losing another husband than of remaining semidetached.

Fitzgerald took this rejection in stride. By now he had enough respect for himself that he was ready to go out into the market again and shop for a wife. He had no trouble conjuring up what the marriage of a Serene Sixties could be like; vivid pictures of it cut across his daily life and worked their way into his lonely sleep.

"I want a woman who can bring her own intellectual and artistic treasures. I'd be open to them, and I'll show her mine. In my fantasy it would be like walking through the galleries of each other's minds, able to appreciate what each other has spent a lifetime collecting and cultivating." He spoke passionately, unapologetically, using declarative sentences for the first time in some years: "I want love. I want companionship. I want sex. I want bodily comfort on a Sunday afternoon, sharing pizza and curling up to watch an old movie. I don't just need a nurse. I feel now I have a lot more in me that I can give."

This was as clear a declaration of emancipation as I've ever heard from a person coming out of a long hard passage. After applauding, I reminded Fitzgerald of what he'd sounded like just a year before.

"But I was an old man a year ago!"

Fitzgerald is not the norm, of course; he is the inspiration. He shook himself out of creeping despair to feel aliveness again. His story reminds those of us who are younger how important it is to begin investing in "a new self" at the beginning of Second Adulthood, so that when we run into the life accidents common to the sixties, we will still have a self-generated passion

to carry us through. That commitment will determine the triumph of aliveness over stagnation.

The more familiar, old-style man in his sixties is depicted by novelist
Joseph Heller in his sequel to *Catch-22*, one of the most influential novels
of the postwar age. His protagonist, Yossarian, the cynical bombardier
whose efforts to avoid flying combat missions cast the heroism of World
War II in a new light, is now up against a more insidious enemy: the incip-
ient depression of aging. Mr. Heller, having reached 72 himself, acknowledges that the sequel's title, *Closing Time,* comes directly from his stage in life
and is meant to signal the dying out of the World War II Generation whose
members are now roughly age 65 to 80.[1]

Yossarian, like Fitzgerald, finds himself living alone for only the second
time in his life, widowed, but helpless to escape his own morbid thoughts
and the "neurotic barrage of confusing physical symptoms to which he had
become increasingly susceptible...." He is like those people one sees in
their sixties anesthetizing themselves with alcohol and still defiantly dragging on cigars or cigarettes, indignantly defensive when their kids plead with
them to stop: "If I have to give up the few things I still enjoy, what's the
point of living?" They slip from benign stagnation into depression; their
health deteriorates, thus confirming their claim that they haven't much time
to live or much else to live for. Their social supports thin out, even close
relations find excuses to stay away, and as they slip further into isolation,
they dig themselves into a tunnel of despair.

Yossarian is desperate for attention but isolated by his own narcissism.
Heller admits that his hero simply "could not learn to live alone. He could
not make a bed. He would sooner starve than cook." So he checks himself
into the hospital for "observation"—the problem is he's in perfect health—
but he is nonetheless able to command a constant round of specialists and
pretty nurses to attend his bedside, dispensing TLC, briefly distracting him
from his fears of stroke, entropy, radiation, and gravity, and allowing him
"budding erections" again.

A busy and successful entrepreneur of 65 I interviewed started out by
saying, "Let me tell you something about the sixties. You are absolutely,
totally unconscious that you are *in* them. You feel like you're still in your
fifties." And today in many ways you are. It seems that a peculiarity of the
change in time sense in the sixties is the way the mind shuttles back and
forth between feeling "old" and a day later feeling obstinately "still young."
The first time the ticket seller at the movie house looks up and says, "Senior
citizen discount?" is one of the first and worst "old" days. A "still-young"

day is when you let go and allow something spontaneous and maybe even magic to happen. "As you get older," a former workaholic told me, "you find more ways to snatch the time to do the *un*necessary and satisfying."

To a large degree we get up and put on the age we feel each morning. Fitzgerald's remark "But last year I was an old man" is indicative. In his desperately lonely, timid, and self-doubting phase, he had shuffled around and smelled of stale tobacco. Now he struts and sparkles with wit and enthusiasm. Depending upon the persona we present to the world—the spring or drag in our step, the lusty laughter or cynical sneer, the lively curiosity or the curmudgeonly indifference we express in conversation—we signal to people how "old" we are, much more than any chronological number. And today it is almost impossible to tell a vital sixtysomething from a phlegmatic 50-year-old.

READY FOR PRIME TIME

The sixties have changed just as dramatically as the earlier stages of middle life. "People who used to be considered old at sixty-five are usually still in their prime at that age today," says Dr. Sanford Finkel, director of the Buehler Center on Aging at Northwestern University.[2] What with beta-blockers and hip replacements, you're as likely to run into a man of 65 Rollerblading in the park as biking along with his youngest child, enjoying the adolescent boy in himself as well as the recycled father. "Don't call me Grandpa!" groans the second-time-around dad to the progeny of his first family. He sees himself as still 40, well, on good days, when he's watching his young son's soccer game and going home to the mirror of a younger second wife.

A profound change in the way we register time accompanies every major passage. But the startling new perspective on time that now characterizes the passage into the third age may not catch up with us until we've settled down to wait for old age to descend. When it doesn't, and only then, do we wake up.

A 61-year-old public relations man walks into Columbia Presbyterian Medical Center's East Side satellite clinic in New York to get the results of an omnibus three-day physical.[3] The lead doctor shows him a video film of his own heart from the inside, beating. He shows him pictures of the inside of his gut, taken by an instrument with a TV camera attached. The results are good. "Now," says the doctor, "we have to think about how we're going to manage the next twenty or thirty years of your life."

The man is stunned. "Twenty or thirty years?"

"It's not that unusual," the doctor says. "You've already made it past sixty, and you have an eighty-nine-year-old mother."

"I never thought of *managing* my life much beyond sixty-five."

"That's right. It's an exercise in management. You make a long-term business plan, don't you? Well, you need to make a body plan, to keep everything up and running smoothly until the last years of your life."

It's an Aha! moment. The dials are suddenly whirring inside the man's head. Thirty more years—this throws off all his calculations. He needs a new life plan. It's at this point, if not before, that a man has to ask himself some tough questions: *Do you really want to spend the next twenty years working at what you've been doing? If you were counting on early retirement, do you really want to spend thirty years watching TV, planting bulbs, and trying to shave ten strokes off your golf handicap?*

"But suppose I get prostate cancer when I'm seventy?" the PR man challenges his doctor. "Do I *want* to live that long?"

"You won't die of prostate cancer."

"Why not?"

"Because when we're older, our cells don't divide that fast. You'll die from something acute, and you probably won't be chronically ill until the last couple of years."

You may recall the new calculation by an NIH medical director: If men can get through to age 60 without dying of heart disease, they can expect to be stronger and less bothered by chronic ailments than women.[4] While a minority of older people suffer from a lifetime of neglect and are in serious need of societal support, the vast majority of over-sixties are quite able, both physically and mentally, to function independently.

> Only 10 percent of Americans 65 and over have a chronic health problem that restricts them from carrying on a major activity.[5]

"It is simply not true that, because of aging, older people are destined to be ill, impoverished, cut off from society, sexually incapacitated, despondent, or unable to reason or to remember," wrote Matilda White Riley, D.Sc., L.H.D., with John W. Riley, Jr., Ph.D., LL.D., on the basis of research conducted in the late 1980s, when she was an associate director of the

National Institute on Aging.[6] "Although death is inevitable, the course of the aging process is not."

Not only are today's retirees far healthier than they have been in the past, but they are also remarkably mobile. *Modern Maturity* magazine claims from its market research that over-50 retirees are hitting the highways or airports for an average of *seven* vacations or personal trips around the United States in the space of a year (only 19 percent of their travel is for business). When they're not being lured to Orlando, Las Vegas, or L.A., they're winging it to Europe or the Caribbean. And for each of these pleasure jaunts they are prepared to shell out an average of nearly $1,500.[7]

Societies have not caught up with the implications of these phenomenal changes in the predictable life course. The proportion of the U.S. population aged 65 and over will reach 12.7 percent in the year 2000.[8] Italy has already tipped the balance scales in the graying of affluent nations, becoming in 1994 the first country in the world with more people over 65 than young people under 15.[9] Not to panic. The economic revolution from a heavy-industry base should ultimately work in favor of the new young-old. If they are well educated—the great dividing line—they can be productive much longer in an information- and service-based economy, where it's possible to tote a personal computer with full-color sales presentations instead of a heavy sample case or to work from home by fax modem instead of commuting to a city office.

Never before have so many been so thoroughly self-governing in their sixties. Not only are people living much longer, but in social welfare societies like America and most of Western Europe, they are also more financially secure than ever. Men 65 and over are the *only* age-group among American males whose money income picture improved over the eighteen years from 1974 to 1992.[10] With liberal Social Security benefits and increases tied to the cost of living, these favored citizens increased in median money income (adjusted to '92 dollars) by 15 percent. And for women 65 and over, hitting Social Security age has been an economic bonanza, moving them up in median money income by 27 percent. Even getting old doesn't present nearly the specter of impoverishment it traditionally did. Since the 1960s in the United States poverty among the elderly has been reduced from an average of 35 to 12 percent.[11]

Clearly the vast majority of American and European women and men now in their sixties have reached the stage where maximum freedom still coexists with a minimum of physical limitations. As a result, the age cues for what it means to be 60 don't match up with people's actual experience.

GROWING BRAIN

Recent research by neurobiologists runs counter to our most basic fears about mental decline with aging. Brain cells don't die off in annual batches of a hundred thousand, as we believed; rather, they shrink or grow dormant in old age, particularly from lack of stimulation and challenge.[12] But even in an older developed brain, "sprouting" can take place, in which new neural processes form additional synapses.[13] Nearly one third of individuals enjoy full mental alertness throughout late age, according to a new study.[14] And some, in their eighties and nineties, surpass almost every other age-group to rank near the top on applied brainpower.

All of the common denominators among sharp-as-a-tack subjects tested in older age-groups are by-products of a lifelong investment in mental challenges: They have above-average educations, they enjoy complex and stimulating lifestyles, and they are married to smart spouses.[15]

Most researchers agree that no functional mental decline occurs before 60 or 65. Short-term memory can become somewhat less reliable. But the vast memory banks in which we have been making deposits over a lifetime continue to grow more sophisticated over the years. What is vulnerable to wear and tear with age is the brain's "hardware"—the billions of telephone line–like connections and relay switches that transmit messages from one brain cell to another,[16] as described by U.S. News & World Report. But some neurologists now believe that we shouldn't concede even this aspect of brainpower to aging. We may be able to boot up the brain's memory with psychoactive drugs that mimic the memory hormones that decline with age.[17] But even without any medical intervention, some mental skills remain relatively undiminished well into old age. One of those is the ability to concentrate, as the next story affirms.

Hugh Downs, the veteran newsman and popular cohost of the TV show 20/20, is one of many who find scholarship to be a most satisfying pursuit of late middle age. Downs had always been fascinated by medicine. "The amateur doctor" his wife called him teasingly. Come his mid-sixties, Downs decided amateur wasn't satisfying enough. He plunged into a post–master's degree program in gerontology and earned his degree while working full-time.

"The whole idea that older people don't learn as well is pure nonsense," he scoffed.[18] "Maybe split-second brain functions slow down after about age forty-eight, but we're talking about microseconds that you wouldn't even notice in a conversation. Mental computation speed is more than offset by

acquired techniques, accumulated wisdom, and *focus.*" He chuckled, recall-
ing the antsiness of his twenties, the horniness, the million-and-one insecurities and distractions that punctuate our attention spans when we're
younger. "My concentration has actually improved," said Downs.

The payoff came when the television star was admitted, at age 70, to
study with medical students in Mount Sinai Medical Center's outstanding
gerontology program. The medical center didn't quite know what to do with
its gerontological wonder boy. It wasn't possible to board-certify him because
he wasn't a physician, but it was decided to give him a diploma anyway. "I
squeaked through, but I did make it." He smiled, his handsome face suffused
with internal satisfaction. Subsequently Downs wrote a practical guidebook
for those who are interested in mapping out their journeys, *Fifty to Forever.*[19]

THE HUNGER FOR HARMONY

The paramount concern of the sixties is: *What will my life add up to? Is it too late
to put more meaning into my life before I'm old? Do I want to be remembered only for this?*

As we draw toward the end of the Age of Mastery in the early sixties, the
shadow of late age begins to fall across our path. But it opens up another
uncharted and deeply meaningful passage, this one to the illumination (or
despair) of the Age of Integrity. Just as in every other major passage, during
late middle age we enjoy a heightened potential for making a leap of growth,
but we can also fall back into entropy or depression or simply ignore the
impulse to change and remain stuck. Erikson conceived of the eighth and
final stage of adult development as a struggle between integrity and despair.
Despair is easy to define: a surrender to the conviction that time is too short
to start another life or try out alternative paths to integrity.[20]

But what does *integrity* really mean? Erikson himself admitted it is difficult to define, suggesting that it is a state of mind assured of order and
meaning, a capacity for postnarcissistic love, and the serenity to bless and
defend one's own life history: "It is the acceptance of one's one and only life
cycle as something that had to be . . . it thus means a new, a different love of
one's parents."[21] Yeats, the great Irish poet, reviewed the two halves of his
adult life in a poem written in his sixties, "A Dialogue of Self and Soul."
After recounting the pain of self-doubts in the first half and the pain of
opposition from his enemies in the second half, Yeats declares his willingness to forgive himself and "cast out remorse." And with that expiation of
guilt and remorse, he is enlivened with sweetness and well-being.[22]

I think of integrity as the work of integration. One of the overarching desires often articulated by men and women I have interviewed in late middle age is for balance—being able to bring all the parts of one's life into harmony, as opposed to incongruity. The need becomes pressing for an emotional integration of all the different roles and the serial identities that have served us through adolescence and middlescence. It is time for *coalescence.* What is the essence of ourselves that we want to leave behind?

An architect, for example, told me he remembered in his hotheaded forties going to work and shouting at people all day, then going home and acting like the good father and the honest husband, then fooling around on the side and lying about it. "It becomes more difficult to lie to yourself as you get older," he ruminated when I interviewed him in his sixties. I asked him if he was trying harder at this stage to achieve a balance between the different parts of his life. "By now I don't feel like I'm playing one role in my work life and another role in my love life and another in my family life and my friendships." A transition from incongruity to harmony sounded right to him. He had an important elaboration to add from the perspective of actually being in his sixties:

"I don't know how to put this . . . you don't want to feel any part of your life is *unauthentic,*" the architect said. "It's not that you have to act the same way in all situations. But whatever is real, whatever you perceive yourself to be, you discover is not endlessly adaptable to circumstance."

The search for your own authenticity—the core self that embodies the values and loyalties for which you stand—begins earlier in Second Adulthood when the false self is first confronted. Much that is false about yourself, tailored to please or perform for others, will already have been sloughed off if you are still developing. What is different about reaching for your own truth in the sixties is that nobody can dictate to you anymore. And there is nobody really to blame. You own your own integrity—or despair—as inescapably as your joys and sorrows are etched into the face that looks back at you from the mirror every morning.

SPECIAL POWERS OF THE SIXTIES

What strengths have we accumulated to take with us into the Age of Integrity? Resilience is probably the most important protection one can have. People who have met and mastered most of the passages and predictable crises of life up to now are, by definition, resilient. Late middle age brings them to the culmination of the developmental gains of the Age of Mastery. The most valuable of these is the ability in any emotional crisis to control their first impulses and unruly feelings. They wait until they can give appropriate and measured responses—"I'll give you my answer tomorrow (or the next day)"—in short, they have attained self-mastery.

An impressive study of the sources of well-being in men at 65 found that by that age the harbinger of emotional health in men was not a stable childhood or a high-flying career. Rather, among older men it was much more important to have developed an ability to handle life's accidents and conflicts without passivity, blaming, or bitterness. "It's having the capacity to hold a conflict or impulse in consciousness without acting on it," concluded George E. Vaillant, a psychiatrist at Dartmouth Medical School, who has been scrutinizing the same 173 Harvard men at five-year intervals since they were graduated in the early 1940s and joined the Grant Study.[23]

Self-mastery also allows us to develop a deeper appreciation for the complexity of human life. As psychologist Thomas Moore writes in his book *Care of the Soul,* "Often care of the soul means not taking sides when there is a conflict at a deep level. It may be necessary to stretch the heart wide enough to embrace contradiction and paradox."[24] The outstretched heart and open mind also seem to be important in the endurance of the centenarians. They view the world with bemused detachment and very little bitterness. Rather than be dogmatic, they are still curious, still absorbing, and accepting of the new.[25]

Time does heal. The Grant Study of Harvard men, done over a period of many years, adds confirmation. Even the most painful and traumatic events in childhood had virtually no effect on the well-being of these men by their mid-sixties, although severe depression earlier in life did predispose some to continuing problems.[26] Traits that turned out to contribute to happiness in the golden years were *not* the same ones that had won friends and influenced people back in their college days: spontaneity, creative flair, and the knack of easy sociability. Instead traits important to smooth functioning as we get older are being dependable, well organized, and pragmatic.

To put it in business terms, people in their sixties are at the subtotal stage. It may still be a long way from the final tally, but people you know are already dying. Their vacancy is a silent reminder that death could crash the party anytime. And with that changed perspective on death, there is a sense of time passing constantly faster.

"Fifteen minutes after fifty you are sixty, and then in ten minutes more you are eighty-five," said Don Marquis, a New York writer.[27]

Not really. Although it does often appear that time passes much faster, there is a great deal going on.

PERMISSION TO PLAY

But let's be honest. "Openness to change" is one of those totems to which we pay lip service. In practice most of my efforts and probably yours, as we slouch toward the third age, go into maximizing our control, trying to know it all, reducing the necessity to change and the inclination to risk. Our efforts are spurred on by commercials promising that if we simply pop enough vitamins, slather on enough cream, flay enough flesh off our thighs, and lube and tune the sexual hydraulic system, we will be armed against the invasions of age. Many people slip into an approach that might be called *life prevention.* And in this grasping for control, something very precious we had as children is lost: the exposure to surprise.

How, if we don't march ourselves out to the end of a limb and jump in new directions now and then, shall we continue to learn? And if we don't continue to learn, how shall we continue to develop? Because children are repeatedly faced with novel and challenging experiences, they are constantly developing the plasticity to deal with them. The quickest way to learn, in my experience, is to interrupt your everyday, predictable existence. Put yourself on the line. Introduce a new task or adventure of the heart, and in that one domain give up some control. The intrinsic reward for putting oneself back into the wobbly-kneed state of a learner is the return of a sense of playfulness and curiosity and the sharp edge of uncertainty. One is simply forced to stop taking oneself so seriously.

For men in particular, "Ennui, emptiness, is the constant enemy that circumvents the ageing man in every sort of way...," as the nineteenth-century artist Eugene Delacroix mused in a letter he wrote at the age of 57.[28] B. J. George of Bernardsville, New Jersey, a law professor before he felt the call to the ministry, is a newly ordained deacon in the Methodist Church at 67 years of age. He told me he sees many of his parishioners in their sixties spending more and more time at home. "I view that as relinquishing what has been meaningful. They start slipping into a spiritual and social isolation."[29]

Paradoxically the problem of regaining playfulness and curiosity is exaggerated for those who have a history of success in the world. Earlier in their careers they could stumble and get away with it. But by their sixties they often find themselves on pedestals and feel apprehensive about stepping off to start something new. They become burdened by the chores of maintaining and polishing their own reputations for posterity. Highly successful people have usually made work central to their lives. They may still enjoy their work, but often they can't seem to figure out how to let themselves play.

THE DESIGNER WHO LEARNED TO PLAY AT 63

"I was doing something I didn't know how to do. And I was learning how to do it."

Aaron Coleman Webb was in a classic early midlife crisis when I first interviewed him for *Passages* (and used the same pseudonym). The supports of success were not holding; for too long he had used his work to avoid scrutinizing what his life was all about. By the 1990s he was virtually canonized as one of the most influential designers of our time, one who had spawned countless disciples and imitators whose very atavistic hunger to replace him had begun to nibble at his own sense of self-worth, not to mention making it more difficult for him to get commissions.

I found Aaron at his studio, as usual, bent over a light board selecting negatives. I reminded him that he was 43 when I first interviewed him about being in midlife.

"What did I know then?" He chuckled. "That was twenty years ago. I'm sixty-three now."

I asked him what 63 feels like.

"I've had great difficulty understanding what sixty means," he said honestly, "outside of the body beginning to fall apart. But I don't *think* sixty. There is no clear correlation between your physical state and your mental state."

People so often make this observation it seems to be a dyssynchrony that defines the sixties. Being a gourmet cook and habitué of the better bistros and cafés in Manhattan, Aaron had an attitude toward diet and exercise of aggressive neglect. The shift in his mental state was something else. Envied for the artistic leaps and juxtapositions of historical styles that were his hallmark, he worried about feeling the first, fatal tugs of caution. "Regardless of the encouragement of risk, which is the cliché of popular psychology," he said, "the fact is there are tremendous punishments for taking risks at this point. People are so eager for others to fail. It's one of the reasons people become frozen in their own development."

The problem is a common one at this stage: Even as we pursue the path of the wiseperson we'd all like to become—that paragon of balance and serenity—we have the sneaking feeling that we're becoming so dignified and encrusted with opinions we run the risk of becoming reruns of ourselves. What about the leftover kid who, more insistently than ever, seems to be knocking on some inner screen door and crying, *Don't forget about me! Can't I come out and play again?* That adolescent, or preadolescent, is the repository of our playfulness and creativity and a reminder of our most primitive pleasures.

It took a heart attack before Aaron could give himself permission to drop out for six weeks in the summer in Tuscany. The windy Italian road looped up to the highest hilltop he and his wife could find, to where the horizon spread out as timelessly as a Renaissance painting. It was withdrawal, exactly what he craved. One day he discovered a little wine and pottery shop at the foot of a voluptuous vineyard. A father and son sat in a shed out back, painting dinner plates. They worked in the traditional Tuscan manner, firing the plates in an old-fashioned brick kiln, but their images were new. Aaron was intrigued.

"Can I come and work here?" he asked.

The artisans shrugged a simple assent. From that day on, Aaron began turning up every morning in old work clothes and painting grapes and nudes and dogs on dinner plates. When the occasional American tourist wandered back to the shed, he pretended to be an old Italian geezer, a day laborer, so he wouldn't have to talk to them. He looked the part, covered with dust and ceramic spittle, sitting in a hot little room without electricity or running water, painting plates. Yet he couldn't wait to get up in the morning and drive down to that shed and spend ten hours a day, every day, until the long light faded. He came home every night deliriously happy.

"I kept thinking, what is this incredible contentment?" he recalled. One day he had a flash of insight. "I was doing something I didn't know how to do. And I was learning how to do it." Everything about the experience was fundamental: the rudimentary colors, the timeless Tuscan landscape, the magic that happens when things are transformed by heat. "I couldn't wait to see the plates come out of the kiln," he told me. "My whole life has been task-oriented. This experience showed me how different it is when you're working for your own pleasure and curiosity. Oh, I got very excited again."

By peeling back down to the simplest existence and letting himself "play," gloriously anonymous, shorn of expectations, able to be an amateur again, he was as free to take risks and make mistakes as a 10-year-old in art class. Aaron rediscovered his greatest joy in life: making things and seeing them transformed into objects of art.

SELF-CONFIDENT SURVIVORS

Women are the greatest beneficiaries of the demographic revolution. Their improved chances of survival into the latest ages is the most significant change in the life cycle. To reiterate, the ordinary woman who reaches 65 can fully expect to make it to 84 or 85.[30] Indeed, for healthy American women today, Second Adulthood may actually last longer than First Adulthood—into their nineties. But to ensure that those extra years are golden, not beholden, women must anticipate as never before the need to garner education, prepare career tracks, build pensions and individual retirement accounts, and demand greater help from society to care for the frail elderly in their families.

> The new reality is this: Women at age 65 today must be prepared to finance an additional two decades of life.[31]

One of the most daunting aspects of the sixties for women is the likely transition to living on their own. While most older males have spouses to lean on when their health fails, most elderly females do not. More than nine million elderly Americans live alone; 78 percent of them are women.[32]

Late divorce or widowhood becomes a transformative event for women of the World War II or Silent Generation, given the early socialization that taught them they could never be complete without men. Liz Carpenter, as strong a Texas pioneer woman as they come, had been a buffer all through the rise and fall of Lyndon Johnson (as Lady Bird Johnson's chief of staff), a founder of the National Women's Political Caucus, and an indefatigable bon vivant through her sixties despite being left, as she puts it, with one of everything: a missing breast, a bum ankle, and "the weakest bladder in Travis County." But widowhood threw her.

"I was in a blue funk after my husband died," she told me. "A friend finally took my hand one day and told me something that turned me completely around. She said, 'Look, Liz, it's like this. Widowhood is a gift. God has given you another life to live.' "[33]

And this new life was to be put to a powerful, if totally unpredictable, purpose. When her brother died, leaving three orphaned teenagers, Liz Carpenter became, at the age of 72, a "born-again parent." With her somber widow's existence torn open as if by a shriek, she found that disaster had catapulted her into the most important role of her life. Liz Carpenter tracks the hilarious road map through unexplored intergenerational terrain in her book *Unplanned Parenthood*.[34] That terrain is populated by a fast-growing sub-culture of grandparents who have had to take over from what she calls the Woodstock Generation. She has a new raison d'être now: "I've told my doctor I've got to live—at least long enough to see them through college."

After grieving for a year, or more likely two, widows who pull out of this painful transition often look upon themselves as survivors. And they are. They have been through a life-threatening passage and didn't die from it. Most will have to get a job (if they don't already have one), which forces them to get out "in the real world," as so many see it. Here is an astounding figure:

> Two thirds of women aged 60 to 64 who are divorced, wid-owed, or not living with spouses are still drawing full-time paychecks.[35]

The "survivors" of late divorce, separation, or widowhood who responded to a survey I did for *New Woman* magazine admitted having to deal with fear and loneliness at times. But each small step toward autonomy further grounds them with a gathering sense of mastery and the "firm sense of self" they have come to late.[36] The dramatic difference between "who I was then and who I am now" is a large part of what makes them look back on their life journeys as special. An Indiana woman spoke for many: "I don't know what old is. I have no idea. I still stand on my head. I love the way I look now. I have my own apartment, I can pay my own rent, I have my first car. I feel like I've re-created myself."

These survivors expect to be even more self-confident as they proceed through their sixties, and most look forward to being serene and ready for new challenges. They name as role models Shirley MacLaine, Maya Angelou, Maggie Kuhn, Jane Fonda (for her body), Katharine Hepburn (for coping with chronic disease), and Debbie Reynolds, but more often they find inspiration from indomitable grandmothers or mothers. Imagining their future selves as 65-year-old women, they see themselves as feisty, nur-turing, and wise. And most feel certain that ten years down the line they will enjoy an even greater sense of inner well-being.[37]

But one cannot passively wait for "another life to live." The women sur-vivors I have interviewed all talk about the importance of breaking taboos, taking risks, bursting out of other people's expectations, being sexually adventurous, and learning to love leading their lives by their own lights. They have to go out and stir up a little trouble to get started again. I ran into a model of this sort at an alumni seminar on "The Meaning of Life" at Duke University.

THE WILEY WIDOW, AGE 60

"I make *the chance."*

Mozelle Nelson, a contemporary 60-year-young widow, decided she would *not* be sequestered with other widows in a canasta-playing, condominiumized, one-sex world. "Nothing bores me more than being with all women." She wrinkled her nose. "I was happily married for thirty-seven years; why would I want to live in a world without men?"

Her home was in Little Rock, Arkansas. The South, she insisted, is relentless about telling widows they must make their new life with other women in the same situation. Mozelle's philosophy of life was "Chances don't come to you." For instance, she has noticed, when you ask people after they've been to a party, "Did you meet so and so?" often the reply is "No, I didn't have a chance." "Well"—she shook her silky white hair and smiled with her very full, brightly painted lips and self-mocking blue eyes—"I *make* the chance."

The first thing she did was to volunteer for the Clinton presidential campaign in the Little Rock headquarters. Nice people but mostly kids. On the premise that one doesn't catch a trout by fishing in a minnow brook, Mozelle looked around for gatherings of intellectually curious people of both sexes and hit upon alumni college seminars. An inspiration! She wrote away to several schools: "Do you have any problem with my attending despite the fact that I don't have an association with your university?" The reply was usually the same: Just bring your money and come.

And so she did. In one year she had been up and down the East Coast, to Washington & Lee University, Dartmouth, University of Virginia, Duke, and Cornell University, for seminars lasting a week or a long weekend. She met all kinds of scintillating company and zeroed in on the few single males who attended such functions. Meanwhile, her mind was pried wide open, and she was learning about *everything*.

By the time I met Mozelle, despite her thirty years at home, she could talk somewhat knowledgeably and certainly engagingly on almost any subject. Watching her make an entrance in her jewel-colored silk dresses with the just-right décolletage and sharpen up her powers of flirtatiousness on the bedazzled men at the seminar was like watching a former professional boxer train a rookie. She had already developed three romantic relationships with single men over the course of the year and fully expected to make her chance to have a husband in her life once again.

"But I can't compromise my standards." She winked. "It *matters* a *lot* who he is. And if a husband isn't to be, well, I still have the most interesting, intelligent male friends a woman could find."

LOVE STORIES OF THE SIXTIES

The most startling aspect of the recent sweeping study of American sex by the numbers is the fact that the researchers studied people only up to age 59, reinforcing the myth that sex after 60 is only a memory.[38]

Yet television is beginning to permit romantic leads who fall crazy in love despite their senior citizen discounts. The images that linger from the miniseries *Armistead Maupin's Tales of the City* on public television here and in Britain are those of a spiritually transformative romance between two over-sixties denizens of San Francisco who open up unexpected parts of each other and accept those parts nonjudgmentally. They meet on a park bench: the charming bohemian landlady who grows pot for her tenants and the old-line Republican tycoon who's just been told he has inoperable cancer. The landlady, played by Olympia Dukakis, doesn't question the Donald Moffat character about his politics. Seeing that he's a man in pain, she opens her heart to him. Immediately he begins to warm up. As she awakens him to the capacity for loving that he thinks he has long since lost, he begins to see her as a goddess figure and unfailingly tells her how beautiful she is. She reveals to him the shocking secret of her past with complete trust that he will accept her just as readily as she has accepted him, a dying man. Without blinking an eyelash, all she asks is "How much time do we have?" Their love is sublime, existing as it does fervently in and for the moment.

Although they approach lovemaking more slowly and tenderly than the usual strip-and-grope Hollywood love scene, we do see them in bed together stroking each other, we watch them stare at each other in public with longing and love, and we see them deeply soul-kissing. It's a new image. Love, including sensual love, is still very much part of the sixties.

. . .

Older men without wives are much more vulnerable than widowed or divorced women. Representative national samples show that men without wives in the 45 to 64 age-group—whether widowed, single, or divorced—suffer almost *twice* the rate of depression as married men. For the first time unattached men of this age have surpassed even the depression levels of the sad young Werthers in their twenties and thirties, reconfirming the fact that middle-aged American males—especially those without wives—are the new at-risk population for depression.[39]

Furthermore, on a variety of psychological and physiological measurements, men who have recently lost their wives are at risk of suffering marked deterioration in physical health. The loss often leads to depression, which may lead to biological changes that render them more vulnerable to heart attacks and other diseases.[40] Men are much more likely than women to follow their spouses into the grave in the first six months to a year after they are alone. Social scientists have finally concluded that the men, having lost their sole confidantes, actually die of grief.[41]

The save-your-life wife often becomes a reality after 60. Joseph Heller was divorced and living alone when he was suddenly paralyzed by a terrifying neurological disease. The author brought his young nurse home from the hospital, fell in love with her while convalescing, and moved to tie the knot. His formerly jaundiced views on marriage have changed drastically. He admitted in an interview that "*Closing Time* treats marriage as an optimum, desirable state."[42]

Another man famously independent who married his nurse and probably prolonged his life, not to mention reviving his aging mind-set, is former Republican Senator Barry Goldwater. When Nurse Susan, thirty years his junior, visited the eightysomething's home to take his blood pressure, he never let her go. Now the man who was the icon of extreme conservatives in the 1960s is fond of speaking out in favor of abortion rights and gays in the military, open in his disgust with fundamentalist Christians who have captured a large portion of the Republican party. His friends attribute his change of heart to the influence of a young wife and a gay grandson.[43]

Even the eternal prince of the *Playboy* magazine empire renounced his vows to hold out for the single life once he had crossed the line into his sixties. It took a year of depression followed by a mild stroke to reverse the lifelong credo of professional hedonist Hugh Hefner. At the age of 62 Hefner asked a 24-year-old model to be Mrs. Playboy, acknowledging "the sense of mortality [has] changed my life."[44]

REKINDLING OLD FLAMES, AGE 77

"I carried a torch for her for fifty-five years!"

One of the curiously repeating stories I hear from both men and women interviewees in their fifties and sixties and even older is how they reconnect, usually accidentally, with old flames. And then what fireworks! Sweethearts long since thought lost to the years and circumstances often turn out to have been Mr. or Miss Right after all. And by this stage there are no meddlesome parents to spoil the match.

If doubt still lingers that love can find a way into the heart of the oldest, least sentimental of men once they are humbled by the specter of their own mortality, there is the story of Dr. William Masters. That's right, the male half of the most renowned couple of sex experts in the world, Masters and Johnson. The clinical half. Dr. Masters and Virginia Johnson were in the process of getting an amicable divorce when I met him at an impotence conference in Washington, D.C. He was 77.

During our formal interview his eyes fixed me with a fishy stare, and he spoke in icy, staccato bursts. His Parkinson's disease was not noticeable, but he walked with a cane and complained about multiple operations on his foot and a long wait for an artificial knee. Once the interview on male menopause was over, I said, "I hear you're planning to remarry."

Suddenly his froggy stare softened, and with no prompting Dr. Masters launched into a heartfelt tale of rediscovering his lost love—after fifty-five years! He had courted Geraldine while he was a poor young medical student at the University of Rochester. When his love came to town to have a breast biopsy, the young swain decided, "She had to have two dozen roses." Nothing less would do. He could find only half a dozen roses in the whole town. "So I took a plane to New York to get another dozen and a half and flew back and gave them to the night nurse. Visiting hours were over. That's how much I loved her."[45]

Dr. Masters sucked in a sob. Tears welled up, and his voice broke several more times as he finished the story. The next day his love went back home and shortly thereafter married a big man on campus. "I was heartbroken. Why? I never knew. I carried a torch for her for fifty-five years!" He then described the heart-stopping accident. One recent day he had stepped onto an elevator in Montreal just as his long-lost love was stepping off.

"My heart almost broke with joy." He purred like a cello. "We recognized each other immediately. I said, 'What happened that day in Rochester, fifty-five years ago?' She looked sad. 'You didn't care enough to come to see me in the hospital,' she said." Oh, cruel destiny. Geraldine had never received his roses.

"The chemistry was there instantly for me, and I think for her too. She'd married the other man! I'd lost out. So of course I still wanted her! We'd never even made love. It was"—he sighed—"wonderful." He pulled out a picture of his love. "I look like an old codger, but she"—his lids flickered in something close to a swoon—"she looks forty-five; she's beautiful!" As we left the restaurant, the old man with limp and cane straightened up. Six months later he married Geraldine Baker Oliver.[46]

RECONCILIATIONS

If we are to achieve the serenity to bless our own life histories as something that had to be, we must find a way to reconcile our hurts and love our parents differently, with compassion for their life histories. Some of the most poignant moments in my interviews with people in late middle age occur when they describe the terrifying outreach to an estranged parent. It requires courage. It demands the honesty to get past the superficial emotion of anger and go beneath to expose the hurt, the longing. We have to feel confident that whether or not a relationship can be rebuilt, we have done what we can to offer love and absolution.

Long after my interview with a late-blooming political consultant in Washington State, Jeanette Fruen sent me a letter with her questionnaire. It had been finished for months, she said, but she was frozen over the item concerning the relationship with one's mother. "My mother and I had an extremely traumatic relationship. It went on for maybe 10 years . . . On the advice of my college counselor, I left home at the age of nineteen, an emotional wreck."

After years of total estrangement from her mother Jeanette had survived a devastating late divorce and gone on to build a cannily successful career doing exactly what she believed in: organizing voters in various state campaigns around women's issues. She had filled her life with people who cared about her and treated her well, and she had finally found some spiritual comfort. Approaching sixty, she took a two-week trip around England to listen to sacred music and meditate. At Salisbury Cathedral near Stonehenge, the cathedral where her ancestors had worshiped, her mind suddenly flooded with vividly detailed memories of a happy vacation she had spent there with her parents when she was very young.

The inner conflict with her mother resurfaced and hung on like a fever. Upon her return she sent a brief note to her mother describing those memories and thanking her for that happy time in childhood. The note opened a window. She accepted an invitation to join her mother for a weekend in Arizona, where they spent time shopping for Jeanette's sixtieth birthday gift, sharing recipes, trading stories of their travels—the normal things that mothers and daughters do together.

"I learned more about how she had been abandoned as a newborn and shunted from foster home to foster home," Jeanette told me. "She had big tears in her eyes as she talked to me. I realized she had never felt loved."

Following a year of efforts to build a new relationship—not between mother and daughter but between two adults with ties of blood and affection—Jeanette was ready to take back her family name, including her mother's given name. She wanted to create a ritual around this passage of reconciliation. The deacon of her Episcopal church was open to a "naming service," and they collaborated on creating an offertory of healing with hymns and dancing and bread and wine, shared with friends and family members in a spirit of thanksgiving. Jeanette said a prayer for being delivered out of the darkness:

> . . . the darkness of staying silent,
> the terror of having nothing to say,
> and the greater terror of needing to say nothing.

Again, I was reminded of the universal importance of reconciliation before we lose the ones to whom we have been closest when I saw the Lincoln Center revival of *Carousel.* This mythical play always stirs people, especially men, because of the things we leave unsaid. The hero, Billy Bigelow, is cursed with a constitutional inability to declare his love. Hidden beneath the rough exterior of this failed fairground barker is a gentler nature, but Billy is so fearful of revealing it that he abuses the only one who loves and trusts him unconditionally, his young wife, Julie Jordan. During Billy's short life the closest either of them has ever come to declaring their hearts was "*If* I loved you."

When the dead Billy is permitted a single day to return to earth and atone for his wasted life, he sings what has always been locked in his heart, but he sings it to his widow, after Julie has spent fifteen sad years as a single mother.

> Longin' to tell you, but afraid and shy,
> I'd let my golden chances pass me by.
> Soon you'd leave me,

> Off you would go in the mist of day,
> Never, never to know
> How I loved you—
> If I loved you.

Turning to look at the audience, I was touched to see the men. They were undone, some of them sobbing. Even certain gunslinging power brokers whose faces I recognized were in tears. Probably they saw in Billy something of their own inability to say what they may never have admitted to themselves they felt. Director Nicholas Hytner has also commented on why men so often cry when the *Carousel* music pierces their heart:

> The words "I love you" are never sufficient, in themselves, to say what any of us feel about those who are dearest to us. . . . We cry for what we have never said, and will never be able to say.[47]

17

MEN: MAKE MY PASSAGE

"Who do you know in Hollywood who is flourishing over sixty?" I asked a friend, producer Irwin Winkler.

"Nobody," he shot back. It was a knee-jerk reaction. He himself had moved on from producing many hit movies to becoming a respected director in his sixties. "Well"—he reconsidered—"Clint."

Clint Eastwood has come to inhabit the American cowboy ideal earlier rendered by John Wayne and Gary Cooper. But those stars of a previous generation stuck unflinchingly to the solitary, stoical, monosyllabic male ideal even as they stiffened and bulked into middle and late-late-middle age. They never changed.

Eastwood is different. He's a real man who eats tofu. He's an authentic working-class movie star who doesn't hang out with the Hollywood elite. Along with James Bond, he helped perfect a new archetype of the solitary, cold-blooded killer who gets the job done with relish bordering on the sadistic. "Go ahead, make my day" has been enshrined in Bartlett's *Familiar Quotations*. As the star of an era of blood-sprayed westerns, Eastwood helped kill some fifty people in *A Fistful of Dollars*. Dirty Harry, the signature character of Eastwood's early midlife acting career, was the cop above the law who used violence to resolve any and all conflicts, the justification being that somebody had to protect a soft-on-crime society from itself—and that was in the Seventies even before the Reagan era. Dirty Harry was a decade ahead of the culture.

Born in May 1930, Clint Eastwood is at this writing 64 years old. Given his worldwide superstar status, he might have been expected to demand more of the same roles and let the studios worry about his aging: *Go ahead, make my passage.* But something changed as he crossed into Second Adulthood.

"I do agree that when you get to a certain stage in life, you change. And you *should* change," he told psychologist Stuart Fischoff, in a rare self-revelatory interview.[1] "As you get older, you try to do things that please you more. . . . I don't want to go and just jump across buildings. You know, shoot nameless people off the top of stagecoaches. . . . That's why *Unforgiven* became a very important film for me, because it sort of summed up my feelings about certain movies I participated in—movies where killing is romantic. And here was a chance to show that it really wasn't so romantic."

He bought the script to *Unforgiven* when he was in his mid-fifties, figuring he would "age into it a bit,"[2] but he became obsessed by it and began exploring the shadows of his own persona. "A man's got to know his limitations" was his telling line in *Magnum Force.* As Eastwood moved through his fifties, he felt free to turn Dirty Harry on his head and expose the human needs and limitations beneath his young-tough code of violence. He seemed to grasp that the old male myths have to be relinquished at a certain stage in order for a man to become something more. "I've played winners, I've played losers who were winners, guys who are cool, but I like reality, and in reality it's not all like that," he said. "There's a frailty in mankind that's very interesting to explore."[3]

His character in *Unforgiven,* William Munny, is a widower in his sixties who, according to the actor, "is really living on the edge of hell."[4] Formerly an alcoholic gunfighter and woman killer, Munny straightened out under the influence of the good woman whose catechisms still direct him from beyond the grave. But it's been three years since her death, and he's lost his sexual confidence (widower's syndrome?). When a prostitute whose life he saves offers him a "free one," he turns it down. As a man who cannot experience his emotional or sexual frailties, he is unable to accept any comfort and ultimately betrays his good deeds by drinking and turning violent again.

Most daring of all, Eastwood openly let his signature character grow older. It used to be that Cary Grant's "character lines" and John Wayne's silvering hair only magnified their appeal as cool, masterful, older men. Dirty Harry isn't aging as well. Eastwood resurrected the Dirty Harry persona in 1993 for *In the Line of Fire,* in which he plays an aging Secret Service agent who has to live with his failure to protect President Kennedy from an assassin's bullet. He also has to work with a young feminist as a partner who can shoot him down with a remark. She challenges him: "What demographics do you represent?"

"White piano-playing heterosexuals over the age of fifty.... There aren't many of us, but we've got a powerful lobby."

As an older man Dirty Harry is increasingly vulnerable, an alienated loner. His independence, which once made him tougher, now renders him weaker, because no man can age well without human companionship. In real life Clint Eastwood has evolved from beefcake actor to celebrated director, from elective politics (where he felt like a fraud) to social work that centers on children and adolescents. He seems to have figured out how to shape a "new self," one that integrates both the masculine and feminine principles. He can express his nurturant feelings with children while using his male energy and power to take action in helping to protect the next generation.

If Clint Eastwood is emblematic of the new integrated man in his prime, his comments to Dr. Fischoff on the appeal of dating girls less than half his age strike an intriguing note: "The prospect of dating someone in her twenties becomes less appealing as you get older. At some point in your life, your tolerance level goes down and you realize that, with someone much younger, there's nothing really to talk about.... [W]hat do you say to her afterwards? If you don't smoke, what do you say? Do you talk about the weather or Jon Bon Jovi?"

He went on to pay homage to women who qualify as grown-ups: "I think we're at a point now where a lot of older women take better care of themselves, compared to the 1940s and '50s when women were programmed to figure it's all over after 30. I find a lot of appeal in a woman if she's kept herself well in her forties and beyond."

In 1993, at the age of 63, Clint Eastwood became a father again. Once more he is a little ahead of the culture.

GRAND DADS

A compulsion to procreate often sweeps over men in the late afternoon of life. And now that the late afternoon stretches into an extended gloaming, more healthy, successful men are able to consider practicing a form of the ancient polygamous privilege of kings. The globe-trotting publisher described in an earlier chapter, who, like many men, was rocked by the first intimation of sexual slowdown in his fifties, felt compelled to chase after women younger than his wife, to couple with them in all their dangerous fertility, to draw potency from them. When he was found out, he recalled, "my first wife put it to me bluntly. 'What this is all about is not sex,' she insisted. 'You want to reproduce.' "

He was stunned by this analysis, but he chose to shrug it off. As if guided by some sociobiological vector, he went on to marry a woman twenty years younger and produced two children, who did indeed make him feel reborn and connected him again to the future.

Fitzgerald had the same "crazy urge to have a child" after his wife died, though it was fleeting. "Especially in a time of stress what a wonderfully satisfying thing to become a father again. It's something that goes with being a young man. Time is pushed backward."

Older men having babies have become a phenomenon in the Southern California movie subculture. Jack Nicholson (playing himself) has done it twice in his late fifties. Warren Beatty, the indefatigable bachelor until he reached age 55, has turned late fatherhood into a fashionable mystique as he and Annette Bening bill and coo over their two babies in one cover story after another. Producer-director Bud Yorkin had a new baby in his mid-sixties and is working on another one. The father of *All in the Family*, Norman Lear, topped them all by bringing forth an offspring from his May–December marriage in his early seventies.

"What better way to prove you're still young than to have a baby?" says producer Irwin Winkler of his friends. But these men also have more time and the inclination to spend a lot of it with their children. "Men, when they're young, are too busy building their careers to be around much as fathers," observes Winkler. "These guys have already made it. So if Clint lives until he's eighty—and he's a healthy, strong guy, he might outlast the statistical average—he'll have given the kid eighteen years of attention. He probably figures that's enough. The others, if they die earlier, will leave these kids very secure financially."[5]

It is not only Hollywood.

Most of us know situations where a man becomes a late-late father and his whole perspective changes. More often than not it's his younger wife's idea. Her biological clock begins to calibrate their lives down to the nanosecond. He may grumble during the period when his determined wife seems only to care about capturing his most important juices in a test tube and rushing them off to the fertility clinic. Once the blessed event occurs, however, you can be sure this man will show off his baby pictures at every opportunity—almost as proof of potency—inspiring the envy and admiration of his peers. Almost universally, it seems, these men do devote much more time and attention to the offspring of their later age then they ever did to the children of an earlier stage.

But these Grand Dads are the exception. Most men in their sixties probably aren't keen to be tied down again or to take on the awesome burdens of saving for college tuition. Many working-class men are likely to have had vasectomies already. Even the most successful men of the current generation in their sixties are likely to have stuck it out with Wife Number One. The possibility of a second family may never have occurred to them, but many are deeply, touchingly, attached to their children's children, their strongest link to immortality.

RETIREMENT: LOVE IT OR LEAVE IT?

Retirement used to be the square that one landed on in the playing board of life roughly five years before one expired, the reward for thirty-five or more years of hard work, when a pencil pusher could enjoy a paid mortgage, a cruise or two, and a golden wedding anniversary while waiting around to die. Today the question is not so much *when* is ideal retirement age as how does one *define* retirement. What association first comes to *your* mind when you hear the word *retirement*? Reward? Release? Being put out to pasture?

Just mention the subject of retirement to most professionals and watch their eyes jump in terror. Retirement, *me*? The notion—when it first becomes real—is burdened with connotations of sudden loss of status, boredom, and encroaching enfeeblement, and it raises fearsome questions: *What do you do when it stops? Who are you when you are no longer defined by your work?*

National surveys confirm that retirement is one of the most troubling passages in adult life for Americans. Forty-one percent of retirees surveyed in New York City in 1993 said the adjustment was difficult.[6] The younger the retiree, the harder the transition. And the higher the status one's work conferred, the steeper the slide to anonymity.

The wife of a legendary American newspaper editor said of his mandatory retirement at 65: "The worst part is not losing the title; it's losing the team. One day he's in feverish contact with a hundred of the best minds in the country, asking what they think about the latest turn in events, and the next day—*silence*. No cross-fertilization. No fevered debates. No phone calls."

The loss of heroic status and the power of command may be hardest for the winners in high-tension, high-stakes fields like the media, entertainment, and Wall Street. Another brilliant media executive with a string of successes behind him confessed to me a few years after he had retired at 65, "I've never been without a deadline to get out a major newspaper. I hate it, having free time to manage. I have no one to give orders to. As a consultant, they can take you or leave you. What you have to get used to is, you're never going to have another hit. You've *had* your fifteen minutes."

After a year or two of this terminal gloom, however, both these men went back to work, and they are going strong into their seventies, one as a national columnist and the other as a regional editor of one of the most successful magazines in the country.

Professionals, managers, and sales workers hang on longest before retiring and are also the most likely to go back to work at some point. Blue-collar workers tend to take their pensions early and run from the monotony of their work.[7]

Retirement spikes for men at age 62 to 64.[8] As people see peers hanging up their gloves, they often feel the social "shoulds" again. After all, the convention since 1950 has been for people to exit from the work force earlier and earlier, driving down the average retirement age from 67 to 63.[9] And the incentives keep increasing. Social Security benefits have been protected from inflation since the 1970s. Population experts say this may be the golden age of the golden years.

But once again the maps in our minds are out-of-date.

Ever since corporations began enticing older employees with early-retirement "windows" and "packages," a huge pool of restless, still-vigorous men and women have been floating around the country, in and out of part-time jobs or self-employed entrepreneurial ventures, in search of the right fit. A growing army of specialists now recommend *serial retirement*, meaning do it in stages.

But Baby Boomers want to do it all at once, and sooner rather than later. Most Boomers—both men and women—say they would like to retire under the age of 50! In the same Gallup poll they indicated that they would settle for retirement at 55. Almost none wants to work after age 70.[10]

Now comes the cold slap of reality: For a couple between the ages of 45 and 54 earning a combined income of $100,000 a year (which is about $70,000 after taxes), Merrill Lynch says they had better be socking away 24.3 percent of their *after-tax* earnings, or $18,000 per year, toward retirement.[11] That's not counting inheritance or pension benefits. *Eighteen thousand bucks per year in the bank or blue-chip investments not to be touched.* Or else what?

Or else they will be forced to accept dramatically lower standards of living during retirement or forget about retirement altogether. The minimum nest egg they need to have by 65 in order to retire then is $483,460—and that's with a traditional pension—or $660, 070 without a traditional pension.[12]

Of course, nobody can really save this much. So people won't be able to live the same way they did, and/or they'll retire later or not at all, or they'll be particularly solicitious of the proverbial rich uncle. In 1994, when Merrill Lynch first commissioned the Stanford University economist Dr. B. Douglas Bernheim to survey the preparedness of Baby Boomers to retire in their midsixties, the recommendation was that the typical Boomer household should triple its rate of savings. A follow-up study revealed that the cost of paying for Social Security and Medicare will saddle these Americans with higher and higher tax burdens, culminating with a net lifetime tax rate on generations yet to be born of—are you ready for this?—*82 percent.* Merrill Lynch then came back with a much more pessimistic assessment: In the worst-case scenarios Boomers are saving less than one tenth of what they would require to avert a lifestyle crash in their sixties.

For single Professional Women there is even more pressure, since they live longer and usually earn less than a man or couple. Ideally by age 55 an unattached woman earning $100,000 a year (pretax) should be setting aside *one third* of her earnings and have no less than $347,150 already saved, exclusive of her pension, if she wants to maintain her current lifestyle after retirement at 65.[13] Boomers shouldn't plan on cashing in at 65 in any case. Social Security age in the United States has already been bumped up to 67 in a phased-in process to begin after the year 2000.

When the issue of retirement came up in my group interviews, it was obvious that people were scrambling to reset their timetables in light of the dazzling changes in the life cycle. The Professional Men in Louisville were applying a lengthened yardstick as they got older.

"I always thought that I'd want to retire at sixty-five," said Dr. David Allen. "Now that really starts to spread out to where I think maybe I'd like to teach till I'm seventy-five."

Bruce Bell, the New Midlife Man with still-young children to support, spoke to the concerns of those still under 50 who are afraid they won't be able to afford to retire at a reasonable age.[14] "I don't see any magic at sixty-five," he said, "because if we're going to live till eighty-five or ninety, that's *twenty or twenty-five years of being retired.* Who wouldn't get tired of that?" But it hasn't registered yet with most Boomers that they will be living routinely up to a quarter century *after* they're pensioned off. In the work force for forty years and out for twenty-five: Does this make sense for the individual? Or society?

One banker, who subscribed to his company's policy of mandatory age cutoffs, told me with nervous bombast, "I'm sixty-four years old and *I don't expect to fail retirement!*" But even former presidents of the United States can fail retirement.

THE BUSH RETIREMENT (NON)PLAN

"I'm unemployed, I'm out of a job."

President George Bush woke up on election day, November 1991, convinced he was going to win a second term, according to his wife, Barbara. Strangely passive throughout the last months of the campaign, he dismissed mounting evidence that the American public was coming to the conclusion he had no economic policy and that he had lied about being up to his ears in the Iran-contra capers of the Reagan era. Stubbornly resisting the prospect of defeat, Bush devoted no time at all to considering his options. Barbara Bush, normally the realist, supported him in this denial of reality. They had no Plan B.

Right up to the day he watched movers cart their possessions out of the White House, Bush had no firm plans for his retirement beyond getting "very active in the grandchild business." Barbara Bush reflects in her biography: "I remember years ago saying to George when we were first married: 'I can't wait for you to retire.' He looked surprised and said that he couldn't think of anything worse and that he hoped he never would. He still feels that way. . . ."[15]

These winter ejectees from the White House, power center of the free world, were suddenly homeless. Their mansion in Maine was not winterized, and their legal residence in Houston was a hotel suite for political convenience. The only inkling of their future life structure was a pocket-size property in suburban Houston, the declared site of their retirement home, a vacant lot.[16]

The greater vacancy was in the life of a man who had always been hyperactive, rarely reflective, and whose identity was closely tied to the current title on his always impressive résumé. When Bush reappeared in Washington in January to receive an honor, a few weeks after vacating the White House, a churchgoer approached him for an autograph. His response spoke volumes about his self-perception: "Oh, no, you don't need my signature. I'm unemployed, I'm out of a job."[17]

And for the next year and a half George Bush dropped out of sight in public life. He did a lot of fishing; he took his family on several cruises; he and Barbara jetted around the world from golf course to golf course.[18] But some of his most loyal political advisers said privately that he seemed to be depressed and befuddled about what to do with his life, as if waiting to be given another mission.

Meanwhile Mrs. Bush seems to have found a second wind. To her fell the task of establishing their new home. It is Barbara who wrote the memoir of President Bush's political career. It is Barbara who's out in public campaigning now, either for literacy or to promote her books. And it is Barbara who appears to be the primary breadwinner in the postpresidential Bush family. After netting a million dollars in royalties for writing her first book about the family dog—money committed to charity since she was still in the White House—the former First Lady claimed the proceeds of her number one best-selling celebrity autobiography as her own money. From a distance it appears that even power and international prestige have not immunized George and Barbara Bush from the accelerated role reversal of the Crossover Crisis.

THE CARTERS' RETIREMENT PLAN

"This is the most important and urgent work I've ever done."

After Jimmy Carter lost his presidency, he returned home to Plains, Georgia, and was faced with himself as a nearly shattered man. His political fortunes had sunk to a nadir, and he found himself near financial ruin, a million dollars in debt with the possibility of losing his farms and even his house. What he saw in his future after "retirement" from the presidency, he later conceded to a reporter, was a "potentially empty life."[19]

Rosalynn Carter, too, was bruised and angry. She pretended to herself that Jimmy would run and regain the White House, although he never joined her in this comforting fantasy. But by their first summer out of office both Carters had book contracts. And just as when Rosalynn had attended cabinet meetings and acted as her husband's chief aide-de-camp, the Carters continued to work in tandem. They run together. They wrote a book together. They established the Carter Center together. They continued to sustain themselves with Christian duty, not only championing the nonprofit Habitat for Humanity but wielding hammer and saw to help construct housing for the poor and homeless.

Still, Jimmy Carter missed having a role in world affairs. Like everyone who has given of himself, he wanted to be appreciated. Friends say it hurt to have been denied the Nobel Peace Prize for his historic role in the Camp

David accords, and he carried on his conscience the weight of the aborted hostage rescue attempt in Iran. What could the Carters do in this forced retirement to put the meaning back in their lives? What might offer a chance for political redemption? That inner struggle went on for nearly a decade—until the Carters were in their mid-sixties.

Late one night Carter jackknifed upright in bed, and out came the words *conflict resolution*.[20] That was the inspiration. He offered his ex officio services to the Republican White House of George Bush. Unlike Ronald Reagan, who had stiff-armed him, Bush did not mind sharing credit. Suddenly Carter seemed to be turning up everywhere that internal conflicts appeared intransigent—Panama, Ethiopia, Nicaragua, Somalia—and playing a more active role in foreign affairs than any former president since Herbert Hoover in the 1930s.

But almost any retiree who creates a role for himself as an independent agent will have to keep working at it. Inevitably, junior people will be wary of the Great Man's shadow. Rivals within the official hierarchy may resent him. When his own party returned to power, Carter was again kept at arm's length, this time by a younger president from the South wary of being tagged "Carter II." With sheer willpower and perseverance, Carter won over Bill Clinton personally. Despite the vehement opposition of top presidential advisers and disdain from the State Department, seemingly overnight, at the age of 69, Jimmy Carter burst forth as President Clinton's foreign policy alter ego. The eyes of the whole world were upon him in the summer of '94, when he single-handedly resolved a nuclear standoff with North Korea that had stymied the Clinton administration. Weeks later the president turned to him again, dispatching Carter to Haiti to stroke the military junta and stave off an unpopular American invasion. When talks stalled, Carter turned for advice to his wife.

"I called Rosalynn and she said, 'Jimmy, you go talk to Cedras' wife," Mr. Carter told a reporter.[21] Sure enough, it turned out to be the dictator's wife who was holding up an agreement. Carter knew how to soften her up, he said, "because I have known for fifty years what it's like to be involved with a strong woman."

Rosalynn Carter has also found a new cause. Having experienced the lonely burdens of helping family members through the throes of lengthy terminal illness, she is sounding the alarm on America's caregiving crisis. She has recently coauthored a book to guide others in this role.[22] And she continues her efforts to destigmatize mental illness through her task force at the Carter Center in Atlanta.

The Jimmy and Rosalynn Carter model—partners in retirement who will not rest until they find a way that their energies can be harnessed and rewarded for meaningful work in the society—is predictive of life in the sixties after the year 2000. Many more Americans aged 65 to 74 than ever before are volunteering for community service or informally helping others on a regular basis.[23] The Silents, who as a generation have always had a tender social conscience, may become a "mentor generation" as they move into their sixties.[24] While they redefine the Age of Integrity for themselves, they will be redefining the concepts of retirement and late middle age for the rest of us.

THE WINNER'S CIRCLE

What does "retirement" hold today for men with the means to design this stage pretty much to their own specifications?

I have been studying one class of Harvard Business School graduates—the Class of '49—at intervals since 1974. These men represent the ultimate stars in business life: More than half became chairmen of the board or presidents, while another third became vice-presidents. Dubbed by *Fortune* magazine "The Class the Dollars Fell On,"[25] it spawned the chief executive officers of Johnson & Johnson, Xerox, Capitol Cities (ABC-TV), Elizabeth Arden, Resorts International, Bloomingdale's, Sonesta Hotels, Hill & Knowlton. Success, however grand, did not exempt these men from going through lapses in vitality and virility as they negotiated the passage from First to Second Adulthood.

By their own admission, when I surveyed and interviewed them in 1979, most of them had gone through a dark or a depressive period sometime between the ages of 46 and 57, when they hit the lowest point in their lives since puberty. A decade later, in 1989, when these corporate winners were at or approaching retirement, they answered a completely new Life History Survey, and I interviewed a representative group of them again.[26] A startling change was almost immediately apparent.

At their thirtieth reunion they had been fat cats. By their fortieth reunion, having attained an average age of 66, the same men had become pussycats. The big switch was from seeking satisfaction *out there*—through the success and status of their business careers—to savoring the pleasures of a return to hearth and home. At this stage they derived their greatest satisfaction from their intimate relationships, with their wives, friends, and children, to whom *they* now look for understanding and support.

Taken as a group, the men at this stage were happier with their lives than they had *ever* been. Their health was remarkably robust; most said their health status hadn't changed over the previous five years, and some said it had improved. Few had given mortality much thought. In fact, on the arithmetic of life they do slow math. At 65 to 67 they were "just beginning to feel middle-aged." More detached and less quick to anger than in their midfifties, they *expected* to mellow out in their seventies at a high plateau.

About their grandchildren they were positively gooey. One questionnaire came in with purple blotches. A note explained, "Grandchildren spilled raspberries from my garden." A few years before, this man had been a powerhouse chairman of the board. His raspberry statement indicated that his primary activities were now growing grapes for winemaking and splitting wood. Like many of the men, he indicated he was able now to open himself to new feelings, including the tender ties to his grandchildren.

It was rare at the turn of the century for teenage grandchildren to know their grandparents throughout their adolescence. Today a typical 15-year-old has a nine out of ten chance of having two or more grandparents still alive.[27] In fact, the affinity between the spry semiretired set and children, who are increasingly left on their own by working parents or abandoned to the streets, should only be enhanced by the graying of society. Shortly beyond the year 2000 mature Americans 55 and over will hold equal weight in numbers with children under 15—each group representing 21 percent of the population (roughly sixty million each).[28] And since the number of years one spends as a grandparent has greatly expanded, it becomes a role that is worth the investment of time and thought to do well.

Most of the Harvard Business School men were still working in their midsixties, many part-time. Some had retired and, finding themselves restless, had gone back to work but in more satisfying, self-directed capacities. Two thirds now classified themselves as self-employed. They were involved in public service, consulting, and serving on boards of directors—often working as hard as ever but usually enjoying it a lot more—although their median income was considerably reduced: down to a mere $127,500. (The peak salary commanded by these stars had ranged between $100,000 and $500,000.)

More and more Americans over 65 are taking part-time jobs: 52 percent of all white men in 1990, compared with 30 percent back in 1960.[29] What these former corporate gunslingers really cared about, however, were entirely new pursuits, like learning how to be gourmet cooks, fanatical gardening, woodworking, restoring antique cars—working with their hands and close to home. The big competition among them at this stage was for who could make the best pasta! And one quarter of them had become learners again—returning to universities for classical studies in music, art, history—for the pure intellectual and aesthetic pleasure of it rather than the instrumental value for their careers.

When they talk about themselves today, they show much greater insight and detachment from their role as businessmen. It is as though they are packing up that whole bundle of risks and rewards, mistakes and failures, and external status represented by their corporate careers and shipping it off to China on a container ship—still a valuable cargo but one that they can now evaluate coolly as only *part* of what is important about their lives. Money was a major incentive in their First Adulthood, and what with all those stock options and golden handshakes they had socked away a lot of it. Half of them now had net worths of over $2 million, and half of them less.

These men were not sure that their earlier obsession with making a lot of money was all that important. In fact, nearly half believed in retrospect that moneymaking was less important than they'd thought. The greater reward from professional life was the high status it had conferred and the chance to leave a mark. Asked if they had it to do over again, would they give more time to family and less to work, half the men admitted "probably not." Others said they would like to *think* they'd have a different set of priorities. But the evidence from the earlier survey was more reliable on this point. Back in their mid-fifties these men simply *thrived* on work. They were consumed with maneuvering into the highest possible positions on the status pyramid before the final shakedown stage. It reminds us that values can change profoundly from one stage to the next.

But even before the era of downsizing, some of those I had interviewed in 1979 spoke of their desire to get out of corporate life before they were "excessed" or ground up in a takeover or merger. Back then the Class of '49 divided right down the middle on those who lit out to try the entrepreneurial life and those who elected to stay with "the security and comfort of working within a large corporation." What happened? Two case histories are instructive.

The first is the archetypal company man.

MR. HAT, THE COMPANY MAN

"Psychologically you never get over the blow."

Under his hat this man's identity was completely subsumed into the corporate identity. Even as a boy he had been a team player, never an individualist. The blocking back in football, the floor man in basketball, he was the feeder, never the top scorer, but usually a respectable second. In business he never aspired to be CEO, but he *did* believe utterly that his thirty years of loyal service to the company would be recognized.

He always wore a hat. Had to. The company's founder always wore a hat. Besides, he was the company's hatchet man. Whenever the company wanted a plant closed, he was the poker face sent in to chop up people's lives and scatter them around the country. The hat, he felt, conferred something of a rabbinical respect on his victims. As his just reward for years of dehumanizing devotion to the company's bottom line, he expected to be named chief financial officer.

A sudden and "violent" change of career disrupted all his plans. He was "given" early retirement. The emotional blow of being told, "Forget it, Mr. Hat, we don't need you anymore," was almost more than he could bear. It struck at the heart of his entire belief in himself as a worthy team player. "That was fourteen and a half years ago," the company man told me precisely, putting down his hat. "Psychologically you never get over the blow."

To look at his position today, as the pro bono chairman of a major world foundation, one would say, "Isn't that worthy?" But when he looks inside, he is shocked. For there, under the heading of "self-esteem," is a blank. He remembers with some awe watching a bolder man tell off the very same boss. The boss was accompanying this man on a client call. The boss said, "You forgot your hat." The upstart told him, "Look, I'll work for you twenty-four hours a day, seven days a week, but I won't wear a hat." And he kept on walking. The boss laughed. He later named the upstart CEO.

"It's indicative of the fact that he was always his own man," concedes the company man. "And me—I still wear a hat."

LATE-AGE ENTREPRENEUR

"I kept saying to myself, Where are your damn guts?"

The alternative path was one chosen by a middle manager who believed that by staying in corporate life, he was losing his manhood. We'll call him Willy because he identified with *Death of a Salesman.*

During our first interview, when he was in his early forties, he had described "feeling myself slipping unalterably into compromising myself in order to keep up the lifestyle." He rationalized like crazy: His money was tied up in stocks; he had his position in the community to think of and the country club he'd just joined. What was truly terrifying for this man, who had bootstrapped himself up from a lower-middle-class background, was the specter of slipping from respectability. Despite the gloss of graduating from Harvard Business School (or perhaps that added to his conflict), he agonized over whether to stay in middle management with a merged firm and become Willy Loman, or to take the first risk of his life.

"I kept saying to myself, *Where are your damn guts?*" he confessed.

Riddled with the normal hurry-up feelings of midlife, he started trying to make money *fast*. The result was, he lost it. So, before turning 50, he gave up his corporate post and took the plunge into starting his own business. This time he imposed a different timetable: *I'm going to look at this project as if I have not three years, not ten years, but a lifetime to make it work.* He tightened his belt, borrowed from the bank, even tapped his friends to be investors, and he didn't sleep a lot. It was an agonizing period. He kept up a confident front, never revealing to anyone, not his wife, or priest or therapist or friends, how terrified he felt. But he was *determined to be his own man.*

Today this late-age entrepreneur is chairman of his own company, which is valued by an independent CPA at $25 million, and he owns it 100 percent. In the last few years, he says, he feels he finally has it all together. About one thing he is absolutely sure: He is *not* retired and does not plan to retire. But just to be ready in case he changes his mind, he is studying piano and voice.

SOURCES OF WELL-BEING IN THE SIXTIES

Not all these winners in business were so satisfied with the way their lives had turned out. In fact, there was a significant minority of men in the Class of '49 who were unhappy. The distinction between those men who hit the top of the well-being scale and those who lagged around the bottom was the most interesting part of the study.

When these men were in their mid-fifties, the distinction was simple and clear: The happiest men were presidents. The *un*happiest men were vice-presidents. By their mid-sixties the predictor of overall life satisfaction had completely shifted.

It's *not* their position in business that makes the difference. Only a handful more of the CEOs and presidents were among the highest well-being group. Vice-presidents were evenly divided between very satisfied and unhappy. Well, then, one would assume, it must be money: The happiest guys had to be the hotshots who hit over the $2 million mark. Wrong again.

There was virtually *no difference in net worth* between those who were satisfied with their lives by their mid-sixties and those who were not. Okay, maybe it was the difference between retiring and still being fully active. Again, just as many of the contented men have left their companies for good as those who still go to the office full-time. However, those of the HBS men who retired completely by their early sixties and have not gone on to do anything productive beyond pleasing themselves do not sound particularly happy.

Would failure explain the difference then? No, almost as many happy men as unhappy ones have failed. The happiest say they are better off for having failed, and they learned a great deal from it. The unhappiest say their failure was destructive. It's a chicken-and-egg argument: If one sees a failure as destructive, it will have a dampening effect on one's outlook on life.

So what *does* make the difference in overall contentment at the subtotal stage?

> The comfort of mature love is the single most important determinant of older men's outlook on life.

Ninety percent of the happiest HBS men are in love with their wives today and say they have grown closer since the children left. In contrast, only half of the unhappiest men have become more intimate with their mates. And we're not talking here about the love of the new young filly or the trophy wife. Of the whole group studied, 88 percent are still married to Wife Number One. Only 9 men out of the 174 had taken a younger second wife, and most of those did say, "She makes me feel terrific," although one man moaned, "She makes me feel old!"

Another huge gap between men at opposite ends of the well-being scale is sexual compatibility with their wives. Most of the men who are savoring mature love with their wives also still enjoy making love to them. *Only one of the high well-being men has lost interest in sex.* But it's not just sex that makes them cherish a wife as a true partner in life at this stage. They are turned on by her intellectual stimulation and her unconditional love.

The low well-being men have long lists of psychosomatic complaints, chiefly insomnia, broken sleep, tiring early, feeling fat, problems with digestion, high blood pressure, and feeling irritable and angry much of the time. Why angry? It's the degree of success they have, or haven't, attained in their careers that gets under their skin. Status in the competitive pecking order is still the primary factor they allow to determine their overall contentment with life. Many feel cheated. Or they endlessly blame themselves for past failures. Perhaps one reason the highs have fewer aches and pains is that they concern themselves with others; many have taken some action to address the country's major social or educational problems. The lows, in contrast, are very involved with themselves.

The grandfather behind the raspberry-stained questionnaire, for example, is a man who cashed in his company stock and invested the money and is now sitting on a nest egg of $5 million. But in retrospect he has mixed feelings about what his life adds up to as a whole. Like others who are completely retired, what he misses most are the *people*—both the colleagues he worked with closely and the business friends who have dropped away. He also misses "working toward a goal." He's dissatisfied with having so much time on his hands. As he notices his friends starting to look old, he dwells more and more on his own mortality. He feels he's lost potency as a high roller in business. Now he fears losing his sexual potency. It's important to point out that his relationship with his wife is not very good.

The wives of these mopey men are by and large frustrated by the reasons (alibis) their husbands give for not being able to change: "Insufficient contacts" or "It's hard to get a good directorship at my age," although a few men admit, "I don't really know why I can't get started again." More than one wife has told her retired husband, "Why don't you go out and get a real job?"

It's almost as though the dissatisfied men believe that because they made a lot of money, they're entitled to coast. *Go ahead, make my passage.* It doesn't work that way.

Continued excitement about life is the other determining factor in high well-being for men at this stage. We have already observed the many new pursuits that bring excitement to men in their sixties. The HBS men who enjoy the highest well-being had reached out for new adventures in half a dozen new directions before any grass grew under their feet. They therefore see semi- or full retirement as an enticing opportunity to add richness to their life balance sheets. The sixties for them are very much a *self-directed stage.*

Thus it is not dollars or titles that are most important to people in their sixties; it is the quality and quantity of meaningful human attachments and having something to be excited about. The high well-being men always take great pleasure in their offspring and often turn to them for comfort. The low-satisfaction men turn to their lawyers. Some admit they were absent or poor fathers.

Obviously all these Harvard men are among the most affluent of Americans. Still, despite the fact that the actual net worth across the board is no higher among the most contented men, *almost half* of the most dissatisfied men are "fearful about not having enough money." Yet money doesn't make up for emptiness in love or estranged children. Money doesn't bring back the juice, not once they've given up on acting to change things for the better in business or marriage or their communities. The low well-being men are much more worried than the highs about advancing age and being abandoned by their wives. Money doesn't make them feel safe. It's never enough.

HOW MUCH IS ENOUGH?

This is a major question of the sixties. As someone said, "If I am what I have, and what I have is lost, who, then, am I?" The British mogul Robert Maxwell must have wondered before he threw himself overboard (or fell or was pushed) in the last twelve hours he spent alone, when he knew his whole house of cards was in collapse. Shortly before he died, Lee Atwater, founder of the "go negative" school of political campaign warfare, was interviewed in *Life.* "The 80's were about acquiring," he said. "I know. I acquired more wealth, power and prestige than most. But you can acquire all you want and still feel empty."[30]

"The more affluent we are, the more the problem of meaninglessness bears down upon us," asserts the author of a book titled *The Search for Meaning,* the former Duke University economics professor Thomas Naylor. "We have too much freedom and the freedom to misuse it, too many choices and not enough discipline or delayed gratification to make the best choices for the long term."

OLD ELEPHANTS' CLUB, AGE 65

"When you've got enough, then what?"

A high-profile athletes' lawyer, whose official tally at the subtotal stage is very impressive, suffered from this crisis of meaninglessness. He invited me to join him at a small private dinner party of sports-world moguls at "21." It was a way of showing off his status.

Bert, I'll call him, came from money and was successful young. He is always in the news, seen making splashy deals for his players and moving people around. He also made himself indispensable behind the scenes to some of the players' unions. His wife has survived breast cancer and had a recent face-lift. He gives every outward appearance of affluence and contentment in his mid-sixties, sitting back in his banquette at "21," his tennis-dark skin contrasting handsomely with his summer-light silk suit. Yet he squirms. Bert cannot refrain from talking about the terrifying emptiness inside: "You're trained for only one thing, getting more. But when you've got enough, then what?"

He conceded that he had always measured his worth as a person by what the money he made could buy: the swimming pool, the fancy foreign car, the deluxe house in the country. Now that he had all the toys he could use, he pondered, "What's the reason? What's the purpose? If you don't have an answer, you just get back on the treadmill because that's all you know."

What do you do when it stops?

Who are you when you're not the boss anymore?

He pushed away the asparagus salad, scolding the waiter for dressing it with something that screams high cholesterol.

"They don't teach us how to do this stage," he continued. "We're all so good at denial. Women can do cosmetic surgery, and they have lots of tricks, but guys, guys don't know how to face this—what do you call it— the last passage?"

Seeing it as the last passage, I said, might make it so. It could also be seen as an opening.

"Well, you're told you have to move off the field and onto the bench and just watch the play, don't interfere—like an old general," he grumbled. Looking back over his life of high-stakes negotiations, he wondered aloud, "What's in it for me at this stage? Where's the meaning, the larger signifi-cance, the fun?"

Bert was terrified of giving up his spot at the top of the "baboon colony," as he calls it. He was critical of other aging agents who abdicate the head-on confrontations to their subordinates. At the same time he is tortured by restlessness. He needs to move on, but where to go from the top, except fade into oblivion? Will Bert have to keep running the treadmill until he drops because he can't think of what else to do if he stops? He's gone sour on New York. He talks it down but doesn't leave. He and his friends recognize their ambivalence:

"We don't want to watch the decay of New York because we don't want to face our own decay," he said. "We're like old elephants, looking for a place to die. But where do you go? Palm Beach? Down there the last thing guys can do to show their power is the WASPs try to keep the new Jews out of the golf club."

This is the sound of a man in the state of despair. The next thing that will probably go is his health.

COMEBACKS FROM HOPELESSNESS

The relationship between physical health and mental health is greatest in later life, as confirmed by Dr. Gene Cohen, National Institute on Aging. "We know, in the face of depression and stress, older people have much more trouble with their health."[31] Even the most apparently famous and indefatigable of men, still plying the trades they love, can tumble into a state of despair and hopelessness.

Mike Wallace, the journalist who created the mold of the hard-hitting investigative TV interviewer during his long tenure on *60 Minutes,* was still apparently going strong in his early sixties after a heart attack and the insertion of a pacemaker. The truth was something else. "I felt like a fake. My life had no meaning." This delayed crisis of meaning threw Wallace into a two-year clinical depression, which he fought off by the age of 65. He has continued working vigorously as a TV journalist well into his late seventies.[32]

One of the common scenarios for men like Bert, the sports agent described above, is to stop feeling much of anything. They drift into chronic depression, without recognizing it, but after some years they turn up with cancer and just don't have the will left to fight it. Our thoughts and feelings do not *cause* cancer or heart attacks, and changing our thoughts and feelings cannot alone *cure* or *prevent* disease. But the emerging science involving the immune system does strongly implicate our feelings as culprits in rendering us *susceptible* to such diseases. Conversely, with the right corrective psychological work, the immune system can be brought up to the fighting strength of a crack Praetorian Guard that fends off viruses and free radicals and cellular aberrations and makes us *resistant* to disease.

Even short-term emotional changes, like feeling happy or sad for twenty minutes, can powerfully affect our immune system. A fascinating study at UCLA by Margaret Kemeny, a Ph.D. psychoimmunologist, used method-trained actors to generate intense emotional states and then measured changes in the number and activity of "killer cells" in their bloodstream.[33] "Killer cells" are the naturally "good" cells that help us fight off disease and eradicate tumor cells if they appear. Now you probably assume, as I did, that being sad or angry would be bad for our health. Not so.

"We found that the effect of the happy state on the immune system was very similar to what we had seen as a result of the sad state," says Dr. Kemeny. Within twenty minutes there was an increase in the killer cells, and they were functioning more effectively. It was the *absence* of emotion that depressed the immune system and predisposed a person to disease. This is what happens when people withdraw or become passive about their lives.

Another professional who deals effectively with this dead-end dilemma is Lawrence LeShan, Ph.D., a research and clinical psychologist considered one of the fathers of mind-body therapy and author of the landmark book *Cancer as a Turning Point.*[34] LeShan's studies have been on psychological means of rebuilding the immune system, the cancer-fighting defense, by rebuilding a person's enthusiasm for life. The following story happens to involve a man diagnosed with cancer, but the principles are applicable to anyone who is battling despair and trying to regain his or her integrity as he or she ages and feels increasingly unwanted.

THE CANCER SURVIVOR

"What's right with you?"

Ted (a pseudonym) was a high-profile businessman whose intelligence, drive, and broad-ranging interests had enabled him to create a retail store with international mystique. He was widely credited with establishing that mystique and the store's phenomenal success in franchising itself. That effort had been his life, ever since he had started in the basement as a young man and worked his way up to vice-president and finally chairman. He was a natural trend spotter, and he loved minding his store, his baby. He got up each morning eager to get in early and check the sales figures on his computer. It gave him a position in his city as an arbiter of taste and an excuse to travel the world on the lookout for exciting influences from other cultures.

The whole structure and context of his life collapsed when his elegant duchess of a store was bought out by a ruthless retail conglomerate. Still a tremendously energetic sixtyish businessman, Ted was persuaded to stay on. It wasn't long before he got fed up with "playing ball" with the new owners, whose only interest was in cutting costs and services and squeezing more profit into the bottom line so they could resell the property. That's what they called his baby: the "property." He felt the integrity of the store, which was inseparable from his own integrity, was being compromised by a thousand tiny cuts.

Not long after he left the store, Ted began to develop some digestive symptoms. He decided that playing well would be the best revenge. He'd fill his life with golf and try to perfect his game. But after a year of playing invitational club tournaments, he realized that his reflexes weren't going to get any keener. The perfect golf game as a goal would become only a measurement of his diminishing abilities. That's when he stopped feeling much emotion of any kind. Something inside him went dark.

He made a stab at starting over. He opened a miniature version of his grand store in a newly developing part of the city. The recession drained away customers, and the area's development stopped cold. Ted was diagnosed with colon cancer. After surgery and a course of chemotherapy he slipped into lethargy. He'd get up in the morning, meaning to go somewhere, but feel a wave of drowsiness overwhelm him and take a little nap; he might not get out of his sweatpants all day, just sit in his chair reading or watching TV. He felt lost. Nothing much interested him. He had no energy or drive.

It wasn't until his wife insisted he see a psychiatrist that he was diagnosed as having been in chronic depression, for several years at least. By the time of our first interview Ted was in his mid-sixties. Now his whole concern was: *How do I keep from having a recurrence of the disease?* In my second interview with Ted I mentioned the work of Dr. LeShan. The retailer said he would be interested in having a consultation with the psychotherapist on how to approach his impending cancer surgery. Although Dr. LeShan has retired from his private practice to train younger psychotherapists in his methods, he agreed to talk to Ted. Highlights of their session were recounted to me.[35]

Larry LeShan is a relaxed, fast-talking 70-year-old psychologist with silver hair and black-rimmed glasses. He has survived a heart attack but projects great vitality and humanity. He greeted Ted at the door of his comfortable West End Avenue apartment wearing casual clothes and slippers. After a brief discussion of the former retailer's upcoming surgery, LeShan jumped the subject ahead to when the man would be fully responsible for his life again.

LeSHAN: Let's suppose the medical treatment is a hundred percent effective. The doctors tell you, "Come back once a year for the next five years; you're fine otherwise." How would your life be different after surgery?

TED: I don't know. I've had a number of disappointments over the last five years in my career.

LeSHAN: Suppose you were given the *ideal* setup. What kind of work would you feel best about doing?

TED: A great retailer is what I wanted to be, always, and I'm pretty good at it. I'm sixty-five years old, and the store I built from the basement up into a franchise is on the block for hundreds of millions today.

LeSHAN: What else could you enjoy doing? Let your imagination go.

TED: The period I was most excited was when I was turning an ordinary store into something unique. It wasn't only the financial success, but the excitement of building a company. I lost that. I've tried that again a couple of times since, most recently buying a store where I've lost a lot of money. Right now I'm a consultant in the retail industry. It's all right; it's not great; I have a layer of corporate executives over me. At least I have something to get up and get dressed for.

LESHAN: You don't sound very enthusiastic about it.

TED: It's very hard for me to see what else I could do successfully. And I find that plunging into the day's activities is a relief to me. I forget about my disease and get excited.

LESHAN: The important question here is, How do you bring back the cancer defense system? Someday we'll do it biologically. Today the only way we know to do it is psychologically—by making a concrete commitment to change things in a way that *will rebuild the enthusiasm for your life.* Ask yourself what you can do that will give you that *good* tired feeling at night, not the blah tired feeling.

TED: I really can't think what it could be. I just don't hear the music anymore.

LESHAN: Okay, you don't know how now. So put the question on the front burner of your life.

TED: My wife and I had our first conversation about that just yesterday, stimulated by reading your book together.

LESHAN: The immune system is kind of feebleminded. It needs concrete stimulation. Now you need to make a commitment between the two of you. You will think about this question every day—like What am I going to wear today? Eat today? Will I take an umbrella? These are front-burner questions. Make this something you worry at, like a dog with a bone. You struggle with it, sulk with it, laugh about it, dream about it. You're saying to your own organism: *"I am so important, I am worth fighting for."* It's as if the immune system looks up and says, *"Oh, I am worth fighting for? Why didn't you say so?"*

Having worked with this technique for more than thirty years, LeShan now says that approximately one half of his patients with poor prognoses (and those of therapists trained by him) have responded with long-term remissions and are still alive. Moreover, the quality of their lives is enhanced. Sometimes, even when no medical treatment is possible, he has seen people recover spontaneously. LeShan always adds a caution: "This stuff is not a *replacement* for medical treatment. It's an *adjunct* to medical treatment." Originally trained as a Freudian to all but genuflect toward Vienna, the psychologist explained why he believes that classical psychotherapy doesn't work in fighting cancer. That's not what it was designed for.

LeShan: We've found you have to have a new strategy—not what's wrong with you but *what's right with you.* What do *you* need to flower most fully? First you and your mate build together the perfect castle in the air. Then you can begin to find a way to put a foundation under it, and then move in. It takes time. But even if it takes you a long time to find out what you could enjoy doing, what is important is that you are working at it all the time. Working at it forces you to keep calling people, reading, traveling, casting in every direction. In all my years of practice, I've never found a person who couldn't come up with an answer—including those with limited education and skills.

Ted: But I seem to be tired all the time. And taking it easy doesn't help.

LeShan: There are different kinds of exhaustion. Chronic exhaustion, the kind you're feeling, is usually caused by a blocked energy flow. You can't take advantage of your *available* energy because you haven't found a way to open channels for your creative expression.

Ted: You're right. Doing nothing is exhausting! I guess I've trained myself with these disappointments to take the blow, not to feel it. Just to focus on finding out what I could do next. Now I know that's not right. *I'm looking for something to give me hope.*

LeShan: Is it possible you have given up hope?

Ted: It may be. I notice when somebody wants me to work, I have a really soaring feeling. When I can't see a future, it drives me down. From one minute to the next, my whole feeling changes.

LeShan: I'll be willing to bet it changes your body chemistry too. The one thing we know depresses your defense system is to believe there is no hope for a meaningful outlet for your creative energies. Then your cancer-fighting mechanism weakens and the disease can take over. If a master bricklayer sees no chance of ever building again, he has lost his hope.

LeShan's final words to the retailer were a ubiquitous prescription for anyone in or near a state of despair: "You've run out of resilience. You and your wife have to keep reminding each other you *will not settle* for filling your life with anything but the *ideal.*" The very process of searching is a healing process, because it's opening up hope.

The retailer and his wife began their search by reviving their many international contacts; she refreshed her language skills and Ted became active with nongovernmental organizations working in foreign countries. That paid for them to travel widely, something they both loved to do. But finding out what he could do *and* make a living, as LeShan had promised, was hard. The retailer went down several blind alleys before he was able to ferret out the essence of what he had loved about his work: It was identifying and developing talented artisans and designers, and then bringing their work to the profitable attention of the outside world. That step alone took him a year.

He heard the State Department was sending a U.S. delegation to China to explore giving privatization grant aid. The old excitement bubbled up, but what did he have to offer? He mulled it over with another retiree from business, who recast Ted's skills in a new light: "Look, a person who has experience in some form of enterprise, coupled with cultural sensitivity, is a very valuable resource to the government."

Fortified with this notion of a new identity, Ted sold himself to the State Department: "What you need in this delegation is an internationally experienced retailer." The trip to China introduced him to a new dimension of thinking. He *was* valuable. Helping other countries to develop local artisans and craftspeople and advising factories on how to design and manufacture their products efficiently for world markets was something that came naturally to him. "The idea of getting away from selling ladies' lingerie suddenly appealed to me greatly."

The cancer survivor and his wife noticed something: Whenever they spent an extended time in another culture, meeting new people and generating ideas with them, they both felt enormously stimulated and energetic. Ted gave almost no thought to the state of his health. Digging into another culture at the grass-roots level was a luxury for which there had been no time when Ted was a busy businessman. But joining government-sponsored trade delegations was a now-and-then thing, not well paid, and in between trips Ted would sometimes slip back into depression.

After several years of working at it, the ideal setup sprang to his mind in the middle of a working trip in Eastern Europe. Why not start his own import-export business? It wasn't the most profitable thing he could do, but it would allow him and his wife to travel the world and spot ideas, and enjoy the artistic fulfillment of bringing them to fruition in the international marketplace.

Today, the importer and his wife work together. They are stretched to their intellectual and physical limits, and they love it. Ted is totally involved and present in his life again. Four years after his cancer surgery, his CAT scan remained clear.

18

WISEWOMEN IN TRAINING

Philosophy is perfectly right in saying that life must be understood backward. But then one forgets
the other clause—that it must be lived forward.

—SØREN KIERKEGAARD[1]

*T*was in for some surprises when I accepted an invitation to the premiere conference on "The New Older Woman" held at the Esalen Institute
in the summer of 1991. A small group of prominent American women
from diverse backgrounds came together to share viewpoints on what it's
like to be energetic, ambitious, optimistic, and over 50 in today's America.
The participants agreed that there had come a point, sometime in their
fifties, when they had to let go of—or at least stop trying to hang on to—
their youthful images and move on. Although painful at the time, they all
had found a source of new vitality and exhilaration—a "kicker." For some
the kicker was a large-scale social mission like AIDS activism or a political
goal like teaching women how to use power. For others it was a more private
challenge: writing a book or pursuing knowledge in a special field for the
pure pleasure of knowing.

A common denominator emerged: The source of continuing aliveness
was to *find your passion and pursue it with whole heart and single mind.*

As peppy and provocative as were the discussions, it was sharing a room
with my 84-year-old roommate that dissolved some of the barriers to my
thinking about "the older woman." When I first encountered this tall, limber lady, Mildred Mathias, she was doubled over, brushing her hair. A
botanist, she had just come in from her daily brisk walk and despite the

foggy weather excitedly displayed a handful of pungent herbs and grasses. At dinner I noticed her laughter was more liquid and full-throated than almost anyone else's. What was the secret of her zest? I wondered.

It turns out that Mildred had retired from her prestigious teaching position in the California University system at the age of 70. She languished for a while, developing ailments and boredom, thinking her life was just about over. A few years later she had an opportunity to take her first field trip down the Amazon River to collect scarce plants with medicinal uses. She dared to step off the precipice. The experience was thrilling. And she felt useful again. She had repeated the trip every year with a commitment bordering on the sacred.

"Each trip down the Amazon, I'm convinced, peels back ten years off my life," Mildred Mathias told me.

Her story brought to mind other women I've known or interviewed who had joined the walking dead, almost dropping out of life for some years, but who revived themselves later by plunging into some new adventure that held both risk and meaning for them. We can learn so much from vital older women. It should be a conscious exercise to pick out those who live their passions with purpose and direction and let them suggest possibilities and guiding principles for our own future self. These are the transformative figures I call Wisewomen.

One Wisewoman who has inspired me over the years is Deborah Szekely, a late bloomer who pioneered in creating fitness spas as a major service industry but whose achievements since she turned 60 bring new meaning to the term *Second Adulthood*.

DREAMER BEYOND DREAMS

"I wanted something to lose sleep over again."

Drawing on Japanese philosophy, Deborah Szekely divides life into three parts. "The first third of life is devoted to being a child, learning in school and at home. The next third is spent working as hard as you're able and being rewarded for it. The final third is perhaps the most important: taking a role in making the world better for the next generation."

In truth there was no imperative for Deborah to do anything, really, by the time she hit 60, except rest on her laurels, enjoy the enduring success of her two world-class spas, stroll around their fabulous gardens, directing others to move this rock or that shrub, and watch her capable son and daughter take over the bottom-line management. She had already lived an exotic life, marked both by tragedy and triumphs. Raised in Tahiti by parents who were fruitarians, she was married off to a charismatic health guru, Edmond Szekely, when she was barely 17.

"He was God," she says of the scholarly philosopher husband who was almost twenty years her senior. Back in 1940 the two of them founded a health camp outside the dusty Mexican border village of Tecate. What began as an adobe hut in the middle of a vineyard, rented for $10 a month, has been nurtured through fifty years of private ownership into the paradisical fitness showplace of the 1990s called Rancho la Puerta.

But for many years, deferring to the Professor and trying to relieve him of the more mundane details of running a business so he could focus on his writings, Deborah worked around the ranch like a hired girl. "He was a gifted authoritarian personality, so I felt very stupid all the time," she says. The Professor didn't want children, so she didn't start her family until her mid-thirties, having made a bargain with him: She would start a spa in the States to provide the financial security for a family.

Very gradually Deborah began to take over the management of the rustic ranch and its more extravagant sister, The Golden Door, founded in 1958 in Escondido, California. When her husband began to spend time with girlfriends, they agreed on a separation. Without bitterness she recalls the period when "my husband began to spend money almost to put us into bankruptcy, just to prove I couldn't manage." Much of the second third of her life was drained by what Deborah calls "the energy of overcoming."

It wasn't until her mid-forties that she found out she was smart. Invited to serve on boards of directors of San Diego's cultural institutions, she began showing what she could do and receiving affirmation from her peers. As the first inklings of an independent identity appeared, she was punished for it. The Professor asked for a divorce. She took the blow with benign defiance. "If I'd had an easy life, I couldn't be the person I am. I'm a great survivor."

She was determined to keep her son and daughter and her two other children—the spas. "My divorce settlement of choice was that he would get all the proceeds from the spas for seven years," she explains. "At the end of seven years the ranch and the Door would then belong to me. But if I missed one payment, he could take everything back. So those seven years were definitely high adrenaline."

She thrived on the dare and turned out to be a naturally gifted entrepreneur. After seven years she was free, and at 50 Deborah was a June bride.

Again, after seven years her life turned over when her second husband pulled the plug on their marriage. He wanted to retire. It was inconceivable to her.

"I decided I would never marry again. Because I'd invested a lot in myself and I wanted to use it. I realized I didn't need a husband. I liked the freedom."

But approaching 60, she was *too* free. The Golden Door had become so polished it was soon to earn the designation of Best Health Spa in the country. To open more Golden Doors would have been to repeat herself, offering no challenge at all. Her son was ready to take over management of the spas. She was bored with parties where she knew beforehand what everyone would say. The dynamic Deborah Szekely was up against an exquisite dilemma: *What do you do when you've exceeded all your dreams?*

"It was like a fantasy to me," she says, a catch of the delicious uncertainty in her voice as she recalls what it was like to cut loose from San Diego and the spas and move herself across the country to Washington to start a new life. "I'd never lived alone. I was married out of my parents' home at seventeen. I'd never been to college. I hardly knew a soul in Washington. I was challenged in every way."

White—this late late bloomer decided that everything in her rented house should be white—the wicker furniture, the white orchid plants hovering on serene single curved stems, the solarium bedroom that would be full of sky and moving white clouds. A beautiful blank slate. Then what to write on it?

"I wanted something to lose sleep over again," she told me.

That comment distilled much of what is missing in the lives of people in their sixties who are proved successes with their dreams mostly behind them. When we're young, we lose sleep over passing tests, over starting our families, over the striving to get ahead in our work, lots of things. Deborah hungered to be totally involved and committed again and compelled to get results. "When you hit fifty, if you're doing well, you have nothing to lose sleep about," she says. "My mom in her fifties was old. Her life was ending, and she hadn't done all the things she'd wanted to do."

After a brief stint of working for the U.S. Information Agency, Deborah campaigned to have herself appointed president and CEO of the Inter-American Foundation, a government agency created to support self-help efforts of the poor throughout Latin America and the Caribbean. Over the next half-dozen years she was endlessly shuttling among twenty-six different countries to oversee their "in-country service" offices, which she set up, and to evaluate innovative programs for which she disbursed $150 million in grants.

One day I visited Deborah in her 1810 Federal town house in George-town, set on a neat apron of brick patio. I persuaded her to try to be reflective for a few moments, instead of what comes naturally: being the perpetual activist. She was about to turn 72. Her contentment glowed through the olive-smooth skin of her full cheeks. Her eyes were like high beams, and she spoke in staccato bursts.

How on earth did she sell the government on hiring a 60-year-old woman who hadn't been in politics? I asked her.

Well, she'd had considerable political clout from years of helping both Democratic and Republican candidates. People had written letters for her. But frankly, she said, the question had puzzled her, too. Years later she asked the young man who had hired her: "There were others much more qualified for the position, even former ambassadors. Why did you put me on the short list?" He said, "Because you wanted it so much."

Then passion is infectious, I suggested.

"Yes." She smiled. "And passion is the right word. It's the same depth and obsession as the erotic passion when you were deeply in love, when you thought about him every minute. Same as when your children were young and always on your mind. The passion takes you above yourself; you don't stew and fret because you're so focused. Therefore, I expect my body and my health to support me."

A lunch of spicy gazpacho, scallops, and steamed vegetables was served by a housekeeper. Deborah lives now with a pair of King Charles spaniels that she finds beautiful company. She is pleasantly rounded and does not make a fetish of fitness. In the solarium is a yawning chaise surrounded by books and plants. But she rarely takes the time to stretch out on it. Occupying a chaise longue runs absolutely counter to her philosophy of successful aging.

In fact, another seven-year cycle having passed, she had felt the wheels turning more slowly and the cutting edge blunted. Her major goals for the Inter-American Foundation had been achieved, and so, in 1990, a fresh idea had sprung from her head. Why not take her experience in seeking out worthy antipoverty projects in Latin America and apply it to the crisis of leadership in America's inner cities? She founded Eureka Communities, a grass-roots effort to train and connect the leaders of the most dynamic inner-city nonprofit organizations that have success stories to share.

Now she travels every week, indefatigably searching out new leaders to serve as mentors and raising funds for her Eureka Fellows to keep their projects going in three different cities. Just the night before, she had been dancing till midnight at the White House at a gala fund-raising dinner for the Ford Theater. People who see this septuagenarian dashing around to do all these things always ask, "Don't you get tired?"

"Of course I get tired!" she exclaimed. "But I'm doing something that needs to be done." She leaned back in her contoured desk chair and propped her feet on the windowsill. "I don't believe that you have to get older," declared this maverick. "You can stay flexible in the head and in the body. We're all going to be living into the high eighties, at least. What that fifty to ninety period is going to be like really and truly depends on what you do at the beginning of the second half. You have to maintain your spirit."

To celebrate her seventy-third birthday, she plans to join her children, once again, in climbing the bouldered slopes of her beloved Mount Kuchumaa at the ranch—five miles straight up the face—and to shout when she comes to the top, "Eureka!"

"What keeps your spirit so alive?" I asked.

"I'm so *curious* about what's going to happen next," she said. "I always think there's more ahead than there was behind."

THE WIT NETWORK

Conversations with Wisewomen like Deborah Szekely and my 84-year-old botanist roommate set me to thinking, How could we harvest the wisdom of the aging process? Out of a creative partnership with Ellen McGrath grew an idea. Why not tap the knowledge of today's pioneering women in postmenopause, especially those who seem to have a knack for living creatively, and invite them to share ideas on how to outwit the culture's programmed model for aging?

"We'll invite them to join a circle—to become Wisewomen."

"But we're not wise yet!"

"Then we'll call it WIT, Wisewomen in Training."

The Flaming Fifties celebration lunch/dinner held in 1993 was the first WIT gathering (see Chapter 10, "From Pleasing to Mastery"). Training to be a Wisewoman probably can't start much before 50, since women have too many other competing priorities before then. Moving into Second Adulthood encourages us to connect in a different way to other people. We become pioneers together in this new territory of life that beckons with possibilities that have been merely glimpsed and rarely lived until recent times. As Dr. McGrath points out, at this point in human history we can no longer rely on external authority, whether it be social science or political authority, to give us the answers. And it's too complicated to figure it out all alone.

We're only just starting to remake the maps in our minds.

By gathering together, we can share our sightings of dangers and delights out on the new frontier and map out some of the safer psychic highways as well as new routes to accomplishment. Creating a WIT circle encourages people to talk more in depth about their experiences and allows them to validate one another. What are they doing that's working and not working?

At one of our WIT councils I met a very down-to-earth Wisewoman model, a school principal from St. Louis, who was approaching her sixtieth birthday. Here is a woman who had never taken hormones but who had come through menopause, hysterectomy, microscopic breast cancer, and widowhood. I'll call her Elise. She is someone worth knowing.

A WISEWOMAN MODEL, AGE 60

"I'm not willing to let a day go by where my life hasn't been touched, or I haven't touched someone else's life."

The way she comes through the door tells a story in itself. She doesn't walk in; she *enters*, with laughter, her tall, limber body an exclamation point on a life fought for and twice saved. One might liken the swirl of short hair to Carol Channing's famous pelt, except that Elise has let the blond go to a light, lustrous gray. Her faintly freckled Scotch-English skin surges to tawny at the cheeks; she exudes health and vigor. There is a teasing twinkle around her eyes, and her mouth opens often into husky laughter.

Remarried at 48, she was too preoccupied with renewing the delights of regular sexual companionship to pay attention to the discomforts of menopause. She ignored the dull ache in her lower regions, even though she had constant vaginal bleeding. Her gynecologist tried the usual corrective procedures, which were unsuccessful. When it was finally suggested she have a hysterectomy, Elise hit the ceiling.

"No way! Not unless I absolutely have to, have to, have to." She had been blessed with a mother who, the day little Elise began to menstruate, dropped what she was doing and poured a drink in celebration: "To being a woman—the best you can be!" It was her magic she was being asked to give up; she couldn't believe she could still be a woman without it. She decided not to take hormones.

The next blow came a year later, when a capillary carcinoma showed up on a mammogram. The surgeon recommended a mastectomy. Again Elise balked. The tumor was still encapsulated inside a milk duct, and no radiation or chemotherapy was recommended. Why couldn't she have a lumpectomy? "Why would I want a mastectomy?" she asked.

"Because then we wouldn't have to worry," the surgeon said.

"It was such a male attitude: Just lop it off so you can forget about it." She grimaced. She found another doctor who was supportive of less radical treatment and vigilant follow-up screening. But then it all seemed to go at once. Her husband became desperately ill with cancer. Precancerous cells were found in her uterus; she ignored them. Her life became consumed by shepherding her husband in and out of hospitals and on the rounds of specialists—that is, in addition to the continuing demands on her as the head of a school who was expected to show up every day to discipline the little darlings and preside over the Christmas pageant and the trustees' dinner. Thank God for that distraction. She couldn't face another hospital, not for herself.

After four years of watching, worrying, and denying, Elise finally surrendered her most carnal organs, as she thought of them. No sooner had she recovered from the hysterectomy than her husband slipped into a ghastly morphine twilight. "Having gone through the menopause thing, and now having lost my uterus, I kept thinking that my life was going to be over along with my husband's," she remembers. She was 55; she felt buried alive.

Except for the horniness. As she tended her husband in a long, laboring death, these anomalous surges became more and more obvious to her, perhaps because she couldn't fulfill them. When she now looks back, she realizes it probably wasn't a total accident that she crossed paths again with a high school sweetheart. Elise was the class correspondent. When Larry's class note arrived from California, she acted on the impulse to call him on her next trip to visit her grandchild in the same city. She found him struggling through a divorce. They talked about loneliness. The next time Larry flew across the country on business he made a point of stopping in St. Louis to take her out to dinner. He looked across the candlelight and said, "You know, you are the girl I wanted to marry but was afraid to ask. I'm not afraid of you anymore."

It wasn't a hot flash that inflamed her cheeks. It was an old-fashioned girlish blush. In no time they were in bed. She was astonished to find that everything still worked. Elise had crossed the dreaded divide of menopause and guess what? "It's not only okay, but better than I thought it would be. Vanity is involved too. You've heard for so many years that you won't be able to find an orgasm, you're going to be bitchy, sweaty, and dried up—and you're not! You're still a woman."

It was an affair of need. It took some negotiating with her guilt, but she decided that at some point the living have to cut loose from the dying. "I just couldn't get enough sex. What a catch I was: a woman who wants no money, can't get pregnant, and asks nothing more than sex and playing. What a dream!" Her prescription for the best posthysterectomy medicine is: "Have a really successful affair with as many orgasms as you can live through and still get up and walk the next day." She laughs at her own "old-lady uninhibitedness." In a more serious vein: "Making a connection with a man at that lowest point was probably the most important thing that's happened to me in the last ten years."

The other man remained a presence through her husband's death a year later and comforted her during the grieving period that followed. A year and a half elapsed before the waves of grief and anger ebbed and the poignant rips in the viscera at the sight of ghosts—anyone who looked like her husband on the street—stopped plunging her back into despair. But during that mourning period Elise made an effort to learn about taking care of herself for the first time. She invested in a trainer and embarked on a strict exercise program. Her bad cholesterol was elevated. Rather than diet strenuously, she retrained her eating habits. *Forget about cheese, Elise,* she told herself. *You might as well just smear Brie on your hips.* A complete lifestyle change to a diet of vegetables and fruit and varied exercise left her feeling exhilarated. For sustenance of the spirit she found a small retreat near water where she could escape for long weekends and sleep for ten hours at a stretch if she needed it.

"Mom, you look younger than you did ten years ago!" Her children marveled. They were right. Elise was a radiant 60. She had not only faced the beast of menopausal cancer but battled with it on both dreaded fronts—breast and womb—and walked away victorious, almost awed at the differentness of her new perspective.

"I'm struck with the lushness and variety of life experience available to me now," she told me. In the last couple of years she has felt an expansiveness that transcends the sort of human relationships she's had in the past. People look at her now as an expert in education, and she feels tremendous respect from her community. "I suppose I've reached a different level of self-confidence," she said. Rather than the need for a primary relationship, an exclusive source of emotional nourishment, as before, this radiant post-menopausal woman finds herself needing, and offering, an ever-expanding *connectedness*.

"My own vocabulary of intimacy has extended. It's like a root system spreading out. It's much more expansive. I've had this intense feeling of being available to many people—women and men—as friends and acquaintances. I'm not willing to let a day go by where my life hasn't been touched, or I haven't touched someone else's life. And I feel very confident about taking risks along with the consequences. When you're younger, you're so strung out with responsibilities, you become very protective of your emotional energy. You think it's finite. It isn't. There's no limit to your emotional availability."

I asked her how long she would like to live.

"Forever!" The word flew up on a gust of laughter.

Then, more thoughtfully: "As long as I can be useful. Especially to other women. The voice of the older woman has been silent in America." She admitted finding the prospect of 60 daunting for a while. Her first thought was: *Less time ahead than already lived.* A second thought followed: *It was thirty years ago when she finished having her children, and that seemed a long time ago.* Then a revelation: "I have thirty years of total freedom *ahead* of me now, to make all sorts of choices. The idea of putting limits on myself, when for the first time I'm without limits, is abhorrent to me."

Her daughter asked her if she'd like a puppy.

"A puppy—no, thanks! Not even a guppy!"

And she laughs like silver rattling in a drawer abruptly opened.

SURVIVOR SEX AND EXTRASEXUAL PASSIONS

You might think the widowed St. Louis school principal an exception, even an aberration. After all, how many movies or novels depict sixtyish heroines enjoying erotic episodes that bring them to new life? It's an American myth that women lose their sexuality by 60, or if they have any, it's a cuddly, decaffeinated, warm socks-by-the-fire prelude to a good night's sleep. One of the great surprises of aging, indeed, one of the more consistent hallmarks of the Wisewomen over 60 I found in my research, was their unanticipated sexual abandon. It seems an internal wildness grows in some women like tropical vegetation, even within the neat borders of conventional marriages.

A white-haired Florida retiree of 75, living with her second and younger
husband, told me matter-of-factly: "Now, sex. As a woman ages, she initiates the sex with her partner more often." I asked how that made her partner feel. "Oh, a man feels flattered," she said definitively, then chuckled.
"And he almost *never* has a headache."

Women at the Esalen conference had talked openly of the sexual passions they enjoyed after passing 50. Sometimes it was a rekindled love with
their husbands. More often than not these stories, like Elise's experience,
concerned a divorced or widowed woman meeting again with an old flame
and being swept up in a spontaneous combustion. In such reencounters the
critical eye surveying the deficits of physical beauty was softened by images
in the memory bank from the time when both partners were young and
beautiful in love together.

I must confess as "the baby" of the conference (being then barely 50), I
was not expecting to see the more dignified specimens in their late fifties,
sixties, and seventies strip down and slip into the famous Esalen hot tubs. It
was even more startling to note that their bodies were still soft-skinned and
feminine in contour. They moved in the water with obvious sensuous pleasure and spontaneity. It struck me that we rarely see older women's bodies
on TV or movie screens, so how would I have known?

The truth is that women are still falling in love in their sixties, seventies,
eighties—some of them for the very first time! It can happen after a long,
dutiful marriage is dissolved by a partner's death. Suddenly the survivor finds
herself passionately, head over heels, scared to death in love, having had no
idea such a state of ecstasy existed. Verification of this phenomenon comes
in the form of thousands of letters received by the Kinsey Institute in
response to a syndicated column published through the 1980s by director
emeritus June Reinisch. Dr. Reinisch shared some of those letters with me:

> I am female, 60 yrs. young. Am having for the first time in my life a most
> satisfying sexual love relationship with a man that I knew when we were
> younger. For almost 2 yrs. We've been having sexual intercourse two or
> three times in a night, when we get together every couple of weeks. I love
> multiorgasms!

This reader wanted to know if she was doing anything injurious to her
health. Often the women who write have been so repressed by their families
or religious proscriptions they can't believe they can enjoy ecstasy over 60

without being punished for it. Others are just getting up the gumption to demand a little ecstasy:

> My wife, Mary Kay, and I have been married forty-one years and have nine children. There has not been any lack of sex, just not always quality sex. Mary Kay has not had an orgasm as yet. She has become more interested in this facet of our sex life [as she's gotten older] and wants something done to give her more pleasure and ultimately an orgasm. Any suggestions? X-rated movies? A vibrator?

And here is a letter from a 70-year-old woman:

> I need to know, *Just what is the feeling of an orgasm?* How can a woman experience this "into orbit" feeling you write about? I have a very concerned new companion who knows I'm not completely fulfilled. I was raised in a family where you just didn't talk about sex. I have had to learn all I know from reading. Now I realize I don't have to settle!

Erotic activities and masturbation are not unusual among women over the age of 65, according to the senior sex researcher and therapist Dr. Helen Singer Kaplan. "In sharp contrast to men, elderly women remain capable of enjoying multiple orgasms . . . [and] 25 per cent of 70-year-old women still masturbate," she writes in *The New Sex Therapy.*[2] "Fantasy and ambience become more important in lovemaking and there is less preoccupation with orgasm."

At another of the WIT dinners, Drs. Patricia Allen and Ellen McGrath and I gathered a varied professional group of Wisewomen in Training to discuss postmenopausal love and sex. Participants compared notes from their various disciplines and agreed they all were seeing or hearing a new trend: women who have been heterosexual all their lives engaging in homosexual relationships after the age of 50 or 55.

"They find female partners more loving and caring but also more accepting of the physical changes of aging," said the psychoanalyst Graciela Abelin-Sas. Dr. McGrath said that psychologists were reporting this trend clinically in many parts of the country. Most of the time the women were first wives, abandoned after twenty or thirty years for younger women or devastatingly widowed. "Again and again, they're turning to other women and having these very satisfying experiences. It can be an antidote to depression."

CONGRATULATIONS, YOU'RE A NEW GRANDMOTHER!

Traditionally the wisdom of the older woman has been concentrated in (or confined to) the role of grandmother. It is one of the prerogatives and pleasures most women can look forward to in the Age of Integrity. But the sudden mutation into grandmother can also be a jolt, challenging her personal identity and her sense of time and future. The anthropologist Margaret Mead described to me her own ambivalence: "Grandparenthood is one life transition over which you have no control. It's done *to* you."[3]

Whatever happened to the bootee-knitting grandma?

Women of the World War II Generation didn't have careers for the most part; everything was invested in their offspring. They never really let go. Almost all they had, after 60, was the phone call or the visit. It's different now. Today's grandmother is not sitting around on call to baby-sit. She could be flying off for a dig on Easter Island or trekking and filming in Tierra del Fuego. She doesn't always answer her phone because she's doing yoga headstands to refresh the electromagnetic currents flowing to her brain so she can stay up half the night learning a new software program on her computer. She's likely to be a drop-in grandmother.

But from the way even the most blasé businesswomen describe the impact of seeing the first new sapling born from their own generational tree, it is still a profoundly soul-shaking, even transforming experience. A media executive nearing 60 couldn't stop talking about it between sets of her highly competitive Saturday morning tennis game. "Grandmother" didn't fit with her image. She was struggling to incorporate her new status.

THE NEW FLY-IN GRANDMOTHER, AGE 56

"When I die, part of me will still be alive . . . it's an incredible experience."

"I've always thought of age as a state of mind, and I guess I saw myself as about thirty," Kay Delaney told me. Sitting there in her tennis shorts and pixie haircut, deeply tanned, with her nose painted in white sunscreen, her body all muscles and sinews from clocking twenty miles on her bike every weekend, Kay did indeed have the silhouette of a 30-year-old. She thought her identity was pretty well set for the rest of her life.

Executive vice-president of a large media company, she is in charge of all international advertising and supervises a division of sixty-some employees. After two decades as a divorced single career mother, she had married again only in her early fifties. It was more like a merger. She and her husband respect each other's separate professional lives. Kay continues to travel all over the world for her job. She's out of the country as often as she's in, and the phone picks up where the jet leaves off. "I don't even count hours. I'll be on the phone at seven A.M. talking to Europe and on the phone at eleven at night talking to Asia. There's no downtime."

A few weeks before, her daughter had produced the first grandchild. "It took me four times of seeing the baby before I could do anything but cry," she said. "I was just overwhelmed by so many emotions." It wasn't easy for her to untangle the jumble of those emotions. "I could see in that little face the whole family—my parents, my aunts and uncles going all the way back to my grandmother, my ex-husband, and his family. I kept thinking: *This child is a continuation of all of these people. He's part and parcel of them. And me, he's part of me.*"

A rush of immortality overwhelmed her. Although raised a Catholic, she found herself looking upon this little pupa as evidence of reincarnation: Matter has neither beginning nor end; it's neither created nor destroyed. There is a continuum, and now she was an integral part of it, "because when I die, part of me will still be alive. I never felt that with my own children. But with a grandchild I definitely felt it, and it's an incredible experience."

The other shock was to be pushed to the front of the generational train. "Since the baby's been born, my whole concept of myself is changing," Kay repeated. "I still saw myself as about thirty, but the birth of the baby . . ." The big blue disks of her eyes widened further, and she spread her hands in a gesture of benign helplessness. "When I first held the baby and saw my hands next to the baby's skin, I thought, *My God, those are the hands of a middle-aged woman.*" The shock was to have that "slow-consuming age" we all try so hard to ignore suddenly telescoped. Kay had no concept that her hands looked that way. "It was like seeing my mother's hands. It dawned on me that I actually was the age that I am."

The passive transformation into grandparent can jump-start the transition to the Age of Integrity. For women or men who had to learn in First Adulthood, painfully, how to compartmentalize their nurturing selves and their achieving selves, grandparenthood is a particularly welcome second chance to bring all the parts of one's life into harmony. For Kay, the new babe brings forth all the feelings of that young, scared, divorced mother with three little children to feed who had to take on the world all alone before she was 35. But by now she can allow these feelings; she doesn't have to suppress her tenderest instincts to forge an image of herself as a fearless businesswoman. With her own kids a working mom longs to be there so *they* don't miss out. With the grandchild she wants to be there so *she* doesn't miss out.

"I am going through this whole questioning thing about changing my life," Kay disclosed. "I'm really getting a sense of my own chronological time frame, which I never had before. Sure, I'm in good health, vital, all the rest of it, but I have a sense that I want to be there as part of this new life. How can I be if I'm running off on planes all the time?"

Does she really want to be a fly-in grandmother? Off before Christmas to Hong Kong and Tokyo and calling up from a hotel room in Singapore to sing the grandchild a lullaby? Kay hears a babble of conflicting voices in her head. *How do I pull out of the achievement track where I've been getting my identity for at least twenty years? There's no external validation by our society for being a grandmother. I can't cut back. I'm too much of a perfectionist and workaholic. And I can't drop out and reenter in two years the way you could when you were twenty-five. But it's such a precious time. I don't want to miss out!*

The question is not really the job, she has decided. "The issue I'm debating is, Who do I want to be *now*?"

NURTURING: THE SECOND WAVE

The prime of the fly-in grandmother may also be cut short by the second wave of nurturing. After the liberation period when the children leave home (unless they come back!), there is likely to be another period of caregiving for aging or invalid parents or for an older, physically vulnerable husband. Some social analysts say that "the average American woman can expect to spend more years caring for her parents than she did caring for her children."[4]

One of the big changes noticed by Deborah Szekely, as she observes people during couples' weeks at her health spas, is that women in their fifties and sixties today who are married to men ten years older appear to belong to two different species. "These women are exploding with energy. They love their husbands, and when they were in their thirties and forties, having an older husband was wonderful. But when you're sixty-five and your husband is seventy-five or eighty, it's a real downer. You regain a child, and you can't go out at night because you don't have a baby-sitter." Indeed, the men of 65 in my Harvard Business School study were asked, "Who thinks and acts 'older' in your marriage?" Although only two or three years actually separate them in age from their spouses, two thirds of the men admitted that they act *older* than their wives.

The Crossover Crisis that often emerges as men and women move closer on the Sexual Diamond was quite evident in the HBS couples over the twenty-year course of the study. In 1974, when I did a survey of these traditional corporate wives in their mid-forties, two thirds were sure some exciting things were going to happen to them. They were right on the money. They were clearly *not* ready to settle. What they seemed to be saying back then was "Look out, world, it's my turn." And off they went, many of them, to all kinds of graduate schools, into the arts, education, urban planning, and into business for themselves. Most did so because they felt uncertain and anxious about their husbands' careers from time to time. Many were also discontent with their marriages.

Those who sought challenges or careers outside the home—usually starting over at 40 to 45—were also the most highly educated of the wives, while the stay-at-homes felt a painful lack of self-confidence. As a result, the gap between the two groups of wives only widened.

By the time they entered their sixties, the women who had shifted to independent activities outside the home were *absolutely certain* they were changing and growing more than their husbands. (Those who remained in the home were painfully aware they were growing less.) Husbands confirmed the disparity in development; 80 percent saw their wives as more independent, and nearly half acknowledged that their wives today are more assertive, competitive, and tougher emotionally.

Women who have never married or spawned children have their own anxieties about the future. They may be worried about having no family members alive to look after them in their own old age. In fact, if one probes just beneath the calm, composed surfaces of the most successful and sophisticated middle-aged women—whether they be wedded, widowed, childless, or never married by choice—one is likely to find they have Bag Lady Fears.

Few events concentrate more professional female star power than the annual Power Lunch for Women at Manhattan's Rainbow Room to benefit Citymeals-on-Wheels. While those in the latest Armani suits pick at their luscious desserts, a film clip is usually shown of the homeless and helpless older women who are the beneficiaries of the $200- to $500-plate luncheon. It was mildly astonishing to hear best-selling author Gloria Steinem, hit filmmaker Nora Ephron, superagent Joni Evans, former high-profile Planned Parenthood director Faye Wattleton, and many others admit that they have fears of finding themselves old, alone, forgotten, or homeless.

They all are probably taking greater notice of the older women at the margins of our society who are invisible to almost everyone else, some of them women who had to quit their jobs and give up health insurance and pension coverage to nurse parents or husbands or in-laws through the long twilight of chronic illness. (Or to nurse themselves through bouts with breast cancer.) They may be faced with the desperate choice of spending their dwindling financial resources on their mothers' old age or saving for themselves for their own third age.

Why? Traditionally women in the middle years have always been depended upon to do the work of unpaid caregiving to the disabled elderly at home. With women in their sixties and seventies today expected to care for people in their nineties, many face a caregiving crisis the second time around. Ninety percent of these caregivers of older Americans are women.[5] But women now fill nearly half the paid positions *outside* the home.

> Twenty-two percent of family caregivers quit paying jobs and give up average earnings of $29,400 per year, in order to spend upward of eighteen hours a day serving as home nurses for no pay.[6]

When they try to reclaim their professional positions or reenter the job market, they run into the wall of ageism. Many end up picking from the dregs of low-pay, no-benefits, high-turnover jobs. As the result of traditional policies of hiring, retirement and pension benefits, health care, and marriage norms—all designed around the typical male life cycle—these same caregiving women are set up for impoverishment in their old age. Many outlive their support systems.[7]

LIFE AND LOVE BEYOND LOSS

On the day her husband died, Genevieve Burke had an experience of profound collapse. "A foggy spiral emitted from me and swirled into the room where he was lying," she told me. "The sensation was so strong I clutched my center to hold myself together. It left me feeling weak and empty."[8] For almost the whole decade of her fifties she had made it her job to keep her disabled husband alive. Now, having "failed," she felt she had nothing more to live for.

The life that doesn't have a sense of responsibility to something broader than oneself is not much of a life. But to practice it intelligently, we need to understand that we can be responsible only in matters open to our control—our own choices and actions, no one else's. We may be able to influence but we cannot control another person's mind or mood. Sometimes a wife despairs because in spite of her best efforts, she cannot stop her husband's self-destructive behaviors or pull him out of chronic depression. Similarly, husbands (like former presidential candidate Michael Dukakis) may feel it's their responsibility to wean their wives off tranquilizers or alcohol. One of the meanings of living responsibly is knowing what we are and are not responsible for and drawing boundaries. Women like Genevieve, who suspend their own lives indefinitely in order to nurse spouses or relatives, may unconsciously be tying themselves up so they don't have to face making the next passage themselves.

In the months following her husband's death, frightened and without focus, Genevieve walked aimlessly around her small town of Winooski, Vermont. At a local pool a woman her age tried to strike up a conversation. Genevieve swam away. But like some guardian angel, the woman called over, "Mrs. Burke, exciting things are going to happen to you!"

The reality was she had to support herself now. She didn't have much time for reeducation. But one doesn't always have to spend years in graduate school to prepare for finding a new dream to enliven the third age. Many older women who chose to stay home and raise their families or care for chronically ill family members do not believe they have the necessary skills to aspire to any position much above working in a supermarket or department store. They don't realize how valuable their life skills, equanimity, and dependability can be to an employer.

Genevieve was, of course, dubious that anyone would hire a 60-year-old woman; nevertheless, she applied for a secretarial position at the state university. "Somehow I found an assertive streak in me," she said, "and within a few days I was hired and began my new life." The shock of being in the working world quickly galvanized Genevieve into realizing that her real responsibility was to find out who she was, not merely an extension of her husband or her children. She took credit courses at the university and self-help classes at the community center, and within a few years she progressed from being a secretary to a business manager to an administrative director.

She found herself by degrees. Apartment shopping, she was surprised when shown a sophisticated condo in a converted woolen mill over a river to find herself suddenly thinking, *Yes, this is where I want to live.* Tall, shapely, and fit, Genevieve puts on jogging gear at the end of her workday and does laps around a track. Then she might change into palazzo pants and a silk shirt. She likes to stand by her window in the woolen-mill apartment, drawing energy from the river below, which might move her to do wild dancing to her records or dream up phrases to describe the nature all around her. Along with her two part-time jobs, she is now a columnist for a new local magazine and is exhilarated by learning to express herself in prose at the age of 72. Her sense of time is altered utterly. She loves being with friends and family but also cherishes being alone. She is not afraid of dying; rather, she finds it imperative to *live* life.

"Today, although I'm the same person, I feel more integrated," she says. "I know *why* I was the way I was, and now I feel like strutting my stuff!"

CARETAKERS OF THE WORLD

More and more older females are putting themselves in training as Wise-women by expanding their knowledge base. More than twelve hundred women aged 50 to 64 are currently studying in the United States for their first professional degrees, seriously applying themselves to law, dentistry, pharmacy, or social psychology or, increasingly, coming out of divinity schools.[9] These highly trained women, with the "sense of mission" that so often solidifies in their sixties, become almost venerated when they return to work in their communities. This is especially true of minority older women.

MASTER OF DIVINITY AT 63

"There's respect for what you're doing at your age and an eagerness to help you succeed."

Generativity—feeling a voluntary obligation to care for others in the broadest sense—was a brand-new notion to Ella Ivey. She remembers reading about it in *Passages* when she first started back to college, a little abashed about being in her fifties. As a mother of three she was especially surprised to read that having children does not necessarily ensure generativity. But Ella Ivey had pulled herself up before by sheer tenacity. As a black woman raised in Blenheim, South Carolina, rather than settle for segregated schools, she had made her way to New York City and finished public high school there. She was the first in her family to have finished college.

In her fifties she began looking for a way to defeat stagnation in later life. This notion of generativity gave her a goal. "I wanted to do more [than a college degree would permit]," she told me. "I wanted to teach instead of being a school secretary." By the age of 59, Ella Ivey had a master's degree in education from Fordham University. (Fordham is one of the forward-looking institutions that has a "College at 60 Program."[10]) And then the best part of the journey began.

Swinging down the street with a book bag on her back, in jeans and san-dals, with metal-framed glasses and salt-and-pepper hair, this tall, deter-mined lady of 60 cut a wide swath through her Bronx neighborhood. She was out to class by ten in the morning and often not home from the library until ten at night. This time she was studying for a master of divinity degree at the New York Theological Seminary. Why another degree? When peo-ple change careers in Second Adulthood, just as when they were in their twenties, they often start by eliminating what they *don't* want to do. Teach-ing in itself did not satisfy Ella Ivey. Having reflected on the joy she took from counseling young people in her Sunday school classes, she finally understood that she wanted to be an ordained minister.

"I found younger people who would act as my mentors," she said. "Some were the ages of my own children!"

This is a pleasant twist on the generativity concept. Younger people who see seniors strenuously attempting something they need almost "adopt" them, help tutor them, and endorse their efforts as worthwhile, in much the way the traditional older mentor nourishes and validates the younger disci-ple. Generativity then becomes reflexive. The older person isn't confined only to the role of teacher, counselor, guru, always dipping into the experi-ence bank to give out; he or she can also feel cared for and cared about by others who, although much younger, may be more experienced in cutting-edge methods and technology.

"There's a certain amount of respect for what you're doing, at your age, and an eagerness to help you succeed at that," Ella Ivey discovered. Her hus-band good-humoredly took over the cooking and keeping tabs on their grown children and nearly a dozen grandchildren. Ella found strengths in herself that had never been there when she was younger.

"Stick-to-itiveness is the big one," she told me. She was also surprised how much easier it was to conceptualize at her age, an observation con-firmed by studies of people educated at late ages. They have also been found to be especially creative in thinking through social problems.[11] The greatest benefit of becoming a scholar in her sixties, said Ella Ivey, was being asked to write out her credo, a thesis of belief required for graduation from the seminary. Composing a personal creed can be an illuminating exer-cise for any of us and can help us arrive at the point where we can bless our own life cycle. The object of the search is to know what you personally believe in and are willing to act upon—a marker of maturity in Second Adulthood.

"It forced me to deal with myself, to understand what I had done to get to that point," Ella said. "I now had a context in which to place my journey."

That journey has paid off. She earned her master of divinity degree at 63 and works now as both an ordained minister and a college professor. Her family and community look upon Ella Ivey almost as on one who walks on water.

LOOKING AHEAD

It is useful to look ahead to the most vital women of age and see how they have met the challenges of later-life passages. Cecelia Hurwich, one of the participants in the Esalen conference, had done a study over time on women in their seventies, eighties, and nineties for her doctorate at the Center for Psychological Studies in Albany, California.[12] The women selected had remained active and creative through unusually productive Second Adulthoods and well into old age. What were their secrets? we all wanted to know.

"They live very much in the present but they always have plans for the future," Dr. Hurwich said. They had mastered the art of "letting go" of their egos gracefully so they could concentrate their attention on a few finetuned priorities. They continued to live in their own homes but involved themselves in community or worldly projects that they found of consuming interest. Close contact with nature was important to them, as was maintaining a multigenerational network of friends. And as they grew older they found themselves concerned more with feeding the soul than the ego.

Surprisingly, these zestful women were not in unusually good physical shape. They had their fair share of the diseases of age—arthritis, loss of hearing, impaired vision—but believing they still had living to do, they concentrated on what they could do rather than on what they had lost. Over the ten-year course of the study, most were widowed. This hardship, like so many others they had endured, they turned into a source of growth rather than defeat. Frequently they mentioned in conversation, "After my husband's death I learned to . . ."

Every one of them acknowledged the need for some form of physical intimacy—not, of course, just with a male. It might be with women friends, grandchildren, young people, but they found it was essential to have someone to touch, to hold, to share affection with. They found love through sharing the most natural of pleasures: music, gardening, hiking, traveling. Several spoke enthusiastically of having active and satisfying sex lives. One woman, asked how she felt about the automatic assumption that women in their seventies and eighties lost all interest in sex, answered after a long pause:

"This is how it is for me. I've become a vegetarian, but every once in a while I want a piece of red meat. And I go out and get it and eat it and enjoy it."

EXPANDING THE WIT NETWORK

Wisdom, or the collective practical knowledge of the culture that we call common sense, has been associated from the time of premodern female healers with older women. We are currently seeing a revival of the concept of the Wisewoman in many different guises. The obsession with angels, particularly guardian angels, has seldom been higher or more commercially successful in this century. Interest is burgeoning in the Earth Mother, an archetype represented in the Bible and in all religions and cultures, and in Sophia, the Goddess of Wisdom, who is also represented in many different religions and personified as a divine figure in the Book of Proverbs.

Scholarly texts now trace the Goddess-worshiping civilizations that flourished in Old Europe between 6500 and 3500 B.C. This was before the hill forts and constant warfare, when peaceful societies were organized around a communal temple guided by a queen-priestess, with her brother or uncle and a council of women as the governing body.[13] Worship of the Goddess is being revived today by renegade religious women even within mainline churches, accompanied, of course, by furious controversy over the very idea of a female aspect of God as blasphemy.

Whatever our religious beliefs, we can probably find agreement around the basic principle of the Earth Mother: We all are parts of a whole. We are not just put on earth for ourselves alone but as part of a higher, mysterious universe and evolutionary process. Some may find comfort in worshiping the Goddess. Most of us need more down-to-earth models.

One way to seek out Wisewomen models in your own community is to form a WIT (Wisewomen in Training) circle. It works best if it is no larger than eight to twelve people. It shouldn't be composed of the same familiar circle of friends or professional colleagues, and it isn't guided by the normal social chitchat. The initiators can each invite one or two stimulating people they know who have shown creative approaches to living in Second Adulthood. Then pick out some dynamic polestars you *don't* know, but would like to, and find out who in your community could contact them for you, so that the gathering will offer something fresh for everyone. The form can be anything from a brunch to a dinner or a weekend retreat. It helps to pass out index cards before the discussion starts and ask a few key questions:

> ❧ What new ventures or adventures can you now dare to try?
> ❧ What old shells can you slough off?
> ❧ How can you best give back?
> ❧ What investments in learning and changes in lifestyle are you willing to undertake to make all the extra years ahead livable?
> ❧ How long do you *want* to live?

As pioneers gathering in WIT groups you are essentially circling the wagons for protection, as Dr. McGrath describes it. "Then, within the safe circle, you 'sit around the campfire' and tell stories from which everybody can learn."

In the future, if women start WIT groups in their own communities, they may be able to link up in a nationwide or even international WIT network. When primitive Wisewomen gathered around stone circles in Ireland and England, sharing secrets of healing and drawing energy from the electrically active crystal in the stones, they had no means of communication with thousands of other such circles. We moderns have TV and the Internet. Those of us eager to be Wisewomen in Training have scarcely begun to tap the wisdom of those old enough to understand life backward.

19

TWO SPECIES OF AGING

At every fork in the journey of my life I have met my mother, the shadow of my age, and silently asked, "What's next?" At 40 she seemed old. But at 50, divorced, she bounced back, started a new business, trimmed down, and took to painting her toenails again. She was courted and married at the age of 53, and, she confided later, celebrated what was surely her sexual peak.

Then, at 64, abruptly, a reckless energy overtook her. She had always smoked, but now she chain-smoked, leaving the butts livid with bright lipstick in defiant little heaps. She took up careless drinking. She ate meats drowned with sauces in death house portions. Her normally sweet and ebullient nature still manifested itself in many acts of kindness, but a certain brittleness at the edges seemed to be hiding a secret desperation. No one could talk to her about the destructive habits she was developing; she became immediately defensive. It was as if she had entered a tunnel beyond the great gray parking lot of middle age and, convinced there was no road beyond, had begun to spin and slam off the walls, determined to inflict upon herself as many little deaths as she could before the controls were taken away from her.

"Don't tell me how to live my life." She sandbagged against my imprecations. "I don't tell you how to live yours." Her statements were punctuated by a shudder of the lungs. "I only have a few years left. What I do with them is none of your affair."

But it was my affair too, of course. We do not alone endure the verdict of our later years. We may sentence mates or children to an unnecessary internment. Not yet broken into my own forties, I found it terrifying to meet myself, in my mother, beyond middle age. *Is this what's next?* Why, I agonized, when she was enjoying a happy marriage and freedom from serious illness, would this lovely woman of 64 drive herself perversely toward an untimely end? She must have settled arbitrarily on a checkout time, I thought.

All at once, a few blocks from the graveyard, at the age of 69, my mother swerved in the opposite direction. She started exercising three times a week: lifting dumbbells, hanging from parallel bars. After being a smoker for fifty years, she awoke one morning and reached for a pack of the old friends and crushed them. No tapering off, no therapeutic programs. Inexplicably my mother had entered her third spring.

Visiting her in her seventy-fourth year, I puzzled aloud over what had revived the sunniness of her nature. What indefinite treaty had she made with the armies of the aging?

She said, "I guess I thought it would be almost over at seventy. Instead I found I was still feeling good. Well"—she qualified her answer—"the emphysema focused for me what I had to do to live longer and still feel good. But I was enjoying the trip. I got excited about it all over again. I wanted an extended itinerary!"

My mother confirmed an attitude that is dangerously common in so many of us. Even though the stage we are in may feel far richer than we had ever anticipated, we look ahead to the *next* stage and know, with an absolute, aggressively uninformed, let's-don't-talk-about-it conviction, that it will be straight downhill from there. Yet if we fail to conspire in our own irreversible deterioration, we will probably arrive at the new stage, rummage around in surprise, and say, "Why, this isn't so bad after all. If only I had known, I would have taken better care of myself."

My mother was traveling with the outdated map of adult life in her mind, and sadly she adjusted her outlook too late. As we age, our perspective on the boundaries of the life cycle and how we define "old" almost inevitably change. An amusing scene was described to me by a 75-year-old man, who was caught out with his own ageist attitudes while attending his mother's hundredth birthday party. Some two hundred members of his mother's extended family were sandwiched under a tent on a summer's day in New England. The son began his toast with this exclamation: "I never thought I'd have a mother who was a hundred!"

His mother cocked her head and challenged him aloud: "I never thought I'd have a *son* who was seventy-five!"

CHOOSING HOW TO AGE

As we grow older, we become less and less alike. The consequences of genes, gender, race, class, marital status, income, and preventive health care (or carelessness) all pile up. But while our genes largely determine our health status and longevity, this holds true only until we reach 60 or 65. After that, if we have escaped catastrophic illnesses during the critical middle life period from 45 to 65, it is our psychological attitude and behavior that more likely determine the quality and duration of our third age.

You will recall Dr. Gene Cohen, now director of the Washington, D.C., Center on Aging, who asserts that the relationship between health and mental health is greatest in later life. Data keep accumulating to show that in the face of chronic depression or stress, biological changes occur that have a negative effect on the immune system and render people more vulnerable to disease. "We're on the frontier of a really fine-tuned understanding of how psychological changes relate to very specific changes in physiology," predicts Margaret Kemeny. She is the research psychologist at UCLA whose study, cited earlier, shows that feeling happy or depressed even for twenty minutes affects the number and activity of natural "good" killer cells in the bloodstream.[1]

People with positive outlooks, who continue to connect themselves to the future and marshal their energies to defeat creeping depression or entropy, are far more likely to extend their Second Adulthoods into healthy and satisfying later lives. But we have to reach for it. It doesn't come to us. We need a new ambition, or, as Deborah Szekely says, something to lose sleep over again. Are you going to sit back and let aging happen to you? Or are you going to continue to make life happen for you? The decision to renew ourselves for a third age—from 65 to who knows?—requires a real investment of faith, risk, and physical discipline.

Increasingly the way that choice is made will create two different species of aging.

Experts in gerontology make a clear distinction between passive aging and successful aging. To engage in successful aging is actually a career choice. Your job is to revive your life energy to make the next passage. That life force is then ready to be applied to whatever current challenges you face or the life accidents that may occur up ahead. Successful aging must be a conscious choice with a commitment to continuing self-education and the development of a whole set of strategies.

Let's don't even call it aging anymore. The very word carries pejorative baggage. Let's refer to successful aging as *sageing*—the process by which men and women accumulate wisdom and grow into the culture's sages.

It struck me how many of the most vital women I was writing about have battled breast cancer. In fact, the disease seemed to act as a wake-up call that committed them to the choice of sageing. Laurie, the Vietnam Generation activist, had her bout with mortality in her forties. It dissolved her illusions about immortality and brought her the inner peace of acceptance that death is a part of life. For the droll Linda Ellerbee, the battle dragged her, doubting and wisecracking, to a spiritual place in her journey. For Gloria Steinem, the diagnosis illuminated what she loved about her life, allowing her to shed some of her female conditioning and begin for the first time to concentrate on taking good care of herself. Elise, the St. Louis school principal, after a lumpectomy and a hysterectomy, felt at 55 buried alive. But at 60, widowed and physically strong, she felt younger than she had at 50 and possessed of unlimited emotional energy to touch other people's lives.

Even Deborah Szekely was diagnosed with breast cancer in her seventieth year. Already caught up in the whirlwind of creating her own foundation, she was stopped in her tracks, stunned and angry. After fifty years of being a health and fitness guru, how could she be betrayed by her body like this? But within weeks she returned to her usual positive, proactive approach, flew back from a trip to Japan, had a mastectomy, and in three days was back to her usual formidable pace. When people asked about her breast cancer, she said, "I don't have cancer. It's in the Dumpster behind the hospital."

By now Deborah is helping define what I like to think of as the Sage Seventies.

"It's the age of confidence," she told me. "By then you know everything about yourself and how you relate to everything else."

As this book has repeatedly shown, when we come to the top of the mountain and look out at the New Territory of Second Adulthood, there is not just a single path down the back side. There is another view, breathtaking, panoramic; for the first time you get a 360-degree view in all directions. Now you can see clearly where you came from, the patterns. Ahead of you lies a course that is neither circular nor linear but, in my view, a spiral. It rises and dips but keeps circling upward. Each new awakening can jump us ahead to a higher curve in the road up the mountain of self-transcendence.

When Erik Erikson and his wife, Joan, were in their eighties, they coauthored a book, *Vital Involvement in Old Age*, that suggested a similar concept. "The life cycle does more than extend itself into the next generation. It curves back on the life of the individual, allowing ... a reexperiencing of earlier stages in a new form."[2]

This spiraling path through Second Adulthood is still largely unmarked. It is not easy to follow. It confronts us with unfamiliar passages to be mastered. Most people don't yet know it exists. But more and more people are discovering it and branching out to open up alternative routes.

It isn't just about increasing our longevity. The simple numerical increase in years-left-to-live does not promise a rich Second Adulthood. That's why people groan as well as cheer when I mention in lectures how long healthy men and women can now expect to live in Second Adulthood. They are imagining those added years only in terms of infirmity and dependency. And of course, without health or a support system, a prolonged third age can be a horror. The added years are merely a blank slate; it's what we write on it that makes the difference.

It's not just having something to live for, but finding something you *have* to live for—like Liz Carpenter, who has to see her brother's orphaned children through college. Or Fitzgerald, who has to see his portraits attain museum quality. Or Mildred Mathias, who has to bring back scarce medicinal plants from the Amazon. Or Jimmy Carter, who has to be ready to drop everything and offer his skills as a political Wiseman to mediate world conflict.

Okay, you say, that sounds like a lot of work. What's the payoff?

RENAISSANCE IN THE ART OF HEALTH

Whether we like it or not, most of us are going to live a lot longer than our parents did. No matter how much money we have, we will live inside the house of our bodies, with heat, light, and energy generated by the brain. If we don't constantly repair and rebuild the body, it will become rickety and weak. If we don't keep "growing" the brain by challenging it, life will become increasingly dull and draining.

In the past, when people developed symptoms or health problems after 60, they usually accepted them as part of an irreversible decline called aging. Their doctors often concurred. A negative cycle would ensue. Their symptoms would multiply, then run out of control, and they would go downhill. Or believing themselves to be sick, they would surrender the power of their minds and allow modern medicine to suppress their symptoms with multiple drugs.

Today the ancient understanding of mind-body medicine is being revived by popular practitioners and adopted all over the world. Americans spent $14 billion of their own money for alternative medicine in 1992 to complement the technology-driven armamentarium of modern medicine. Yet even today, when older patients complain of feeling dizzy or depressed or their memories are foggy or their balances are off, doctors often ascribe these secondary symptoms to old age when, indeed, they may be side effects of drugs. These are the conclusions of a recent study published in the *Journal of the American Medical Association*, which shows that one in four of elderly patients receives the wrong drugs.[3]

But a symptom doesn't necessarily represent the human organism's collapse in the face of stress or infection. Rather, it can be seen as the best possible defense the body can muster on the basis of its present resources. And people today are much more likely to nip a problem in the bud and stop it from getting out of control. There are so many natural ways to bolster the body's self-healing apparatus. Modifying your diet, using nutritional supplements, committing yourself to regular exercise, cutting out cigarette smoking, and learning various techniques to reduce stress can help not only to avoid drugs that may suppress your own immune response but, if they become habits, to help ensure that you will be less subject to disease when you reach later life.

And later life may be much longer than you think.

Although death is inevitable, the way in which we age is not. It has long been accepted as immutable fact that the human being is genetically programmed to die after seventy-five to eighty-five years. Important islands within the scientific community are departing from that traditional "time bomb model," which held that the human body self-destructs when it reaches a certain age, and considering instead a new "spaceship model," whereby the body, like a spaceship engineered to reach a particular goal, can be retrofitted to go farther.[4] Research projects supported by the National Institute on Aging have swung the balance toward the new view that there may be no end in sight to the ever-increasing human life span.[5]

Researchers in the exciting new field of structural biology, who are beginning to understand at a molecular level how to decode RNA messages, believe they will be able to inhibit bad cell actions, like cancer, or get cells to mimic good actions. Skin, for example, ages prematurely when overexposed to sunlight. Treatment with Retin-A is often able to reverse these effects of aging. Why? It reactivates genes that had been turned off by sunlight, thereby turning on the skin's production of collagen and plumping out the wrinkles. Similar reversals may become possible with all organ systems, including the brain. We have already learned that our thinking spans can be increased even in advanced age. The brain is as dynamic as any other organ of the body, and if high stimulation is regularly provided to an older brain, it begins to "sprout" new connections.

Dr. William Haseltine, one of the early researchers on the human genome project, believes that for every tissue in the body there are "growth factors"—a protein that makes that tissue grow or slow down. "In a very few years I believe we will identify the majority of those growth factors for every tissue," he says, "and once we identify them, we will be able to manipulate them to speed up tissue growth, or slow it down." As our knowledge of the genes involved in the normal processes of tissue repair and maintenance expands, biotechnologists will be able to use that knowledge to repair damage that accumulates by aging. We will go into a clinic or hospital for the routine *maintenance* and *regeneration* of organs.[6]

For more predictions I checked with Caleb ("Tuck") Finch, a brilliant neurobiologist I first met in New York in the Seventies, when he was a whiz-kid researcher who predicted that hormone replacement therapy would revolutionize aging in women. Today, older (like all of us), 53, his long beard striped in several shades of gray, Tuck is still grandly perspicacious. I found him at the University of Southern California, where he is principal investigator at the Alzheimer Disease Research Center. We talked about how children of the future will be given genotype assessments, even before they reach three months of fetal life.

"This will in the long run make a significant dent in AIDS-related diseases and therefore in the health of people of later years," he predicted.

"How long do *you* expect to live, Tuck?" I asked him.

"Probably ninety to one hundred," he said casually. He confirmed that it is totally plausible to modify aspects of human development so that some cells can replace themselves throughout life. "There is no part of an organism that can't be manipulated in some way these days, given the understanding of genetic information."

"It's the equivalent of the Italian Renaissance in art," claims Purnell Choppin, president of the largest private medical research facility in the world, the Howard Hughes Medical Institute.

The odds on increased longevity keep increasing exponentially. In 1950 the chance that a 65-year-old American would reach the age of 90 was only

7 percent. Forty years later, in 1990, the probability was up to 25 percent. But it's not up 25 percent for everybody. For example, a 65-year-old white woman in good health with an adequate income can look forward confidently to fully functioning for twenty to thirty years, right up to nearly the end of her life. For many lower-income women, particularly those of minority backgrounds whose educations and life expectancies are foreshortened, the prospects for life after 65 are fairly bleak. And as Information Age societies become more divided between highly educated and poorly educated citizens, we may increasingly see two tiers of health care perpetuating the divisions between two species of aging.

SHARPENING UP FOR THE
SAGE SEVENTIES AND BEYOND

The mental skills of people over 70 are sharper than they think, according to recent research.[7] But because most seniors accept outdated cultural prejudices about "dotty old people," they underestimate their mental skills, which are particularly high in reasoning and verbal expression, and try to evade intellectual tasks—exactly the opposite of what they should do to stay sharp. Their pessimism often leads to a premature and unnecessary dependence on others—spouses or children or their doctors.

People who develop the discipline of daily mental exercise—reading newspapers instead of only passively ingesting TV news, noodling over the crossword puzzle every day, keeping journals, balancing their checkbooks, and reading the fine print on insurance forms, etc.—are preparing themselves to graduate from the Sage Seventies into the Uninhibited Eighties. The most successful octogenarians I have come across seem to share a quality of directness. Robust and unaffected, and often hilariously uninhibited in expressing what they really think, they are liable to live with a partner rather than get married or to pick up an old sweetheart and marry despite their kids' disapproval. They do all kinds of things they wouldn't have dared at earlier stages. They have nothing left to lose.

Those who make the passage into the next decade can become distinguished today by belonging to the new aristocracy of successful aging. They acquire the nobility of the nineties. These added years offer an opportunity to display a great generosity of mind and soul, to forgive former enemies, or to show a dignity of conception in composing a thought, a poem, an expression of any sort that helps illuminate the path for others coming behind them. Members of the Noble Nineties have earned the right to be cared for and cherished.

Given the genetic manipulations and hormone therapies that may keep us living longer and fitter, the best investment today is in our own personal health portfolio. I asked an exercise physiologist who works with severely depressed patients as well as healthy wealthy resort dwellers, "In all your experience, what is the single greatest difference between those who begin to fall apart as they get older and those who stay healthy and fit and seem to go on forever?"

Christine Grimaldi didn't have to stop and think. "Mental stimulation," she said. "People who keep themselves active and don't isolate themselves as they get older are the ones who keep their mind-body connection working to stay healthy. Even if it's just attaining one small goal for the day, it works. The ones who get sicker and sicker are the ones who surrender themselves to doctors and drugs and keep having the message reinforced, You're sick."

Just that morning she had arrived to give an exercise workout to a wealthy, talented 65-year-old woman who was on a combination of Prozac and lithium. The woman was still in bed at eleven-thirty. Christine woke her up. She was in a deep depression.

"First of all," Christine told her, "you have to be your own best friend, not your enemy. If you don't support yourself, nobody else will. Try to remember this is a temporary situation and you're going to come out of it."

The woman got dressed, and Christine started her moving aerobically, joking with her. After half an hour the woman said, "Why do I feel so much better?"

The exercise had oxygenated her sluggish blood and probably released her body's natural mood-elevating endorphins. She was engaged instead of isolated. But perhaps most important was the fact the woman was doing something *for herself*. The reason doctors had taken over her life was that she had given up fighting for it.

Your immune system needs to be signaled that you believe your life is worth fighting for. Again, even if you don't know what will give your life meaning at this stage, the very process of searching and working at it, every day, is a healing process, because it is opening up hope.

Fine, you say, but how do you keep mentally stimulated once aging begins to limit some of the pleasures and opportunities that lent flavor to your earlier life? It takes time and imagination to create new opportunities to stay active and to grow mentally and spiritually. Just as people are advised to develop financial portfolios, Dr. Cohen suggests that people start early in midlife to work on building a "social portfolio"—a range of different activities they will be able to draw upon in their later years: some that can be done alone and some with others, some that take a lot of energy, and others that can be enjoyed in a more sedentary way.

Exercise appears to be the single most effective nonmedical elixir to retard aging. Orchestra conductors, who are compelled to do vigorous aerobic exercise, are notable for their longevity.[8] People in the performing arts in general, where intense mental and physical discipline is demanded, offer some of the most remarkable examples of old age. Pianist Vladimir Horowitz retired for a number of years, outgrew his neuroticisms, and took up touring again. He enjoyed an autumnal period when he played the piano at home, no longer to prove anything but to have a good time. Shortly after his eighty-sixth birthday he began recording at home pieces he had never done—still taking risks. Following the last recording session, in the same year, while sitting in a chair making dinner plans with his wife, he quietly slipped out of life.[9]

Long daily walks are part of the job of successful aging. Men and women who walk at least half an hour every day cut their mortality rates in *half* compared with sedentary people of both sexes. That was among the striking results of a massive study on thirteen thousand men and women who performed treadmill tests over an eight-year period at the Cooper Institute for Aerobics Research in Dallas, Texas. Nobody has to sweat out miles on the treadmill. The most impressive improvement came from fairly modest levels of activity, noted Dr. Steven Blair, director of epidemiology and clinical applications at the institute. Someone who walked thirty minutes a day six days a week enjoyed a mortality rate almost as low as someone who ran thirty or forty miles per week.[10]

We are never too old to benefit from exercise, it seems. In another groundbreaking study, men and women who appeared to be typical of frail nursing home residents worked out vigorously on exercise machines for forty-five minutes three times a week to strengthen their legs. After only a few weeks residents in their late eighties or their nineties could get around more quickly, climb stairs better, and sometimes even throw away their walkers.

"People have an unduly negative attitude about what can be done with those at the end of their lives," said the study director, Dr. Maria A.

Fiatarone of the U.S. Department of Agriculture's Human Nutrition Center at Tufts University. "We need to be more optimistic." Not only does working out strengthen aging muscles, but that extra strength improves people's lives in other important ways. Those octogenarians who started exercising were also less depressed and more likely to walk around on their own and take part in social activities.[11]

CELEBRATORY CENTENARIANS

With people over 90 constituting the fastest-growing age-group in America, percentage-wise, we are seeing and hearing much more these days about what the oldest can teach us. In an interesting sociological survey of those over 90 who looked back, what these men and women remembered most vividly about their lives—the periods that still lived in Technicolor for them—were not their successes or their failures. They were the times they took risks.[12]

Sociologists who study centenarians are inevitably struck by their strong attachments to freedom and independence. Throughout their lives centenarians tend to avoid being held back by constraints. Traditionally they have tended to be their own bosses. They prize autonomy, and they do not retire early.[13] Look what they get for their boldness and self-support: They can celebrate breaking the bonds of ordinary mortality.

The word researchers apply most frequently to centenarians is *adaptable.* All have suffered losses and setbacks. But even the most intense loss, such as that of a spouse after fifty or sixty years of marriage, was mourned, and then the person moved on. There was also a marked lack of high ambition.[14]

Other characteristics of healthy centenarians, garnered from a number of studies, are these: Most have high native intelligence, a keen interest in current events, a good memory, and few illnesses. They tend to be early risers, sleeping on average between six and seven hours. Most drink coffee, follow no special diets, but generally prefer diets high in protein, low in fat. There is no uniformity in their drinking habits, but they use less medication in their lifetimes than many old people use in a week. They prefer living in the present, with changes, and are usually religious in the broad sense.

All have a degree of optimism and a marked sense of humor. Life seems to have been a great adventure.[15]

THE PRESENT NEVER AGES

Your soul, and its nurturing and crafting, is something only *you* have control over. Even if your life of getting and spending may have been less than a success, you still hold the power to shape the nature of your soul. What is the soul anyway? Let's look at it this way: It is the sum total of your essence, what you have done in the world, what is special about you. When you die, the soul represents who you were up to the moment you passed on. It is the residual you leave on earth—the influence you hold over your children, friends, colleagues, community—and it can be enormously powerful. For a doctor, it's the impact on his or her patients; a writer, on his or her readers; a teacher, on students; etc. Willa Cather, one of my favorite writers, described the soul as an essential spirit, an expressive and inviolable self. She saw the task of every life to fashion an existence that would "free the expressive self."[16]

In American and most Western European societies people are led to believe the spirit is separate from the mind and body. The spirit is an area of growth most of us set aside, half hoping the day will come when some soul-stretching peak experience will lift us out of our ordinary consciousness for a glimpse of the sacred and eternal. But we have to prepare our consciousness for taking such a path. And that requires another level of letting go. We need to change the way we measure time and to relax our insistence on control.

The Age of Integrity is primarily a stage of spiritual growth. Instead of focusing on the time running out, it should be a daily exercise in the third age to mark the moment. The present never ages. Each moment is like a snowflake, unique, unspoiled, unrepeatable, and can be appreciated in its surprisingness. Fitzgerald found his time sense completely "rejiggered" once he developed a new dream. The 63-year-old designer Aaron Coleman Webb spoke to the conscious choice of letting go of future time. "The one clear sense you do have is that you must stop postponing. You want to live in the moment as much as you possibly can."

And instead of trying to maximize our control over our environment, a goal that was perfectly appropriate to the earlier Age of Mastery, now we must cultivate greater appreciation and acceptance of that which we cannot control. Some of the losses of Second Adulthood are inconsolable losses. To accept them without bitterness usually requires making a greater effort to discern the universal intelligence or spiritual force that is operating behind the changes and losses we now notice daily.

Dr. Deepak Chopra, a pioneer in reviving the ancient mind-body medicine approach called *ayurveda*, offers scientific evidence in his book *Ageless Body, Timeless Mind* to show that as long as we constantly try to relieve old hurts, escape old fears, and impose control over the uncontrollable, we will continue to accumulate stress and accelerate the aging process that chronic stress chemicals produce.[17] The attitude that works is the one Fitzgerald ultimately adopted: "... learning to accept your life not as a series of random events but as a path of awakening."[18]

If every day is an awakening, you will never grow old. You will just keep growing.

Acknowledgments

reat editors are rare, and I feel blessed that several of the best cared
enough to extend themselves on behalf of this book. I cannot begin to
acknowledge my gratitude to Robert Loomis, distinguished executive editor
at Random House. Five years ago Bob jumped with me off the edge of the
known world of adult development. He remained the constant intellectual
companion who kept me from drowning in a sea of material. Although one
deadline after another came and went, Bob never blew a whistle on me. Each
time I asked anxiously, "But how much longer do you think this will take?"
Bob smiled his serene little smile and said, "It will take as long as it takes.
The important thing is that it be the best book it can be."

I am also grateful to Joni Evans, who believed in this book when it was
only a concept and originally signed it up for Random House while she was
publisher. George Hodgman, the talented editor with whom it is my pleasure to work at *Vanity Fair,* took time to read endless drafts of the book and
offer the fresh perspective of a wise man in First Adulthood. And then
there is the editor whose support and encouragement always gets me
through the day, the months, the years—the editor I live with and who lives
in my heart, my husband, Clay Felker.

I am indebted to my friends among the top social scientists at the U.S.
Census Bureau for providing subtle analyses of data and working with me
to develop the generational profiles: Arthur Norton, chief of the Population Division, and Paul M. Siegel, Martin O'Connell, Arlene Saluter, and
Amara Bachu; Donald J. Hernandez, chief of the Marriage and Family

Statistics Branch; Edward Welniak, chief of the Income Branch, and Paul Ryscavage, Chuck Nelson, and Jack McNeil; Suzanne Bianchi, assistant chief of Social/Demographic Statistics; Campbell Gibson, and Alfredo Navarro.

To my whip-smart assistant for three years on this project, Leora Tanenbaum, I want to express boundless thanks; through the learning process she has grown into a freelance writer herself. I am grateful to Clare McElhinney, who has been an unfailingly loyal editorial assistant through the final writing, editing, footnoting, and proofreading crunch. My agent, Lynn Nesbit, has contributed both personally and professionally in immeasurable ways.

I'm grateful to my research partner in developing and analyzing the surveys, Carin Rubenstein, Ph.D. Thanks are also due to the men and women who volunteered to coordinate the group interviews: Beth Struever, Erica Spaberg, Susan Campbell, Dick Fitts, James Sniechowski, Jim and Alice MacMahon, Pam Catlett, Myra Madnick, Leonard Doran, Clementine Pugh, Suzanne Schut, Becky Brown, Carol Waters, and Betty Merton.

I also want to express my pleasure in working with the extraordinarily talented designer Nigel Holmes and with the expert staff at Random House led by publisher Harold Evans, notably Carol Schneider, Sally Hoffman, Amy Edelman, Barbé Hammer, and copy editor Pearl Hanig. Thank you, Noah Green, for creating our unique database and Tom Keough for precise transcriptions. As always we are sustained by tea and sympathy from Ella Council.

APPENDIXES

Appendix 1

LIFE HISTORY SURVEY

1. Please write in your age. _____ years old

2. Please write in below how old you feel and how old people think you are.

    I feel _____ years old   People think I am _____ years old

3. Please rank the following age periods in life from most satisfying to least satisfying. Write in a "1" next to the age period that was the most satisfying. Then write in a "2" next to the second most satisfying age period. Please continue until you have ranked all the age periods appropriate to you. Do not use a number more than once. Be sure to rank all age periods up to your current one.

    18 to 22 years old ...._____   40 to 49 years old ...._____
    23 to 29 years old ...._____   50 to 59 years old ...._____
    30 to 39 years old ...._____   67 to 69 years old ...._____

4. In your opinion, how much control do you have over the *good* or *pleasant things* that happen to you? *("X" only one.)*

    Almost no control...-1 ☐
    Mostly not under my control ....-2 ☐
    About half the time I can control the good things .....-3 ☐
    Mostly under my control...................................-4 ☐
    Almost total control..-5 ☐

5. In your opinion, how much control do you have over the *bad* or *unpleasant things* that happen to you? *("X" only one.)*

    Almost no control...-1 ☐
    Mostly not under my control ....-2 ☐

About half the time I can control the bad things........-3 ☐
Mostly under my control...-4 ☐
Almost total control ....-5 ☐

6. **About how much of the time do you feel "bored"?** *("X" only one.)*

Constantly ....-1 ☐   Monthly..................................-4 ☐
Every day ....-2 ☐   Almost never..........................-5 ☐
A few times a week ....-3 ☐

7. **Do struggles that used to claim much of your emotional life seem to have subsided now?** *("X" only one.)*

Yes, not as anxious/angry or depressed..........................-1 ☐
Emotional life is the same ....-2 ☐
Struggles are still there, but use less
   destructive defenses ....-3 ☐
No, worse than ever ....-4 ☐

8. **How often do you enjoy what you are doing professionally?** *("X" only one.)*

None of the time..................-1 ☐   Most of the time..................-4 ☐
Almost none of the time ....-2 ☐   All of the time......................-5 ☐
Some of the time..................-3 ☐

9. **How often do you feel that the work you do is "useful" to others?** *("X" only one.)*

None of the time..................-1 ☐   Most of the time..................-4 ☐
Almost none of the time ....-2 ☐   All of the time......................-5 ☐
Some of the time..................-3 ☐

10. **Looking back at your original dream or aspiration, how do you feel at this point in your career?** *("X" only one.)*

I have never had a clear dream or aspiration..................-1 ☐
I will probably never achieve my original dream............-2 ☐
I am just beginning to shape my dream...........................-3 ☐
I am on my way to achieving my dream ....-4 ☐
I have achieved my original dream and have
   generated a new one ....-5 ☐
I have achieved my original dream and haven't
   generated a new one ....-6 ☐

11. **Have you *ever* changed careers?**

Yes...-1 ☐   No→SKIP TO Q.#13........-2 ☐

12. **Write in the age at which you changed careers.**

First major career change ...._____ years old
Second major career change ...._____ years old
Third major career change......................_____ years old

13. Would you like to make a major career change but feel you can't?

Yes ....-1 ☐   No→SKIP TO Q.#15 ....-2 ☐

14. Which of the following best describes why you feel you can't make a major change in your career? *("X" all that apply.)*

Loss of income...-1 ☐
Fear of failure in trying something new.........................-2 ☐
No decent opportunities at my age................................-3 ☐
Loss of security...-4 ☐
Family wouldn't approve...-5 ☐
Have to wait for retirement benefits ....-6 ☐
Other...-7 ☐

15. Did you have (or do you have) a mentor—an older, non-parental person in your profession who has helped to guide, encourage, and inspire you? *("X" only one.)*

Yes, one mentor..-1 ☐
Yes, more than one mentor.......................................-2 ☐
No, no mentors ....-3 ☐

16. At this stage of your life, who is your *primary* source of intimacy? *("X" only one.)*

Spouse or partner ....-1 ☐   Parent.........................-5 ☐
Same-sex friend ....-2 ☐   Sibling...........................-6 ☐
Opposite-sex friend..............-3 ☐   Therapist........................-7 ☐
Child................................-4 ☐   Don't have one ....-8 ☐

17. Write in the number of close friends you have, that is, friends in whom you can confide almost anything. If none, write in a zero.

Number of close friends..........................._____

18. Did you include your partner in the number of your close friends?

Yes..................................-1 ☐   No ....-2 ☐

19. What do you value *most* in a loving relationship right now? *("X" only one.)*

Companionship......................-1 ☐   Being with someone
Intimacy and trust ....-2 ☐   younger...................-5 ☐
Regular, safe sex ....-3 ☐   Passionate sex ....-6 ☐
Novelty...................................-4 ☐   Other...........................-7 ☐

20. Which of the following best describes your family when you were growing up? *("X" only one.)*

Poor ....-1 ☐   Upper middle class ....-4 ☐
Lower middle class ....-2 ☐   Rich.............................-5 ☐
Middle class...........................-3 ☐

21. **Are one or both of your parents alive?** *("X" only one.)*

      Both are still living ....-1 ☐

      Mother is alive ....-2 ☐

      Father is alive..-3 ☐

      Both deceased→SKIP TO Q.#24 ....-4 ☐

      Don't know→SKIP TO Q.#24.............................-5 ☐

22. **How dependent are you on your parents?** *("X" all that apply.)*

      I'm still living with parent(s).............................-1 ☐

      I need some financial help from my parents ....-2 ☐

      I'm somewhat emotionally dependent

        on my parents ....-3 ☐

      I'm completely independent from my parents ....-4 ☐

23. **How dependent do you think your parent(s) are on you?** *("X" all that apply.)*

      One or both parents (or in-laws) live with me ....-1 ☐

      My parent(s) need some financial help from me ....-2 ☐

      My parent(s) are somewhat emotionally

        dependent on me ....-3 ☐

      My parent(s) are completely independent from me .....-4 ☐

24. **For each activity listed, *write in* the number of hours you spend doing each in an average day. Be sure to write in a number next to each activity.**

      Work..._____ hours a day

      Work-related travel (commuting,

        business trips, etc.).............................._____ hours a day

      Housework..._____ hours a day

      Time with your children ...._____ hours a day

      Time with your spouse or lover........_____ hours a day

      Time to yourself (reading, thinking,

        walking, etc.) ...._____ hours a day

      Time volunteered to help others ......_____ hours a day

      Time socializing with friends............._____ hours a day

      Exercise or sports..............................._____ hours a day

      Watching TV/playing on

        the computer ...._____ hours a day

      Creative or craft activities.................._____ hours a day

      Sleeping..._____ hours a day

25. **How satisfied are you with this allotment of your time?** *("X" only one.)*

      Very satisfied...-1 ☐

      Somewhat satisfied..-2 ☐

      Somewhat dissatisfied ....-3 ☐

      Very dissatisfied..-4 ☐

26. **In general, how have you been feeling about your life as a whole during the past *six months*?** *("X" only one.)* **Then, indicate how you think your part-**

ner has been feeling about his or her life during the past *six months.* *("X"* *only one.)*

	SELF	PARTNER
Terrible......................................	-1 ☐	-1 ☐
Unhappy....................................	-2 ☐	-2 ☐
Mostly dissatisfied...........................	-3 ☐	-3 ☐
Mixed (equally satisfied and dissatisfied).............................	-4 ☐	-4 ☐
Mostly satisfied..............................	-5 ☐	-5 ☐
Pleased...	-6 ☐	-6 ☐
Delighted....................................	-7 ☐	-7 ☐
No partner		-y ☐

27. For each of the following aspects of your life, tell how you have been feeling during the *last six months.* *("X" only one.)*

	TERRIBLE	UNHAPPY	MOSTLY DISSATISFIED	MIXED—EQUALLY SATISFIED AND DISSATISFIED	MOSTLY SATISFIED	PLEASED	DELIGHTED	NO FEELINGS
Your work or primary activity	-1 ☐	-2 ☐	-3 ☐	-4 ☐	-5 ☐	-6 ☐	-7 ☐	-8 ☐
Your love relationship/marriage	-1 ☐	-2 ☐	-3 ☐	-4 ☐	-5 ☐	-6 ☐	-7 ☐	-8 ☐
Children and being a parent	-1 ☐	-2 ☐	-3 ☐	-4 ☐	-5 ☐	-6 ☐	-7 ☐	-8 ☐
Recognition/success	-1 ☐	-2 ☐	-3 ☐	-4 ☐	-5 ☐	-6 ☐	-7 ☐	-8 ☐
Your financial situation	-1 ☐	-2 ☐	-3 ☐	-4 ☐	-5 ☐	-6 ☐	-7 ☐	-8 ☐
Your health and physical condition	-1 ☐	-2 ☐	-3 ☐	-4 ☐	-5 ☐	-6 ☐	-7 ☐	-8 ☐
Personal growth and development	-1 ☐	-2 ☐	-3 ☐	-4 ☐	-5 ☐	-6 ☐	-7 ☐	-8 ☐
Your sex life	-1 ☐	-2 ☐	-3 ☐	-4 ☐	-5 ☐	-6 ☐	-7 ☐	-8 ☐
Your partner's happiness	-1 ☐	-2 ☐	-3 ☐	-4 ☐	-5 ☐	-6 ☐	-7 ☐	-8 ☐
Friends and social life	-1 ☐	-2 ☐	-3 ☐	-4 ☐	-5 ☐	-6 ☐	-7 ☐	-8 ☐
Your athletic skills	-1 ☐	-2 ☐	-3 ☐	-4 ☐	-5 ☐	-6 ☐	-7 ☐	-8 ☐
Your body and physical attractiveness	-1 ☐	-2 ☐	-3 ☐	-4 ☐	-5 ☐	-6 ☐	-7 ☐	-8 ☐
Making a contribution to others	-1 ☐	-2 ☐	-3 ☐	-4 ☐	-5 ☐	-6 ☐	-7 ☐	-8 ☐

28. Which *one* of the following is *most* important to you today? *("X" only one.)*

Independence (autonomy)	-1 ☐
Achievement	-2 ☐
Social change (setting things right).............................	-3 ☐
Romance..	-4 ☐
Family commitment...	-5 ☐
Financial security..	-6 ☐
Recognition, fame	-7 ☐
Search for meaning...	-8 ☐
Intimacy	-9 ☐
Creative or intellectual pursuits................................	-0 ☐

29. **Indicate below how much power you have to make things happen the way you want them to go.** *("X" only one for each.)*

	VERY LITTLE POWER	SOME POWER	A LOT OF POWER
With your spouse or partner...............	-1 ☐	-2 ☐	-3 ☐
With your children.............................	-1 ☐	-2 ☐	-3 ☐
At work...	-1 ☐	-2 ☐	-3 ☐
In your community.............................	-1 ☐	-2 ☐	-3 ☐

30. **At this stage of your life, what does your greatest fear center on?** *("X" only one.)*

Others will find out I'm not as good as they think ....-1 ☐

I will find out I'm not as good as I thought I was...-2 ☐

Lack of recognition...-3 ☐

Not advancing fast enough ....-4 ☐

Time running out ....-5 ☐

No longer being physically attractive.....................-6 ☐

Loneliness ....-7 ☐

Messing up my personal life ....-8 ☐

Being "locked in," unable to freely change my way of life ....-9 ☐

Being surpassed by younger people in my field ....-0 ☐

Not having enough money...-x ☐

Being abandoned by spouse or lover ....-y ☐

Declining physical capabilities, illness ....-1 ☐

Other..-2 ☐

I have no major fear ....-3 ☐

31. **Thinking about your stage of life, indicate below how secure you feel about being able to maintain or grow in *each* of the following areas.** *("X" one box for each area.)*

	NOT AT ALL SECURE	SOMEWHAT SECURE	VERY SECURE
Your financial future	-1 ☐	-2 ☐	-3 ☐
Career advancement................................	-1 ☐	-2 ☐	-3 ☐
Your physical health	-1 ☐	-2 ☐	-3 ☐
Your physical strength or allure	-1 ☐	-2 ☐	-3 ☐
Your spiritual strength.........................	-1 ☐	-2 ☐	-3 ☐
Your sexual prowess................................	-1 ☐	-2 ☐	-3 ☐
Your judgment.......................................	-1 ☐	-2 ☐	-3 ☐
Your power and status in the world....	-1 ☐	-2 ☐	-3 ☐
Memory/mental alertness	-1 ☐	-2 ☐	-3 ☐
Optimism, serenity................................	-1 ☐	-2 ☐	-3 ☐
Physical attractiveness	-1 ☐	-2 ☐	-3 ☐

32. **How do you typically react to rough spots, serious problems, or crises in your life?** *("X" all that apply.)*

Devote more time and energy to work ....-1 ☐
Devote more time and energy to recreation ....-2 ☐
Develop physical symptoms (headaches, ulcers,
    diarrhea, insomnia, etc.) ....-3 ☐
Do more drinking, eating, taking tranquilizers, etc.....-4 ☐
Seek new romantic and/or sexual involvements...........-5 ☐
Pretend publicly that the problem doesn't exist............-6 ☐
Depend on friends and associates to pull
    me through...-7 ☐
See a counselor or therapist ....-8 ☐
Mostly wait until the problem solves itself...................-9 ☐
Carry on with regular activities while trying
    to solve the problem...-0 ☐
Other..-x ☐

33. **Which of the following have been true of you in the last year?** *("X" all that apply.)*

Frequent headaches...................-1 ☐	Irrational fears.........................-1 ☐
Stomach ulcers...........................-2 ☐	Crying spells.............................-2 ☐
High blood pressure..................-3 ☐	Often feeling lonely ....-3 ☐
Insomnia ....-4 ☐	Feeling fat, gaining
Constant worry and anxiety ...-5 ☐	weight ....-4 ☐
Chronic constipation/	Lack of interest in sex...........-5 ☐
diarrhea..............................-6 ☐	Eating disorder........................-6 ☐
Tiring easily ....-7 ☐	Feeling of worthlessness.......-7 ☐
Trouble concentrating..............-8 ☐	Poor appetite ....-8 ☐
Often feeling guilty ....-9 ☐	Dizziness..................................-9 ☐
Sometimes feeling that	Heart palpitations.................-0 ☐
you just can't go on ....-0 ☐	

34. **Which of the following do you do to maintain your health and physical appearance?** *("X" all that apply.)*

Nothing...-1 ☐
Gave up smoking or drinking..-2 ☐
Eat a healthy or low-fat diet ....-3 ☐
Have massages, see a chiropractor ....-4 ☐
Have regular mammograms or prostate exams.............-5 ☐
Exercise regularly, play a sport ....-6 ☐
Color hair..-7 ☐
Do yoga or meditate...-8 ☐
Take hormones ....-9 ☐
Have plastic surgery...-0 ☐
Other..-x ☐

35. Are you devoted to some cause or project outside yourself and larger than yourself?

      Yes...............................-1 ☐   No ....-2 ☐

36. If you are devoted to some cause or project outside yourself and larger than yourself, please write it in below.

_____

37. Indicate below how many hours a day you spent thinking about, pursuing, or engaging in sex while you were in your twenties. Then indicate how many hours a day you think about sex now. ("X" only one under each column.)

	TWENTIES	NOW
Nearly 24 hours a day	-1 ☐	-1 ☐
At least 12 hours a day..................	-2 ☐	-2 ☐
A few hours a day............................	-3 ☐	-3 ☐
One hour or less................................	-4 ☐	-4 ☐
Still in my twenties............................		-5 ☐

38. Over the last six months, about how often have you had sexual intercourse? ("X" only one.)

More than 6 times	Once a week ....-4 ☐
a week.....................................-1 ☐	Once or twice a month ....-5 ☐
4 to 6 times a week................-2 ☐	Less than once a month........-6 ☐
2 to 3 times a week................-3 ☐	Never.......................................-7 ☐

39. Have you ever become seriously depressed or discontented for an extended period of time? ("X" only one.)

Yes, once.....................-1 ☐	Yes, several times ....-3 ☐
Yes, twice...................-2 ☐	No→SKIP TO Q.#41........-4 ☐

40. If so, how old were you the first time you became seriously depressed or discontented for an extended period of time?   _____ years old

41. Which one of the following best describes your feelings about death? ("X" only one.)

      I am afraid of death ....-1 ☐
      It troubles me, but I don't fear it...................................-2 ☐
      I haven't thought much about it...-3 ☐
      I am working toward accepting it ....-4 ☐
      I have come to accept it ....-5 ☐
      I am not afraid of death...-6 ☐

42. Thinking about how happy you are now, indicate below how happy you expect to be in the next 10 years. ("X" only one.)

Much happier ....-1 ☐	Somewhat less happy.............-4 ☐
Somewhat happier ....-2 ☐	Much less happy....................-5 ☐
About the same as now.........-3 ☐	

43. Looking back at your life so far, has it been:

Extraordinary........................-1 ☐   Ordinary...................................-3 ☐
Interesting..............................-2 ☐   Dull...-4 ☐

44. OPTIONAL: On a separate sheet of paper, explain why you described your life this way.

45. Which of the following describes what turning 50 means/would mean to you? *("X" only one.)*

Too late to accomplish what I haven't already...............-1 ☐
An optimistic, can-do time of life ....-2 ☐
A fearful time..-3 ☐
Time for me ....-4 ☐

IF YOU HAVE NOT YET TURNED 45, SKIP TO THE "ABOUT YOU" SECTION AFTER Q.#53.

---

46. Since you turned 45, are you:

A. Less competitive..-1 ☐
   More competitive ....-2 ☐
   The same ....-3 ☐
B. Less interested in close relationships......................-4 ☐
   More interested in close relationships....................-5 ☐
   The same ....-6 ☐
C. Less concerned with just getting by........................-7 ☐
   More concerned with just getting by ....-8 ☐
   The same ....-9 ☐
D. Feeling more competent at managing
   the complexities of life...-0 ☐
   Feeling less competent at managing
   the complexities of life ....-x ☐
   The same ....-y ☐
E. More interested in sex ....-1 ☐
   Less interested in sex...-2 ☐
   The same ....-3 ☐
F. More accepting of what you can't change...............-4 ☐
   Less accepting of what you can't change.................-5 ☐
   The same ....-6 ☐
G. More involved with friends ....-7 ☐
   Less involved with friends..-8 ☐
   The same ....-9 ☐
H. More spiritually involved ....-0 ☐
   Less spiritually involved..-x ☐
   The same ....-y ☐

47. **How close did you come to achieving your vision of your ideal self by your mid-forties?** *("X" only one.)*

    I exceeded my expectations ....-1 ☐
    I worked harder to achieve my original ambitions ....-2 ☐
    I adjusted my aspirations downward...............................-3 ☐
    I changed course altogether..-4 ☐

48. **Indicate below the *three best* things about being over 45.** *("X" only three.)*

    Can really rely on my experience...................................-1 ☐
    Don't have to compete so hard.......................................-2 ☐
    Live by my own lights, stop trying
       to please everyone ....-3 ☐
    Feel in command...-4 ☐
    Have more time for myself..-5 ☐
    Easier to connect to people...-6 ☐
    Less anxious and angry ....-1 ☐
    Clearer now about what is truly important in life ....-2 ☐
    Have a richer spiritual life ....-3 ☐
    More fun, less friction in marriage.................................-4 ☐
    Enjoying my adult children...-5 ☐
    Taking pleasure in deepening friendships......................-6 ☐
    Other..-7 ☐

49. **Indicate below the *three worst* things about being over 45.** *("X" only three.)*

    Feeling invisible or irrelevant ....-1 ☐
    Feeling tired, running out of gas ....-2 ☐
    Too late to accomplish what I'd hoped ....-3 ☐
    Overwhelmed by responsibility for both
       children and parents...-4 ☐
    Being professionally handicapped by aging ....-5 ☐
    Worried about spouse's health ....-6 ☐
    No longer able to take my own health
       for granted...-7 ☐
    Having more trouble finding sexual partner ....-8 ☐
    Worried about losing my sexual desirability.................-9 ☐
    Can't stand looking old..-0 ☐
    Other..-x ☐

50. **Do you believe that there is a "male menopause" or a time of reduced vitality and potency for men?**

    Yes...-1 ☐   No ....-2 ☐

51. **Have you yourself experienced menopause? (Answer whether you are a man or a woman.)** *("X" only one.)*

    Yes, I am going through it now ....-1 ☐
    Yes, I finished with it ....-2 ☐

No, not yet..-3 ☐
No, I don't expect to.....................................-4 ☐

52. Do you feel prepared for your own menopause? *("X" only one.)*

Yes, I have already experienced it.......................-1 ☐
Yes, I'm prepared but haven't experienced it...........-2 ☐
No, I'm not prepared ....-3 ☐
I don't believe I'll have one ....-4 ☐

53. Has your life been affected by your partner's menopause? *("X" only one.)*

My partner experienced menopause,
and made my life better................................-1 ☐
My partner experienced menopause,
and made my life worse...............................-2 ☐
My partner experienced menopause,
and I was not affected...............................-3 ☐
My partner has not yet experienced menopause ....-4 ☐
I have no partner ....-5 ☐

ABOUT YOU

I. Gender:

Female ....-1 ☐   Male ....-2 ☐

2. Do you work full-time or part-time for a wage? *("X" only one.)*

Yes, full-time (35 hours a week or more)...............-1 ☐
Yes, part-time (less than 35 hours a week) ....-2 ☐
No, I do not work outside my home
for a wage→SKIP TO Q.#4 ....-3 ☐

3. Which of the following best describes your occupation? *("X" only one.)*

Professional with advanced degree (doctor, lawyer,
pharmacist, radiologist, chiropractor, etc.)...............-1 ☐
Teacher, counselor, social worker, nurse.................-2 ☐
Managerial, administrative, business ....-3 ☐
White-collar (sales, clerical, secretarial)...............-4 ☐
Artist, writer, designer, craftsperson ....-5 ☐
Full-time homemaker ....-6 ☐
Technician, skilled worker............................-7 ☐
Service worker or office temp.........................-8 ☐
Student ....-9 ☐
Unemployed...-0 ☐
Other..-x ☐

4. Have you gone back to school in the last 5 years?

Yes..............................-1 ☐   No→SKIP TO Q.#6 ....-2 ☐

5. Below are reasons for going back to school. For each reason that applies to you, write in how old you were when you started.

To finish high school................................._____ years old
To take college courses............................_____ years old
To get a college degree ...._____ years old
To get an advanced degree......................._____ years old
Required by employer..............................._____ years old

6. What is your marital status? ("X" only one.)

Single..-1 ☐
Living with a lover ....-2 ☐
Married for the first time.......................................-3 ☐
Remarried once..-4 ☐
Remarried more than once.....................................-5 ☐
Separated...-6 ☐
Divorced..-7 ☐
Widowed..-8 ☐

7. Write in the number of times you have been divorced or widowed. If you have not been widowed or divorced, write in a zero.

Divorced.............._____ times   Widowed............._____ times

8. Write in the number of years you have been married to your current partner.

Number of years married to current partner............_____

IF YOU DO NOT HAVE CHILDREN, SKIP TO Q.#13.

9. Write in the number of children, stepchildren, or adopted children you have. If you do not have any in that category, write in a zero.

Children ....._____   Stepchildren......._____   Adopted children......._____

10. Which one of the following describes how you feel about the number of children you have? ("X" only one.)

Content with the number of children I have ....-1 ☐
If I had to do it over, I'd have fewer children.................-2 ☐
If I had to do it over, I'd have more children.................-3 ☐
I still hope to have more children ....-4 ☐

11. Do you have children from a former marriage?

Yes...-1 ☐   No→SKIP TO Q.#14........-2 ☐

12. How often do you see your children from your former marriage? ("X" only one.)

One (or more) lives with me ....-1 ☐	Once a month ....-3 ☐
	Several times a year ....-4 ☐
Nearly every week ....-2 ☐	Hardly ever ....-5 ☐

13. If you do not have children, indicate below why. ("X" all that apply.)

Not ready ....-1 ☐	Pursuing career first..............-5 ☐
No partner ....-2 ☐	Prefer independence..............-6 ☐
Physically unable ....-3 ☐	Don't want children ....-7 ☐
Partner unable........................-4 ☐	Other.......................................-8 ☐

14. What is the highest level of education you have completed? ("X" only one.)

Some high school or less ....-1 ☐
Graduated high school...-2 ☐
Some college..-3 ☐
Graduated college..-4 ☐
Some post-graduate or professional school..................-5 ☐
Received a graduate or professional degree ....-6 ☐

15. Indicate below your personal annual income for the current year, before taxes. ("X" only one.)

Less than $20,000.................-1 ☐	$40,000 to $44,999..............-6 ☐
$20,000 to $24,999 ....-2 ☐	$45,000 to $49,999..............-7 ☐
$25,000 to $29,999 ....-3 ☐	$50,000 to $74,999..............-8 ☐
$30,000 to $34,999 ....-4 ☐	$75,000 to $99,999..............-9 ☐
$35,000 to $39,999 ....-5 ☐	$100,000 or more.................-0 ☐

16. Indicate below your total estimated household income before taxes for the current year for all family members. Be sure to include your own income as well as that of all other household members. Income from all sources such as wages, bonuses, profits, dividends, rentals, interest, etc., should be included. ("X" only one.)

Less than $20,000.................-1 ☐	$45,000 to $49,999..............-7 ☐
$20,000 to $24,999 ....-2 ☐	$50,000 to $74,999..............-8 ☐
$25,000 to $29,999 ....-3 ☐	$75,000 to $99,999..............-9 ☐
$30,000 to $34,999 ....-4 ☐	$100,000 to $149,999.........-0 ☐
$35,000 to $39,999 ....-5 ☐	$150,000 or more.................-x ☐
$40,000 to $44,999 ....-6 ☐	

Appendix 11
___

PROFESSIONAL WOMEN'S
AND MEN'S SURVEYS

The 687 questionnaires from women and 110 from men in this sample supplied a larger context for the texture and humanness of the group interviews.

The 687 Professional Women attended conferences sponsored by women's organizations around the country: Central California Women's Conference, Fresno, California (September 17, 1992), CentraState Medical Center in Freehold, New Jersey (April 15, 1992), International Women's Forum in San Antonio, Texas (April 29, 1993), Center for the American Woman and Politics Conference of Women State Legislators, San Diego, California (November 14, 1991), International Alliance of Business and Professional Women, Rochester, New York (October 27, 1991), League of Women Voters National Convention, Boston, Massachusetts (June 17, 1992), and hospital-sponsored events: Center for Women's Medicine at Florida Hospital, Orlando, Florida (May 4, 1993), co-sponsored event in Des Moines, Iowa, by Mercy Hospital and WHO-TV (May 18, 1993), Swedish Medical Center, Seattle, Washington (October 8, 1993).

Respondents completed a 103-question Life History Survey; 313 of them also answered a 24-question supplemental survey for women over 50.

These women ranged in age from 23 to 75; half were older than 46, and their average age was 50. The women came from nearly every state in the country, including 21% from New York, 17% from California, and 13% from Kentucky. Two thirds were married, and four in ten had been separated, divorced, or widowed at some point. Most of these women—78%—had at least one child. Four in ten had graduate degrees and another 37% were college graduates.

Seven in ten of these women worked either full- or part-time. One third held managerial, administrative, or business jobs; 18% were in teaching, counseling, or nursing; 14% were professionals with an advanced degree. One third had annual family incomes of more than $100,000, but only 7% earned that much on their own. Two in ten earned between $50,000 and $100,000 a year.

The 110 Professional Men were from focus groups I conducted nationwide in 1993; they answered a Special Questionnaire for Men in Second Adulthood.

The men ranged in age from 40 to 65; on average, they were 52. Most (87%) were married, but only 40% of them were still in first marriages, 20% were in second marriages, and 13% in third marriages.

Two thirds of these men had some graduate training or graduate degrees, and the majority earned more than $50,000 a year. Among those, 28% earned more than $100,000, 10% earned $75,000 to $100,000, and 28% earned $50,000 to $75,000.

Appendix 111

FAMILY CIRCLE SURVEY

Family Circle maintains a reader's panel that is weighted to approximate a representative national sample, excluding the very rich and very poor. In November 1993, *Family Circle* randomly distributed 2,000 of my Life History surveys to members of this reader's panel. Of the 1,024 who responded, 630 were women, 394 were men. The total number of couples who returned surveys together was 385.

Women: ranged in age from 18 to 85; on average, 45 years old (295 of them answered the special section for women over the age of 45). Most of these women (76%) were married (31% had been divorced), and 81% had at least one child. The majority of these women, 67%, had not graduated from college.

About six in ten of these women worked either full- or part-time: One third were white-collar workers, 20% were teachers, counselors, social workers, or nurses, 19% were managers or administrators. Only 2% held a professional job. Two thirds earned less than $25,000 a year; half had an annual family income of less than $40,000.

Men: ranged in age from 22 to 86; on average, 47 years old (200 men answered the special section for men over the age of 45). Most of the men (94%) were married and had at least one child; 26% had been divorced. The majority (61%) were not college graduates.

Eight in ten of these men worked full- or part-time; 31% were technical or skilled workers, 26% were managers or administrators, 11% held a professional job. While 30% earned less than $25,000 a year; 21% earned more than $50,000 a year.

None of my research or the major longitudinal studies cited in the book include people still struggling for survival: the illiterate, the seriously ill, or those at poverty level.

Appendix 1V

NEW WOMAN SURVEY

The Original Survey on Aging, conducted in 1993 by Gail Sheehy and Carin Rubenstein, Ph.D., was published in *New Woman* (November 1993). A total of six thousand women responded to the survey. They ranged in age from 18 to 85; on average, they were 44 years old (45% answered a special section for postmenopausal women). Four in ten of these women were married; 39% were divorced, separated, or widowed; 12% had never married. Slightly more than half (56%) were not college graduates.

Seven in ten of these women worked full- or part-time; 49% had white-collar jobs; 15% held professional jobs. The majority, 57%, earned less than $30,000 a year; 24% earned more than $40,000 a year. One third were divorced, many others were in remarriages, and a number remained steadfastly single or lived with a lover, either male or female.

Appendix V

SUGGESTED READINGS
ON MENOPAUSE

BOOKS ABOUT MENOPAUSE
(IN ADDITION TO *THE SILENT PASSAGE*)
RECOMMENDED BY WOMEN'S HEALTH CENTERS
AROUND THE COUNTRY

Penny Wise Budoff, *No More Hot Flashes* (New York: Warner Books, 1984).

Janine O'Leary Cobb, *Understanding Menopause* (Toronto: Key Porter Books, 1989).

Winnifred B. Cutler and Celso-Ramon Edwards, *Menopause: A Guide for Women and the Men Who Love Them* (New York: W. W. Norton, 1992).

Vicki Hufnagel, M.D., *No More Hysterectomies* (New York: Penguin, 1988).

Ruth Jacobowitz, *150 Most-Asked Questions About Menopause* (New York: William Morrow, 1992).

Susan Lark, *The Menopause Self-Help Book* (Berkeley: Celestial Arts, 1990).

Alice MacMahon, *Women and Hormones: An Essential Guide to Being Female* (Maitland, Fla.: Family Publications, 1990).

Lila Nachtigall and Joan Rattner Heilman, *Estrogen* (New York: HarperPerennial, 1991).

Morris Notelovitz and Diana Tonnessen, *Menopause and Midlife Health* (New York: St. Martin's, 1993).

L. Ojedo, *Menopause Without Medicine* (Reading, Mass.: Addison-Wesley, 1992).

Rosetta Reitz, *Menopause: A Positive Approach* (New York and London: Penguin, 1977).

Notes

NOTE FROM THE AUTHOR

1. Gail Sheehy, *The Silent Passage* (New York: Random House, 1992).
2. The life expectancy at birth for white Americans in 1900 was 47 to 49. For other than white Americans, the life expectancy at birth was shockingly low: only 33 to 34. From Cynthia M. Tauber, *Sixty-Five Plus in America*, 1992. Bureau of the Census, Current Population Reports, Special Studies, Table 3-1, "Life Expectancy at Birth and at 65 Years of Age, by Race and Sex; Selected Years 1900 to 1989."
3. Gail Sheehy, *Passages* (New York: E. P. Dutton & Co., Inc., 1976).

BOOK ONE: FIRST ADULTHOOD
PROLOGUE: OH, PIONEERS!

1. Thomas R. Cole, *The Journey of Life: A Cultural History of Aging in America* (Cambridge: Cambridge University Press, 1992), p. 3.
2. Evelyn Mann, "Children Ever Born—1940–1990," unpublished report, based on PUMS data.
3. Robert Lowell, "Day by Day," *The Oxford Book of Ages*, ed. Anthony and Sally Sampson (New York: Oxford University Press, 1985).
4. Brian Knowlton, "The Changing Face of European Families," *International Herald Tribune*, March 25, 1989.
5. Author's interview with Dr. Kenneth Manton, demographer at Duke University, spring 1993.
6. Evelyn Mann, "Life Expectancy at Birth, at Age 50, at Age 60," unpublished report. Sources used were Tables 106 and 107 from the U.S. Bureau of the Census's 1980 *Statistical Abstract of the United States;* Tables 115 and 116 from the 1990 *Statistical Abstract.*
7. Patricia Aburdene and John Naisbitt, *Megatrends for Women* (New York: Villard, 1992), p. 138.
8. U.S. Department of Commerce Bureau of the Census, Current Population Reports. Life Expectancy at Birth and at Age 65, by Race and Sex: 1950 to 2080, Table B-5.

9. Mann, "Life Expectancy."

10. David Gergen, "Sixty Something: Part I," *U.S. News & World Report*, April 16, 1990, p. 64.

11. Gina Kolata, "Study Challenges Longevity Theory," *The New York Times*, October 16, 1992.

12. Gina Kolata, "New Views on Life Span Alter Forecasts on Elderly," *The New York Times*, November 16, 1992.

13. New York: Basic Books, 1992.

14. Michael Waldholtz, "Fountain of Youth May Not Be Fairy Tale, Study Finds," *The Wall Street Journal*, October 16, 1992.

15. Erik Erikson, *Childhood and Society* (New York: W. W. Norton, 1963 ed.), Chapter 7. Erik Erikson, ed., *Adulthood* (New York: W. W. Norton, 1978), p. vii.

16. Daniel J. Levinson, *Seasons of a Man's Life*, ed. Charlotte N. Dorrow, Edward B. Klein, Maria H. Levinson, and Braxton McKee (New York: Alfred A. Knopf, 1978). For more about Erikson, see Sheehy, *Passages*, Chapter 5, "If I'm Late, Start the Crisis Without Me."

17. Evelyn Mann, "Percent Change in Median Money by Sex, United States, 1974–1992," unpublished report, based on U.S. Bureau of the Census, Current Population Reports, *Consumer Income Series*, P60-184, Table B-15.

18. Evelyn Mann, "Percent Change in Median Earnings of Full-Time and Full-Time Year-Round Workers by Sex, United States—Various Time Periods," unpublished report, based on U.S. Bureau of the Census, Current Population Reports, *Consumer Income Series*, P60-184, Table B-16.

19. Susan Faludi, *Backlash: The Undeclared War Against American Women* (New York: Crown, 1991), p. 67.

20. Gina Kolata, "Reproductive Revolution Is Jolting Old Views," *The New York Times*, January 11, 1994.

21. Václav Havel, "The New Measure of Man," speech delivered at Independence Hall, Philadelphia, July 4, 1994.

22. Study by Daniel Yankelovich, Inc. (1973), cited in Sheehy's *Passages*, Chapter 1, "Madness and Method."

PART ONE: WHATEVER HAPPENED TO THE LIFE CYCLE?

I. MAPPING LIVES ACROSS TIME

1. See Sheehy, *Passages*, Chapter 3, "Breast to Breakaway."

2. Evelyn Mann, "Persons in the Military, 1990," unpublished report, based on 1990 unpublished Census Bureau data.

3. Evelyn Mann, "Trends in Real Income and Earnings 1970–1992," unpublished report, based on U.S. Bureau of the Census, Current Population Reports, *Consumer Income Series*, P60-184: "Money Income of Households, Families, and Persons in the United States," issued September 1993.

4. Author's interview with Paul Ryscavage, November 1993.

5. General Louis B. Hershey, then director of the U.S. Selective Service, quoted in 1940s *Time* documentary *March of Time*.

6. Evelyn Mann, "World War II Generation," unpublished report, based on PUMS data.

7. *Time* magazine documentary *March of Time*.

8. Ibid.

9. Mann, "World War II Generation."

10. See James Lincoln Collier, *Jazz: The American Theme Song* (New York: Oxford University Press, 1993).

11. Evelyn Mann, "16 to 19 Year Olds from World War II to the Safety Generation," unpublished report, based on PUMS data.

12. Evelyn Mann, "The Silent Generation," unpublished report, based on PUMS data.

13. Evelyn Mann, "Children Ever Born and the Percent of Childlessness at the End of Childbearing," unpublished report, based on PUMS data.

14. Mann, "The Silent Generation."

15. Campbell Gibson, "The Myth of the Homogeneous Baby-Boom Generation," U.S. Bureau of the Census, October 1993, Table 6.

16. William Manchester, *The Glory and the Dream: A Narrative History of America, 1932–1972* (New York: Bantam, 1975).

17. Sloan Wilson, *The Man in the Gray Flannel Suit* (New York: Morrow, 1955).

18. Gibson, Table 2.

19. Mann, "The Silent Generation."

20. Ibid.

21. Ibid.

22. Ibid.

23. William Strauss and Neil Howe, *Generations: The History of America's Future, 1584–2069* (New York: Morrow, 1991), p. 281.

24. Wade Greene's comment, cited ibid., p. 281.

25. Evelyn Mann, "School Enrollment of Women 40 and Over, Educational Achievement of World War II, Silent, and Vietnam Generations," unpublished report, based on PUMS data.

26. Evelyn Mann, "Fall Enrollment in Institutions of Higher Education by Level and Attendance Status of Student Females, Age 40 and Over, 1991," unpublished report based on U.S. Department of Education, National Center for Education Statistics, Integrated Postsecondary Education Data System, "Fall Enrollment, 1991" survey.

27. Judith Hole and Ellen Levine, *Rebirth of Feminism* (New York: Quadrangle/New York Times Books, 1971), p. 123.

28. Strauss and Howe, p. 282.

29. According to Terry Banks, former director of England's Third Age Inquiry, in interview with author, September 1992.

30. This is the observation of Thomas Kiley, Massachusetts pollster.

31. Katharine Q. Seelye, "With Fiery Words, Gingrich Builds His Kingdom," *The New York Times,* October 27, 1994.

32. Cited in Manchester, pp. 1,110.

33. This was how Dorothy Rodham described her daughter's dream to me in an interview I conducted for a *Vanity Fair* profile that appeared in May 1992.

34. Interview with Hillary Rodham Clinton, February 1992.

35. Gail Sheehy, "What Hillary Wants," *Vanity Fair,* May 1992.

36. Manchester, pp. 1,107.

37. Gibson, Table 6.

38. Ibid.

39. Evelyn Mann, "The Vietnam Generation," unpublished report, based on PUMS data.

40. Ibid.

41. Mickey Kaus, "Confessions of an Ex-Radical," *Newsweek,* September 5, 1988, p. 24.

42. Paul Leinberger, a California management consultant, cited in Walter Kiechel III, "The Workaholic Generation," *Fortune,* April 10, 1989.

43. Author's interview with Susan Hayward of Yankelovich Partners, September 1992.

44. Tom Wolfe, "The 'Me' Decade and the Third Great Awakening," *New York,* August 23, 1976.

45. John Greenwald, "Baby, You're a Rich Man, Still," *Time,* May 14, 1990, p. 72.

46. Lynn Barber, "McInerney Rising," *New York Observer,* June 1, 1992.

47. This was a study for an article in *Glamour* magazine. Gail Sheehy, "The Happiness Report," April 1989.

48. Evelyn Mann, "The 'Me' Generation," unpublished report, based on PUMS data.

49. Clifford Adelman, "Women at Thirtysomething: Paradoxes of Attainment," U.S. Department of Education publication, July 1992, p. 1.

50. Ibid.

51. Evelyn Mann, "Never Married—Trends and Projections, United States, 1940–1990," unpublished report, based on PUMS data.

52. Mann, "Children Ever Born and the Percent of Childlessness at the End of Childbearing."

53. Florence Kaslow, "Thirty-Plus and Not Married," in *Gender Issues Across the Lifecycle*, ed. Barbara Rubin Wainrib (New York: Springer, 1992), p. 92.

54. Mann, "Trends in Real Income and Earnings 1970–1992."

55. Gibson, p. 12.

56. Author's interview with Susan Hayward.

57. Gibson. The paper was popularized in an article for *American Demographics*, November 1993, titled "The Four Baby Booms."

58. Census Bureau data amassed by analysts Jessie Allen and Cynthia Taueber, "Women in Our Aging Society: A Demographic Outlook," *Women on the Front Lines: Meeting the Challenge of an Aging America*, ed. Jessie Allen and Alan Pifer (Washington, D.C.: Urban Institute Press, 1993), pp. 11–40.

59. Author's interview with Susan Hayward.

60. Mann, "Trends in Real Income and Earnings 1970–1992."

61. Gail Sheehy, Preface, in Allen and Pifer, p. xiv.

62. The MONITOR study, 1986 and 1991, from Yankelovich Partners, Table 68. The question asked by Yankelovich was: "Is there a need to restore some romance and mystery to modern life?" Among women 25–34, 39.7 percent said, "Moderately," in 1986. In 1991 the number jumped to 48.2 percent for this cohort.

63. Mark Landler, "Move Over Boomers: The Busters Are Here—and They're Angry," *Business Week*, December 14, 1992.

64. Handout by Nancy Reuben at Friends Seminary AIDS assembly, March 12, 1987.

65. "Facts in Brief: Teenage Sexual and Reproductive Behavior," 1993 fact sheet from the Alan Guttmacher Institute, New York, New York.

66. Marcia Kramer, "Forty Teens Here Have AIDS: Say No to Sex, City Urges in New Ads," *New York Daily News*, November 11, 1987.

67. Gabrielle Glaser, "What About the New Chastity?" *Mademoiselle*, March 1994.

68. Leslie Ansley, " 'It Just Keeps Getting Worse,' " *USA Weekend*, August 13–15, 1993. The results of the survey are based on the written answers of 65,193 sixth through twelfth graders who responded individually or as classes to a questionnaire printed in the April 23–25 issues of *USA Weekend* and in the Classline Today teaching plan and distributed by the National Association of Secondary School Principals.

69. Landler.

70. Bob Herbert, "The Hate Game," *The New York Times*, February 9, 1994.

71. Ellen McGrath, "New Treatment Strategies for Women in the Middle," *Gender Issues Across the Lifecycle*, ed. Barbara Rubin Wainrib (New York: Springer, 1992), p. 130.

72. According to Dr. Myrna Weissman, a psychiatric epidemiologist at the New York State Psychiatric Institute and Columbia Presbyterian Medical Center, who directed the first international study of major depression. The study revealed a steady rise in the disorder worldwide. Daniel Goleman, "A Rising Cost of Modernity: Depression," *The New York Times*, December 8, 1992.

73. Mann, "16 to 19 Year Olds from World War II to the Safety Generation."

74. Evelyn Mann, "The Safety Generation," unpublished report, based on PUMS data for 1990. These figures encompass whites, blacks, Hispanics, and Asians for 1990, age 20–24.

75. Personal interview with Arthur Norton, March 1992, at the U.S. Bureau of the Census.

76. Donald L. Barlett and James B. Steele, *America: What Went Wrong?* (Kansas City: Andrews and McMeel, 1992), p. xiv.

77. Neil Howe and Bill Strauss, "Hey, Boomers: Share the Wealth, Dudes," *The New York Times*, September 26, 1993.

78. Alan Riding, "In a Time of Shared Hardship, the Young Embrace Europe," *The New York Times*, August 12, 1993.

79. Evelyn Mann, "Age of Householder by Tenure, United States, 1970–1980–1990," table utilizing data from: U.S. Census, Subjects Reports, Family Composition, Table I (1970); U.S. Census Summary, Metropolitan Housing Characteristics, Table A-10 (1980); U.S. Census of Population and Housing, Summary Tape File 3-C (1990).

80. Evelyn Mann, "Living Arrangements of Unmarried Persons Age 20 to 34 by Sex," based on unpublished PUMS data and Current Population Reports P20-468. Of males 25–34, 39.4 percent still live with their parents or other relations.

81. Ibid.

82. "Ratio of Unmarried Men per 100 Unmarried Women by Age," U.S. Bureau of the Census, "Marital Status and Living Arrangements: March 1992," Series P20-468, December 1992.

83. Author's interview with Vivian Young, May 1994.

84. Mann, "Never Married—Trends and Projections, United States, 1940–1990."

85. Arthur Norton and Louisa Miller, "Marriage, Divorce and Remarriage in the 1990's," U.S. Bureau of the Census Special Studies, Series P23-180, October 1992, Table E.

86. Ibid., Table C. This projection is based on the difference between the 1985 to 1990 experience and 1975 to 1980 experience which produced the "one-in-two" statistic.

87. Author's interviews with Kathleen Malley, Boston University, November 1993; and Susan J. Frank, psychologist at Michigan State University, October 1993.

PART TWO: THE FLOURISHING FORTIES

2. THE VIETNAM GENERATION HITS MIDDLESCENCE

1. According to Alan Causey, director of social analysis at Ammirati & Puris/Lintas advertising agency, New York City. Author's interview, May 1994.

2. Douglas Jehl, "Weary Clinton Takes Break from His Own Frenetic Style," *The New York Times*, August 15, 1993.

3. Garrison Keillor, "A Baby Boom President Young Enough to Be (Gasp) Me," *The New York Times*, December 17, 1992.

4. These comparative results of over-45 and under-45 men come from a national survey of 1,024 men and women conducted by Sheehy in 1993 for *Family Circle* magazine, with the assistance of Carin Rubinstein, Ph.D.

   In November 1993 *Family Circle* mailed out surveys to 1,000 women from the magazine's reader's panel; an extra survey was included in each packet so the women could give it to a "significant other." Surveys were returned by 1,024 people, 630 of them women and 394 men. (Among them were 385 couples who mailed back surveys together.)

5. Sheehy's Life History Survey of 110 Professional Men who attended her men's group interviews. See Appendix II, for full explanation.

6. *Family Circle* national survey results.

7. Combe, Inc., a New Jersey–based company that makes Just for Men hair-coloring products, conducted a survey of five hundred men in 1992. More than 44 percent said they felt at least ten years younger than their chronological ages.

8. From author's interview with Burt Manning, CEO of J. Walter Thompson.

9. Nancy Collins, "Hey, Mike, What's with the Beard?" *Vanity Fair*, November 1994, pp. 78–91.

10. Ibid.

11. William Grimes, "The Melody of His Voice Lingers On," *The New York Times,* September 26, 1993.

12. Mervyn Rothstein, "Ann Beattie's Life After Real Estate," *The New York Times,* December 30, 1985.

3. MEN REDEFINING SUCCESS

1. Report from the Organization for Economic Cooperation and Development, Paris, September 1994; and author's interview with David Aaron, American ambassador to the OECD.

2. Sylvia Nasar, "More Men in Prime of Life Spend Less Time Working," *The New York Times,* December 1, 1994.

3. Patricia Edmonds and Richard Bendetto, "Angry White Men," *USA Today,* November 11, 1994.

4. Author's interview, July 1994.

5. Latest figures (July 1994) from Cognetics, Inc., an economic research firm in Cambridge, Massachusetts, with a database of ten million American companies. David Birch, Cognetics's president, confirmed that 6 million people are employed at Fortune 500 companies out of a work force of 120 million. Peter F. Drucker was counting overseas employment by the Fortune 500 when he cited a reduction of 30 percent to 13 percent in an interview with T. George Harris, "The Post-Capitalist Executive," interview with Peter F. Drucker, *Harvard Business Review* (May 1993).

6. Harris.

7. Author's interview, July 1994.

8. Harris.

9. See C. Z. Gove, "Multiple Roles and Happiness," *Spouse, Parent, Worker,* ed. F. Crosby (New Haven: Yale University Press, 1987), pp. 126–37.

10. Matilda White Riley and John W. Riley, "The Lives of Older People and Changing Social Roles," *The Annals of the American Academy of Political and Social Science,* May 1, 1989, pp. 14–28.

11. Nasar.

12. Ibid.

13. Yankelovich MONITOR study. Table 74, 1986 and 1991.

14. Cited in Lisa Grunwald, "Is It Time to Get Out?" *Esquire,* April 1990.

15. New York: Pocket Books, 1982.

16. From the preface to the 1921 edition of *The Song of the Lark.* Cited in the Introduction to *Willa Cather,* an anthology of some of her works (New York: Gramercy Books, 1994), p. vii.

17. According to research from the University for Human Development, University of California, Berkeley, discussed in Dorothy Eichorn, John Clausen, Norma Haan, Marjorie Honzik, and Paul Mussen, eds., *Present and Past in Middle Life* (Berkeley: University for Human Development, University of California, 1981). See Chapter 8, "Paths to Psychological Health in the Middle Years: Sex Differences."

18. Deborah Tannen, *You Just Don't Understand* (New York: Morrow, 1990).

19. Debra Goldman, "Baby Boomerangers Back Home," *Adweek,* September 2, 1991.

4. OUT-OF-SIGHT WOMEN

1. Ellen McGrath, *When Feeling Bad Is Good: An Innovative Self-Help Program for Women to Convert Healthy Depression into New Sources of Growth and Power* (New York: Henry Holt, 1992), pp. 51–71.

2. Sheehy, *Passages,* Chapter 13, "Catch-30."

3. Gibson, pp. 36–40.

4. Ibid., p. 12.

5. Mann, "Trends in Real Income and Earnings 1970–1992."

6. Gibson, p. 12.

7. Jane Gross, "Divorced, Middle-Aged and Happy: Women, Especially, Adjust to the 90s," *The New York Times*, December 7, 1992.

8. "Median Total Money Income in 1992 of Females Ages 18 to 64 by Work Experience, Marital Status, Race and Hispanic Origin," from PUMS data:

	Total Money Income	Married, Spouse Present	Married, Spouse Absent	Widowed	Divorced	Never Married
White women, 25–44 (all)	$15,079	13,376	11,530	16,290	18,491	19,070
(Full-time workers)	$23,368	23,008	19,273	22,430	23,651	24,807
White women, 45–64 (all)	$13,567	11,920	12,031	14,508	19,072	20,497
(Full-time workers)	$24,267	23,506	21,919	24,979	25,232	28,478

9. "The New Female Confidence," results of a *McCall's* magazine survey, November 1993, p. 96. *McCall's* joined with Yankelovich Partners, the marketing and social research firm, to launch a landmark study exploring confidence in American women. They questioned women of all ages, representing a cross section of the United States.

10. Nancy Bartley, "Prayer Heals, Says Doctor," *The Seattle Times*, October 9, 1993.

5. THE FANTASY OF FERTILITY FOREVER

1. Author's interview, 1992.

2. Ibid., June 1994.

3. Ibid., March 1992.

4. Author's interview, April 1994.

5. New York: Morrow, 1994.

6. Anne Taylor Fleming, *Motherhood Deferred: A Woman's Journey* (New York: Putnam, 1994).

7. Author's interview with Dr. Richard Marrs, Santa Monica, California, May 1994.

8. Terry McMillan, *Waiting to Exhale* (New York: Viking Penguin, 1992), pp. 10–11.

9. Interview with Dr. Marrs.

10. Cited by Jamie Grifo in author's interview, April 1992.

11. Telephone interview with Dr. Jamie Grifo, July 1994.

12. Barbara Grizzuti Harrison, "Fetal Distractions," *Mirabella*, May 1994.

13. According to Mark Sauer's clinic, University of Southern California Reproductive Group. Author's interview, December 1994.

14. "Never Too Late," a segment hosted by Ed Bradley on *60 Minutes*, May 8, 1994.

15. "Never Too Late," *Prime Time Live*, September 10, 1992.

16. Joan Juliet Buck, "The Annette Effect," *Vanity Fair*, June 1992, p. 158.

17. "Never Too Late," *Prime Time Live*.

18. Robin Marantz Henig, "Can't Win for Losing" (a review of *Women as Wombs: Reproductive Technologies and the Battle over Women's Freedom* by Janice Raymond), *The New York Times Book Review*, February 6, 1994, p. 25.

19. Susan Peterson, "Twin Miracles, Age 1," *The Orange County Register*, November 7, 1993.

20. Kolata, "Reproductive Revolution Is Jolting Old Views."

21. Tamar Lewin, "Adopted Youths Are Normal in Self-Esteem, Study Finds," *The New York Times*, June 23, 1994.

6. PERPETUAL MIDDLESCENCE

1. Daniel Rudman, Axel G. Feller, Hoskote S. Nagraj, et al., "Effects of Human Growth Hormone in Men over 60 Years Old, *The New England Journal of Medicine*, vol. 323, no. I (July 5, 1990), pp. I–6.

2. Richard Kirkland, "Why We Will Live Longer . . . and What It Will Mean," *Fortune*, February 21, 1994, pp. 66–78.

3. Gloria Steinem, *Revolution from Within: A Book of Self-Esteem* (Boston: Little, Brown, 1992).

4. Gross.

5. Ibid.

6. Ibid.

7. See Sheehy, *Pathfinders*, Chapter I, "Hunting the Secrets of Well-Being," and Myers, *Pursuit of Happiness: What Makes A Person Happy and Why* (New York: Morrow, 1992).

    The link between marriage and high well-being has also been confirmed by University of Washington psychologist John Gottman. See his book *Why Marriages Succeed or Fail* (New York: Simon & Schuster, 1994). Also see John Gottman, "Predicting the Longitudinal Course of Marriages," *Journal of Marital and Family Therapy*, vol. 17 (January 1991), pp. 3–7, 25–32; John Gottman and Lowell Krokoff, "Marital Interaction and Satisfaction: A Longitudinal View," *Journal of Consulting and Clinical Psychology*, vol. 57 (February 1989), pp. 47–52; John Gottman, "What Makes Marriage Work?" *Psychology Today* (March/April 1994), pp. 38–43.

8. Cited in "Marriage: Men Happier. Guys Wed for Better; Wives, for Worse," *USA Today*, October 11, 1993.

9. Gottman, *Why Marriages Succeed or Fail.*

10. Quoted in "Marriage: Men Happier."

11. Quoted ibid.

12. Quoted in Gross.

BOOK TWO: SECOND ADULTHOOD

PROLOGUE: A BRAND-NEW PASSAGE

1. Steven Schiff, "New York Story," *Vanity Fair*, July 1990, pp. 96–99, 124–26.

2. Author's interview with Dr. Edward Schneider, director of Andrus Gerontology Center at the University of Southern California, November 1991.

3. According to Robert Blancato, executive director of the White House Conference on Aging, at the Fifty Plus Expo held in New York City, April 1994.

4. Author's interview with Dr. William Haseltine, chairman and chief executive officer of Human Genome Sciences, September 1993.

5. Evelyn Mann, "Population Projections of the United States by Age, Sex, Race and Hispanic Origin 1993 to 2050," unpublished report, based on Current Population Reports P-25 1104, U.S. Bureau of the Census.

6. Carl Gustav Jung, "The Stages of Life," *Collected Works of C. G. Jung*, tr. R. F. C. Hull (Princeton: Princeton University Press, 1969), vol. 8, pp. 398–99.

7. Charlotte Painter, *Gifts of Age* (San Francisco: Chronicle Books, 1985).

8. Dr. Jack Rowe, president of Mount Sinai School of Medicine, who with his colleagues did a study of thirteen hundred healthy men and women whose average age was 75. Cited in Daniel Goleman, "Mental Decline in Aging Need Not Be Inevitable," *The New York Times*, April 26, 1994.

9. Ecclesiastes 3:1–8.

10. Author's interview with Dr. Aryeh Maidenbaum, Jungian analyst and director of the New York Center for Jungian Studies. Address: 121 Madison Avenue, Suite 31, New York, NY 10016, (212) 689-8238.

11. Eichorn, Clausen, Haan, Honzik, and Massen.

12. *havel havalim . . . hakol havel*. The Hebrew word *havel* can be translated as "meaninglessness," "futility," "nonsense," or "breath," which implies insubstantiality. *Tanakh: The Holy Scriptures*, tr. Jewish Publication Society (New York: JPS, 1985).

13. Jeffrey Burke Satinover and Lenore Thomson Bentz, "Aching in the Places Where We Used to Play," in *Quadrant: The Journal of Contemporary Jungian Thought*, volume XXV:1 (1992), pp. 21–57.

14. "Remarks of the First Lady at Liz Carpenter's Lectureship Series," University of Texas in Austin, April 7, 1993.

15. Lloyd Grove, "First Lady of the World Stage," *The Washington Post*, July 12, 1993.

16. Howell Raines, *Fly Fishing Through the Midlife Crisis* (New York: Morrow, 1993).

17. These are the women I surveyed through my Life History Survey. About half of these older women (47 percent) have goals they didn't achieve earlier but intend to accomplish now; 75 percent also say they have *not* discarded dreams from their forties. They believe that they have, on average, nineteen years left to complete their missions. Women of high well-being expect to live to the age of 87; lows expect to live to age 83.

18. John Lahr, "Dead Souls," *The New Yorker*, May 9, 1994, p. 94.

19. Eichorn et al.

20. Daniel Hart, *Becoming Men: The Development of Aspirations, Values and Adaptational Styles* (New York: Plenum, 1992), Chapter 6, "Adaptational Styles," pp. 159–84.

PART THREE: PASSAGE TO THE AGE OF MASTERY

7. THE MORTALITY CRISIS

1. Stanley Fisher and James Ellison, *Discovering the Power of Self-Hypnosis: A New Approach for Enabling Change and Promoting Healing* (New York: HarperCollins, 1992).

2. Albert Camus, *The Myth of Sisyphus and Other Essays* (New York: Vintage, 1955), p. 122.

3. Chuck and Peggy Downes, *Dialogue of Hope: Talking Our Way Through Cancer* (Carmel, Calif.: Sunflower Ink, 1992).

4. Camus, p. 15.

5. Dr. Jerome Bruner of New York University in particular has studied the way people tell their life stories. See explanation of his research in Gail Sheehy, *Character: America's Search for Leadership* (New York: Morrow, 1988), p. 34.

6. *Søren Kierkegaard's Journals and Papers*, tr. Howard V. Hong and Edna H. Hong (Bloomington: Indiana University Press, 1967), vol. I, p. 450.

7. See Buhler, "The Course of Human Life as a Psychological Problem," in *The Process of Child Development*, ed. Peter Neubauer (Northvale, N.J.: Jason Aronson, 1983).

8. Margaret Morganroth Gullette, *Safe at Last in the Middle Years: The Invention of the Midlife Progress Novel: Saul Bellow, Margaret Drabble, Anne Tyler, John Updike* (Berkeley: University of California Press, 1988).

9. New York: Knopf, 1985.

10. Updike is cited in Gullette, p. 60.

11. New York: Harcourt, Brace, 1993.

12. B. Cohler, "Personal Narrative and the Life Course," in *Life-Span Development and Behavior*, ed. P. B. Baltes and O. G. Brim (San Diego: Academic Press, 1982), vol. 4, pp. 205–41.

13. John Dunne, *A Search for God in Time and Memory* (New York: Macmillan, 1969), p. viii.

14. Sophocles, *Oedipus at Colonus,* tr. with notes by Mary W. Blundell (Newburyport, Maine: Focus Information Group, 1990).

15. Camus, p. 123.

16. Author's interview with Eric Kandel at Columbia Presbyterian in 1989.

17. Nashville, Tenn.: Abingdon Press, 1994.

18. San Francisco: HarperSanFrancisco, 1993, p. 11.

19. Quoted in Sogyal Rinpoche, *Tibetan Book of the Dead* (San Francisco: HarperSan Francisco, 1993), p. 35.

PART FOUR: FLAMING FIFTIES: WOMEN

8. WOMEN: PITS TO PEAK

1. Edward Albee, *Three Tall Women, American Theatre,* September 1994, pp. 39–53.

2. Maureen Orth, "The Lady Has Legs," *Vanity Fair,* May 1993, pp. 114–21.

3. Thomas Moore, *Care of the Soul* (New York: HarperCollins, 1992), p. 63.

4. Linda Witt, Karen M. Paget, and Glenna Matthews, *Running as a Woman* (New York: Free Press, 1994).

5. Of Silent Generation women aged 50–54 in 1990, only 16.7 percent had four years of college or more.

6. Sally Squires, "Rapid Increase in Gravely Overweight American Adults Alarms Researchers," *The Washington Post,* July 20, 1994.

7. In the *Family Circle* survey, 43 percent of those who measured on the lowest end of the well-being scale have an annual family income of less than $30,000, compared with 30 percent among those in the highest well-being quadrant.

8. These observations are based on responses from the women who answered the *Family Circle* survey.

9. Evelyn Mann, "Labor Force Participation Rates," unpublished report based on data derived from PUMS file 1940–1990. At ages 50–54, fully 68.3 percent of women are in the labor force (three quarters of whom employed full-time). At ages 55–59, their labor force participation drops only to 56 percent (70.2 percent of whom are employed full-time).

10. Mann, "Silent Generation."

11. Women between 45 and 54 are predicted by the Census Bureau to increase their ranks in the work force from 14,160 in 1992 to 18,411 in the year 2000. The second-largest increase in job holders will be among women ages 55–64, whose ranks will swell by over 100 percent. Unpublished report based on the American Workforce: 1992–2005, U.S. Department of Labor, Bureau of Labor Statistics, Bulletin 2452, April 1994, Appendix Table A-1 and A-2.

12. According to the American Psychiatric Association, the term *involutional melancholia* was expunged in 1980 from the *Diagnostic and Statistical Manual,* No. 3.

13. Author's interview with Dr. Frederick Goodwin, then director of the National Institute of Mental Health, June 1993.

14. From recent epidemiological data cited by Dr. Goodwin in author's interview.
    Ellen McGrath, the psychologist who chaired the American Psychological Association's Task Force on Women and Depression, verifies from her research that "most older women have less dissatisfaction and psychological stress than at any other time in life." See her book *When Feeling Bad Is Good,* p. 176.

15. Leo Srole and Anita Kassen Fischer, "The Midtown Manhattan Longitudinal Study vs. 'The Mental Doctrine,' " *Archives of General Psychiatry,* 1980.

16. Leo Srole, Thomas S. Langner, Marvin K. Opler, and Thomas A. C. Rennie, *Mental Health in the Metropolis,* vol. 1, *Midtown Manhattan Study* (New York: McGraw-Hill, 1962).

17. Jean Baker Miller, *Toward a New Psychology of Women* (Boston: Beacon Press, 1976); Nancy Chodorow, *The Reproduction of Mothering* (Berkeley: University of California Press, 1978); Judith Bardwick, "The Seasons of a Woman's Life," in D. McGuigan, ed., *Women's Lives: New Theory, Research, and Policy* (Ann Arbor: Center for the Education of Women, University of Michigan, 1980); Carol Gilligan, *In a Different Voice: Psychological Theory and Women's Development* (Cambridge, Mass.: Harvard University Press, 1982); Ellen McGrath, *When Feeling Bad Is Good;* Kathleen Day Hulbert and Diane Tickton Schuster, eds., *Women's Lives Through Time: Educated American Women of the Twentieth Century* (San Francisco: Jossey-Bass, 1993).

18. Eichorn et al., Chapter 8, "Paths to Psychological Health in the Middle Years: Sex Differences."

19. Ravenna Helson and Paul Wink, "Personality Change in Women from the Early 40s to the Early 50s," *Psychology and Aging*, vol. 7, no. 1 (1992).

20. P. Wink and R. Helson, "Personality Change in Women and Their Partners," *Journal of Personality and Social Psychology*, September 1993.

21. David Gutmann, *Reclaimed Powers: Toward a New Psychology of Men and Women in Later Life* (New York: Basic Books, 1987).

22. Sheehy, *Pathfinders.*

9. WONDER WOMAN MEETS MENOPAUSE

1. Gail Sheehy, "Is George Bush Too Nice to Be President?" *Vanity Fair*, February 1987, pp. 48–53, 119–25.

2. Barbara Bush, *Barbara Bush: A Memoir* (New York: Scribner's, 1994), p. 135.

3. Gail Sheehy, "The Silent Passage—Menopause," *Vanity Fair*, October 1991.

4. "Resident Population Estimates by Age, Sex, Race and Hispanic Origin," Table A, U.S. Bureau of the Census.

5. Joan Swirsky, "Menopause: New Research and Treatment," *The New York Times*, June 6, 1993.

6. Sheehy, *Silent Passage*, p. 7.

7. Lois Banner, *In Full Flower: Aging Women, Power and Sexuality* (New York: Knopf, 1992), p. 273.

8. Swirsky.

9. Gill Harley, "Suffering in Silence," *Sunday Express*, September 29, 1991.

10. According to public health expert Lewis Kuller, as cited in Sheehy, *Silent Passage*, p. 23.

11. Bush, pp. 135–36.

12. According to Phyllis Kernoff Mansfield, a veteran researcher of female cycles at Penn State, quoted in Sheehy, *Silent Passage*, p. 9.

13. Cathy Perlmutter, Toby Hanlon, and Maureen Sangiorgio, "Triumph over Menopause," *Prevention*, August 1994, pp. 78–87, 137, 142.

14. Author's interview with Dr. Patricia Allen, November 1994.

15. According to a lecture by Dr. Sherry Jackson, assistant professor of clinical medicine, Columbia Presbyterian Medical Center, given at the International Women's Forum Tenth Annual Conference, October 6, 1994, Memorial Sloan-Kettering Cancer Center, New York, New York.

16. According to Dr. C. B. Ballinger, an eminent Scottish psychiatrist, academic researcher, and consultant at Royal Dundee Liff Hospital, cited in the revised paperback edition of Sheehy, *The Silent Passage* (New York: Pocket, 1993), p. 114.

17. Perlmutter et al. Also author's interview with Dr. Estelle Ramey, professor emeritus of physiology at Georgetown University School of Medicine, October 1994.

18. Author's interview with Dr. Ramey.

19. Melinda Beck, "The New Middle Age," *Newsweek*, December 7, 1992, pp. 50–56.

20. Amanda Spake, "The Raging Hormone Debate," *Hippocrates*, February 1994, pp. 33–41.

21. Author's interview with Valerie Ryan, senior marketing analyst, Wyeth-Ayerst Laboratories, January 1995.

22. Women's Health Initiative Program Advisory Committee meeting, March I, 1994.

23. *Ob.Gyn. News,* January 15, 1995.

24. Author's interview with Ryan.

25. Author's interview with principal investigator for PEPI, Dr. Trudy Bush, November 1994.

26. Mary Ann Howkins, "Diet and Breast Cancer: Exploring the Link," *Glamour,* June 1994, p. 46.

27. Perlmutter et al.

28. According to Dr. Eric Poehlman at "Women and the Hormones in Their Lives" symposium, Baltimore, October 8, 1994. Sponsored by the Women's Health Research Group, Department of Epidemiology and Preventive Medicine, University of Maryland School of Medicine.

29. Jane Brody, "New Therapy for Menopause Reduces Risks," *The New York Times,* November 18, 1994.

30. According to Dr. Judith Reichman, gynecologist at Cedars-Sinai Medical Center, Los Angeles, as stated at the Women's Health Initiative Program Advisory Committee Meeting, Washington, D.C., March I, 1994.

31. Wulf H. Utian and Isaac Schiff, "NAMS (North American Menopause Society)—Gallup Survey on Women's Knowledge, Information Sources, and Attitudes to Menopause and Hormone Replacement Therapy," *Menopause: The Journal of the North American Menopause Society,* vol. I, no. I (1994), pp. 39–48.

32. According to Dr. Mary Corretti, assistant professor of cardiology and director of transesophageal echocardiography, University of Maryland Hospital. Lecture at University of Baltimore symposium "Women and the Hormones in Their Lives," October 8, 1994, Omni Harbor Hotel, Baltimore, Md.

33. Jane Brody, "Hormone Replacement Study Answers Questions, But Not All," *The New York Times,* January 18, 1995.

34. Dr. Judith Reichman, Women's Health Initiative Program Advisory Committee Meeting, March I, 1994.

35. Ibid.

36. Author's interview with Dr. Ruth Merkatz, director of Office of Women's Health, Rockville, Md., and Dr. Sol Sobel, chief of the FDA's Division of Endocrine and Metabolic Products, January 1995.

37. Author's interview with Dr. Trudy Bush.

38. Sources for natural micronized progesterone in the United States are only a few pharmacies: Two are in Madison, Wisconsin: Women's International Pharmacy (800) 279–5708; and Madison Pharmacy Associates (800) 558–7046. It is also available through College Pharmacy in Colorado Springs, Colorado (800) 888–9358 or Bajamar Women's Health Care in St. Louis, Mo. (800) 255–8025.

39. Author's interview with Dr. Merkatz and Dr. Sobel, January 1995.

40. Spake.

41. John R. Lee, M.D., "Osteoporosis Reversal—The Role of Progesterone," *International Clinical Nutrition Review,* vol. 10, no. 3 (July 1990).

42. John R. Lee, M.D., *Natural Progesterone—The Multiple Roles of a Remarkable Hormone* (Sebastopol, Calif.: BLL Publishing, 1993), pp. 53–70.

43. Author's interview with Dr. Barbara Sherwin, November 1994. Also see Barbara Sherwin and Diane L. Kampen, "Estrogen Use and Verbal Memory in Healthy Postmenopausal Women," *Obstetrics & Gynecology,* vol. 83, no. 6 (June 1994), pp. 979–83.

44. According to Dr. Bruce S. McEwen, a neurobiologist at Rockefeller University in New York, cited in Natalie Angier, "How Estrogen May Work to Protect Against Alzheimer's," *The New York Times,* March 8, 1994.

45. Annlia Paganini-Hill and Victor W. Henderson, "Estrogen Deficiency and Risk of Alzheimer's Disease," *American Journal of Epidemiology,* vol. 140, no. 3 (1994), pp. 256–61. Also see Henderson, Paganini-Hill, et al., "Estrogen Replacement Therapy in Older Women," *Archives of Neurology,* vol. 51 (September 1994), pp. 896–900.

46. Anna Quindlen, "Birthday Girl," *The New York Times*, November 21, 1993.

47. Carnegie Corporation report cited in Karen Peterson, "The Terrible Tweens," *USA Today*, verified by Peterson in December 1994.

48. According to Anne Peterson, dean of the College of Human Development at Penn State, cited by Karen Peterson.

49. Lyn Mikel Brown and Carol Gilligan, *Meeting at the Crossroads: Women's Psychology and Girls' Development*, (Cambridge, Mass.: Harvard University Press, 1992), p. 39.

10. FROM PLEASING TO MASTERY

1. Of the women surveyed about the best thing about being over 45, 43 percent of the women in the *Family Circle* and 39 percent of the Professional Women said this was so. The *New Woman* survey did not ask this question.

PART FIVE: FLAMING FIFTIES: MEN

11. THE SAMSON COMPLEX

1. John Updike, *The Afterlife* (New York: Knopf, 1994).

2. Michael Murphy, *Golf in the Kingdom* (New York: Arkana Books, 1972), p. 51.

3. Howell Raines, *Fly Fishing Through the Midlife Crisis* (New York: Morrow, 1993).

4. Ibid., pp. 111–12.

5. Ibid., p. 296.

6. Eichorn et al., p. 211.

7. "Advanced Report of Final Mortality Statistics 1991," National Center for Health Statistics, a division of Centers for Disease Control and Prevention (Hyattsville, Md.: Public Health Service, 1993), vol. 42, no. 2, Supplement.

   The difference between life expectancies between the sexes was 6.9 years in 1991.

8. D. C. Kimmel, *Adulthood and Aging* (New York: John Wiley, 1990), p. 14, cited in McGrath, Chapter 6, "Age Rage Depression."

9. "Advanced Report of Final Mortality Statistics 1991."

10. From 1,195 men age 45–49 in 1979 to 1,614 in 1991, according to the Centers for Disease Control in Atlanta, Georgia. In recent years the death rate of all causes has been 40 percent higher for men than for women.

11. Sheehy's *Family Circle* survey.

12. Jane Brody, "Strength Workouts Can Help Keep Aging at Bay," *The New York Times*, August 10, 1994. A study reported in *The New England Journal of Medicine* by Tufts University researchers showed that strength training can help even the frail and elderly to increase markedly their walking speed and stair-climbing ability, allowing them to remain active and independent.

13. "Lack of Doctor-Patient Communication in Older Men," a news release of the American Medical Association, October 17, 1991, reported on a Gallup poll in which one in four men "cited embarrassment as the No. 1 reason for not discussing sexual dysfunction or depression. 'Threat to masculinity' was the second reason most often cited."

14. According to the *Seer Cancer Statistics Review 1973–1990* (Bethesda, Md.: U.S. Department of Health and Human Services), Table XXII-6.

15. Dr. Kenneth Goldberg, *How Men Can Live as Long as Women* (New York: Summit, 1994).

16. Author's interview with Dr. Kenneth Goldberg, December 1994; Eric Lax, "Is Your Husband Dying of Embarrassment? The Truth About Prostate Cancer," *Family Circle*, July 20, 1993.

17. Dean Ornish, M.D., is the president and director of the Preventive Medicine Research Institute as well as the author of four books, including *Dr. Dean Ornish's Program for Reversing Heart Disease* (New York: Random House, 1990), and *Eat More, Weigh Less* (New York: HarperCollins, 1993).

12. FALL GUYS OF THE ECONOMIC REVOLUTION

1. "By the Numbers: Year's Hottest Jobs for Women" (no byline), *The San Diego Union-Tribune*, September 7, 1993. Excerpted from the July 1993 issue of *Working Woman* magazine. The U.S. Census Bureau's latest report on Discretionary Income finds 44 percent is in households where the head is over 50.

2. U.S. Bureau of the Census, Household Wealth and Asset Ownership, 1991; compiled from Survey of Income and Program Participation conducted February to May 1991.

3. E.P.M. Communications market newsletter, Research Alert, August 20, 1993.

4. Ann Cooper, "A Lighter Touch for the Gray Market," *Adweek*, July 19, 1993.

5. Louis Uchitelle, "Male, Educated and Falling Behind," *The New York Times*, February 11, 1994.

6. Evelyn Mann, "Median Earnings of Males Ages 45 to 54 Who Have Completed Four Years of College Education, United States, 1987 to 1992 (in 1992 Dollars)," unpublished report, based on unpublished Census Bureau Data, compiled from the March Current Population Survey Files from 1989 through 1993 by Paul Ryscavage, which reported on income of respondents from 1987 through 1992.

7. Author's interview with Marilyn Puder-York, former staff clinical psychologist for Citibank, December 1994.

8. Author's interview with Robert Sind, corporate restructuring expert, August 1994.

9. Author's interview, January 1994.

10. Author's interview, November 1993.

11. Timothy Egan, "Triumph Leaves No Targets for Conservative Talk Shows," *The New York Times*, January 1, 1995.

12. Tony Horwitz, "Jobless Male Managers Proliferate in Suburbs, Causing Subtle Malaise," *The Wall Street Journal*, September 20, 1993.

13. U.S. Census Bureau table from 1990 Census, Social and Economic Characteristics, N.S. Summary, Table 19.

14. Amanda Bennett, "More and More Women Are Staying on the Job Later in Life Than Men," *The Wall Street Journal*, September 1, 1994. The labor-force participation rate among men over the same period, from 1978 to 1993, dropped nearly seven percentage points to 66.5 percent.

15. Actual figure is 30 percent, reported by Janet L. Fix: "More Couples See Earnings Power Shift," *USA Today*, October 17, 1994.

16. Ibid.

17. According to author's interview, September 1994, with David L. Birch, president of Cognetics, Inc., an economic research firm that maintains a database on ten million American companies.

18. Author's interview, January 1995. According to the U.S. Department of Labor, in December 1994 out of the total labor force today of 131,725,000, 5.4 percent were reported unemployed, or 7,239,000.

19. Marc Levinson, with William Burger and Bill Powell, "Can Anyone Spare a Job?" *Newsweek*, June 14, 1993.

20. Author's interview, July 1994.

21. Harry Levinson, "Easing the Pain of Personal Loss," *Harvard Business Review*, September–October 1972.

22. Sheehy's pilot study of 110 Professional Men, 1993.

13. THE OPTIMISM SURGE

1. Sheehy survey of Professional Men; 63 percent feel "very secure" in their sense of optimism and serenity; 72 percent feel "very secure" about their judgment.
2. Sheehy survey of Professional Men: 60 percent feel more optimistic and a sense of serenity.
3. Author's interview, January 1993.
4. Sheehy surveys. Two thirds of the Professional Men over 45 feel closer to their wives.
5. Eichorn et al., pp. 216–17.
6. From research at University for Human Development, University of California, Berkeley, discussed ibid., Chapter 8: "Paths to Psychological Health in the Middle Years: Sex Differences."
7. Author's interview, January 1995.
8. "For, Brother, What Are We?" by Thomas Wolfe. From *Of Time and the River.*
9. Bernie Zilbergeld, *The New Male Sexuality* (New York: Bantam, 1992), pp. 28, 9.
10. Rosalind Barnett, Nancy Marshall, and Joseph Pleck, "Study of Full-Time Employed Dual-Earner Couples," *Journal of Marriage and the Family* (1992), vol. 54, pp. 358–67. Also see Ronald F. Levant and William S. Pollack, eds., *Toward a New Psychology of Men* (New York: Basic Books, 1995).
11. Levant and Pollack, op. cit.
12. Jon Katz, "The Good Father: Defining Dad in 1994," *Family Life*, May–June 1994, pp. 47–56.
13. Ibid.
14. Levant and Pollack, op. cit.
15. Aaron Latham, "Fathering the Nest: The New American Manhood," "*M*," May 1992, pp. 67–75.
16. Ibid.
17. In 1984 the Catalyst research organization launched a landmark study on parental leave policies in the nation's largest fifteen hundred companies (based on annual sales). According to the study results, 37 percent of these companies offered paternity leaves. A 1990 survey by the recruitment firm Robert Half International (Menlo Park, California) showed that 31 percent of the thousand companies queried offered some form of paternity leave.
18. Latham.

14. THE UNSPEAKABLE PASSAGE: MALE MENOPAUSE

1. Quoted in Randi Hutter Epstein, "Do Men Go Through Menopause?" *Frontiers*, July 1992, p. 31.
2. Author's interview, May 1993.
3. Cary Grant quoted in photo caption from *People's* Special Tribute to Audrey Hepburn issue, January 1993.
4. Author's interview, October 1992.
5. Author's interview, November 1991.
6. Doctors Malcolm Carruthers and John Moran are the foremost practitioners in Great Britain of hormone replacement therapy for men. In their London clinic, the Hormonal Healthcare Centre, they have prescribed male hormone to more than four hundred men, accompanied by counseling and diet and lifestyle education.
7. According to Dr. Georges Debled, chief urologist at the St. Pierre Hospital in Brussels. Dr. Debled was speaking at a conference, March 25–28, 1993, in Rye Brook, New York, sponsored by the Broda Barnes, M.D., Research Foundation (Connecticut).
8. Ibid.

9. John Cheever, *The Journals of John Cheever* (New York: Ballantine, 1991), pp. 147–49.

10. Ibid.

11. "National Institute on Aging Launches Initiative to Study New Hormone Therapies for Preventing Frailty," National Institute on Aging press release, October 13, 1992.

12. Lawrence Altman, "Study Suggests High Rate of Impotence," *The New York Times*, December 22, 1993.

13. Author's interview with Dr. Irwin Goldstein, January 1993. Dr. Goldstein was also an author of the Massachusetts Male Aging Study reported in the January 1994 issue of *The Journal of Urology.*

14. Altman.

15. U.S. Bureau of the Census, "Population Projections of the United States, by Age, Sex, Race, and Hispanic Origin: 1993 to 2050," Current Population Reports, pp. 25–1104, pp. 38–39.

16. Celia Hall, "Celibate Life for Many Older Men," *The Independent*, March 26, 1993.

17. "Putting the 'Men' into Menopause," *The Week in Germany*, July 15, 1994, p. 7.

18. Sheehy survey for *Family Circle.*

19. Ibid. Of the men in my sample 56 percent over 45 say male menopause exists; 62 percent say they won't go through it; 28 percent say they are now experiencing it or already have been through male menopause.

20. Author's interview, January 1993.

21. Sheehy *Family Circle* survey.

22. Sheehy survey of 110 Professional Men.

23. Author's interview, November 1992.

24. Author's interview, February 1993.

25. Author's interview, September 1992.

26. According to Dr. Debled, two large-scale studies show that the frequency of impotence rises with age. The striking thing is how greatly the incidence of impotence has increased in twenty-four years.

In 1948: *Incidence of impotence in a series of 4,108 patients:* cited in A. C. Kinsey, W. B. Pomeroy, and C. E. Martin, *Sexual Behavior in the Human Male* (Philadelphia: W. B. Saunders Co., 1948).

Age in Years	Percent Impotent
40	1.9
45	2.6
50	6.7
55	6.7
60	18.4
65	25
70	27
75	55
80	75

In 1972: *Incidence of impotence in 2,801 men:* cited in C. K. Pearlman and L. I. Kobashi, "Frequency of Intercourse in Men," *The Journal of Urology*, vol. 107 (1972), pp. 298–301.

Age in Years	Percent Impotent
40–49	5
50–59	11.3
60–69	35.6
70–79	59
80+	85

27. The Massachusetts Male Aging Study was a federally funded study of 1,709 men in eleven areas of Massachusetts. Results of the report are found in the January 1994 issue of *The Journal of Urology.* Also reported in Altman.

28. Author's interview with Dr. Irwin Goldstein, January 1993.

29. Samuel and Cynthia Janus, *Janus Report on Sexual Behavior* (New York: Wiley, 1993).

30. *Impotence: NIH Consensus Statement*, National Institutes of Health Consensus Development Conference, Bethesda, Md., December 7–9, 1992.
31. Ibid.
32. *Random House Dictionary of the English Language.*
33. Author's interview, December 1992.
34. New York: Summit, 1994.
35. Author's interviews with Boston urologist Dr. Irwin Goldstein, January 1993; and San Francisco urologist Dr. Tom Lue, June 1994.
36. New York: Dell, 1991.
37. Author's interview, August 1994.
38. Author's interview, January 1993.
39. Author's interview, July 1994.
40. Author's interview, January 1992.
41. Kenneth Goldberg, "Impotence Is Often a Sign of Greater Ills," *The Dallas Morning News*, September 7, 1992.
42. Karen Schmidt, "Old No More," *U.S. News & World Report*, March 8, 1993, pp. 67–73.
43. Ibid.
44. "Male Menopause: Could a Testosterone Patch Turn Back the Clock?" *Men's Confidential*, July 1993, pp. 6–7.
45. Altman.
46. According to Dr. Debled, who explained during the Barnes Foundation conference that testosterone has a direct action on the nucleus of a cell. It is implicated not only in the metabolism of all proteins but in the conversion of blood sugar and fat. He said, "Every three years you are a different man, because your molecules have changed. The protein structures are constantly rejuvenating."
47. It is very difficult to define a "normal" level of testosterone. Dr. Tom Lue describes a broad band of normality (300 to 1,200 nanograms per deciliter). Dr. Debled, the Brussels physician, says 300 to 1000. At the Highland Park Hospital outside Chicago, the laboratory considers a normal testosterone level to be 225 to 900 nanograms/deciliter. Even though a man's testosterone levels may measure within these wide parameters, there is usually a decline in his *free* testosterone as he ages. That means the sex hormone that the body can actually use. "Young men have twice as much *available* testosterone as older men," says Dr. Stanley Korenman, a reproductive endocrinologist at the UCLA Medical School. "I think what happens to men is that their brain ages. Older men become relatively insensitive to sexual stimuli because available testosterone goes down with age, so the tissues are less stimulated and testosterone receptors in the brain don't respond as well."
48. Epstein.
49. Rudman et al., pp. 1–6.
50. Ibid.
51. Rick Weiss, "A Shot at Youth," *Health*, November–December 1993, pp. 38–47.
52. Emiliano Corpas, S. Mitchell Harman, and Marc R. Blackman, "Human Growth Hormone and Human Aging," *Endocrine Reviews*, vol. 14, no. 1 (1993), pp. 20–39.
53. Stephen E. Borst, William J. Millard, and David T. Lowenthal, "Growth Hormone, Exercise, and Aging: The Future of Therapy for the Frail Elderly," *Journal of the American Geriatric Society*, vol. 42 (May 1994), pp. 529–35.
54. Weiss. After the first six months, the cost is $2,400 for a three-month supply, or $9,600 per year.
55. Weiss.
56. Author's interview and according to Dr. David Jacobs, chief of endocrinology at Lenox Hill Hospital, New York City.
57. Borst, Millard, and Lowenthal.
58. "National Institute on Aging Launches Initiative to Study New Hormone Therapies for Preventing Frailty," National Institute on Aging press release, October 13, 1992.

59. Author's interview, July 1994.

60. Arlene J. Morales, John J. Nolan, Jerald C. Nelson, and Samuel S. C. Yen, "Effects of Replacement Dose of Dehydroepiandrosterone in Men and Women of Advancing Age," *Journal of Clinical Endocrinology and Metabolism*, vol. 78, no. 6 (February 25, 1994). The team studied the effect of a replacement dose of DHEA in thirteen men and seventeen women, 40 to 70 years of age. A randomized placebo-controlled crossover trial of nightly oral DHEA administration (50 mg) of six-month duration was conducted.

15. MEN AND WOMEN: THE NEW GEOMETRY OF THE SEXUAL DIAMOND

1. Research on human brains has shown that the fibrous "switchboard" that connects the two sides of the brain (corpus callosum) is larger in women than in men, particularly in the areas responsible for language. Scientists speculate that this may explain why women experience more "cross talk" in their thinking process; why, for instance, in the middle of an abstract problem-solving exercise, a woman can suddenly pick up a signal about another person's needs—an intuition. These findings, of UCLA neuroscientist Roger Gorski and his colleague Laura Allen correlate with previous observations of other researchers, particularly neuropsychologist Sandra Witelson of McMaster University in Hamilton, Canada. See summary of findings to date in Thomas Maugh, "New Homosexuality Link Found in Brain," *Los Angeles Times*, August 1, 1992.

    Dr. Gorski also told me in an interview that the "splenium of the corpus callosum is more bulbous in women." He and his colleagues confirmed this observation using MRIs.

2. A series of cross-cultural studies done in the 1970s by anthropologist David Gutmann. For further information see his *Reclaimed Powers: Men and Women in Later Life* (Evanston, Ill.: Northwestern University Press, 1994).

3. Ibid.

4. Kevin Starr, *Inventing the Dream: California Through the Progressive Era* (New York: Oxford University Press, 1985).

5. Gail Sheehy, "California Dreamin'," *Vanity Fair*, June 1994.

6. Sheehy, *Pathfinders*, Chapter 9, "Best of Male and Female Strengths."

7. Meg Lavigne, "The Secret Mind of the Brain," *Columbia Magazine*, December 1983, pp. 12–17.

8. Natalie Angier, "How Estrogen May Work to Protect Against Alzheimer's," *The New York Times*, March 8, 1994.

9. Author's interview with Roger Gorski, Ph.D. See L. S. Allen and R. A. Gorski, "A Sex Difference in the Bed Nucleus of the Stria Terminalis of the Human Brain," *Journal of Comparative Neurology*, no. 302 (1990); Allen and Gorski, "Sexual Dimorphism of the Anterior Commissure and the Massa Intermedia of the Human Brain," *Journal of Comparative Neurology*, no. 312 (1991); and P. E. Cowell, L. S. Allen, N. Zalatimo, and V. H. Denenberg, "A Developmental Study of Sex and Age Interactions in the Human Corpus Callosum," *Developmental Brain Research*, no. 66 (1992).

10. Lawrence Wright, "Women and Men: Can We Get Along? Should We Even Try?," *Texas Monthly*, February 1992, excerpted in the January/February 1993 issue of *Utne Reader*.

11. Author's interview with P. K. Siiteri. The endocrinologist first established this principle, with P. C. MacDonald, in "The Role of Extraglandular Estrogen in Human Endocrinology," *Handbook of Physiology*, ed. S. R. Geiger, E. B. Astwood, and R. O. Greer (New York: American Physiological Society, 1973).

12. Sheehy, *The Silent Passage*, rev. ed., quoting Dr. Howard Judd, professor of obstetrics and gynecology at UCLA.

13. Confirmed by Dr. Siiteri.

14. Angier.

15. According to Dr. Georges Debled. See Chapter 14, note 7.

16. James O'Neil and Jean Egan, "Men's and Women's Gender Role Journeys: A Metaphor for Healing, Transition and Transformation," *Gender Issues Across the Lifecycle*, ed. Barbara Rubin Wainrib (New York: Springer, 1992), p. 31.

17. Author's interview, August 1993. Her first book was *Workforce America! Managing Employee Diversity as a Vital Resource* (Homewood, Ill.: Irwin Publishing, 1991).

18. Sheehy, *Pathfinders*, Chapter 10, "A Certain Age."

19. Sheehy's survey of 110 Professional Men.

20. Ernest Becker, *The Denial of Death* (New York: Free Press, 1973), p. 162.

21. Robert T. Michael, et al. *Sex in America: A Definitive Survey* (Boston: Little, Brown, 1994). Survey is based on a study of 3,432 men and women aged 18 to 59, conducted in 1992 by the National Opinion Research Center at the University of Chicago.

22. Natalie Angier, "For Men, Better Wed than Dead," New York Times Syndicate, 1990.

23. Ibid. See also Maradee Davis, John Neuhasu, et al., "Living Arrangements and Survival Among Middle-Aged and Older Adults in the NHANES I Epidemiological Follow-up Study," *American Journal of Public Health*, vol. 82, no. 3 (March 1992).

24. Davis and Neuhasu.

25. Gullette.

26. Gross.

27. Ibid.

28. Sheehy's Survey on Aging for *New Woman*.

29. See Christopher Hayes, Deborah Anderson, and Melinda Blau, *Our Turn: The Good News About Women and Divorce* (New York: Pocket, 1993). Of the 352 respondents who filled out questionnaires, 46 percent were in their fifties and early sixties and had married during the 1950s; another 54 percent were in their forties and had married in the 1960s.

30. Sheehy's Survey on Aging for *New Woman*.

31. Mann, "Living Arrangements of Unmarried 45- to 64-year-old (White, Non-Hispanic) Males."

32. Ibid.

33. O'Neil and Egan.

PART SIX: PASSAGE TO THE AGE OF INTEGRITY

16. THE SERENE SIXTIES

1. Joseph Heller, *Closing Time: The Sequel to Catch-22* (New York: Simon & Schuster, 1994).

2. Christopher Farrell, "The Economics of Aging," *Business Week*, September 12, 1994, pp. 60–68.

3. Author's interview with patient.

4. Ruth Kirschstein, director of NIH's National Institute of General Medical Sciences, quoted in Aburdene and Naisbitt.

5. "Current Estimates from the National Health Interview Survey, 1992," published by the National Center for Health Statistics, Illness and Disability Branch.

6. Riley and Riley, pp. 20–25.

7. Profile of the twenty-two million readers of *Modern Maturity*, the magazine sent free to all members of the American Association of Retired Persons, analyzed by Simmons Market Research Bureau, 1991 report.

8. U.S. Bureau of the Census Population Projections of the United States by Age 1993–2050, Table P-25-1104.

9. Alan Cowell, "Affluent Europe's Plight: Graying," *The New York Times*, September 7, 1994.

10. U.S. Bureau of Census, Current Population Reports, *Consumer Income Series*, P60–184, Table B-15.

11. Cynthia M. Taeuber, "Women in Our Aging Society: Golden Years or Increased Dependency?" *USA Today* magazine, September 1993. Taeuber is chief, Age & Sex Statistics Branch, U.S. Bureau of the Census.

12. Author's interview with Dr. Dale Purves, chair of Neurobiology Department at Duke University Medical Center, November 1991.

13. Gerald M. Edelman, director of Neurosciences Institute at the Scripps Research Institute. See *Bright Air, Brilliant Fire.*

14. Douglas Powell, Harvard University psychologist, in his book *Profiles in Cognitive Aging* (Cambridge, Mass.: Harvard University Press, 1994).

15. K. Warner Schaie, pioneering cognitive scientist, who designed the Seattle Longitudinal Study.

16. Joannie M. Schrof, "Brain Power," *US. News & World Report,* November 28, 1994, pp. 89–97.

17. Ibid., citing neurologists at Harvard University.

18. Author's interview, June 1993.

19. Hugh Downs, *Fifty to Forever* (Nashville, Tenn.: Thomas Nelson, Inc., 1994).

20. Erikson, *Childhood and Society,* p. 269.

21. Ibid., pp. 268–69.

22. Dunne, pp. 159–60.

23. George E. Vaillant and Caroline O. Vaillant, "Natural History of Male Psychological Health, a 45-Year Study of Predictors of Successful Aging at Age 65," *The American Journal of Psychiatry,* vol. 147 (January 1990), pp. 31–37. For summary, see Daniel Goleman, "Men at 65: New Findings on Well-Being," *The New York Times,* January 16, 1990.

24. Moore, p. 14.

25. Author's interview with *20/20* host Hugh Downs about the centenarians he has studied.

26. Vaillant and Vaillant, pp. 31–37.

27. Sampson and Sampson, p. 161.

28. From a letter to Charles Soulier, written August 6, 1855. Quoted in Sampson and Sampson, p. 107.

29. Author's interview, September 1994.

30. Vital Statistics of the United States Annual and unpublished data. Selected Life Table Values, *Statistical Abstract of the United States, 1993,* Tables 115 and 116.

31. Taeuber, pp. 42–44.

32. Ibid.

33. Author's interview, August 1993.

34. New York: Random House, 1994.

35. Evelyn Mann, "Labor Force Participation Rates, Full-Time Employment," unpublished report, based on 1990 PUMS data. The percentages are 73.5 divorced, 60.7 widowed, 70.8 not living with a spouse, for an average of 66.3 percent.

36. Sheehy's survey on aging for *New Woman.*

37. Ibid.

38. Robert T. Michael, John H. Gagnon, Edward O. Laumann, and Gina Kolata, *Sex in America: A Definitive Survey* (New York: Little, Brown, 1994).

39. NIH Epidemiological Catchment Study, 1990, a representative national sample of 22,000 men surveyed by direct intensive interviews. The study was described to me by Dr. Goodwin of the NIH, September 1994.

40. Bill Moyers, *Healing and the Mind* (New York: Doubleday, 1993), pp. 195–211: Interview with Margaret Kemeny, Ph.D., in psychoneuroimmunology, whose research at the University of California, Los Angeles, explores the relationship between emotions and the immune system.

41. Edward Dolnick, "Why Do Women Outlive Men?" *The Washington Post,* August 3, 1991.

42. Barbara Gelb, "A Conversation with Joseph Heller," *The New York Times Book Review,* August 28, 1994.

43. Timothy Egan, "Goldwater Defending Clinton: Conservatives Faint," *The New York Times,* March 24, 1994.

44. Robert Reinhold, "Hefner Says Playing Days Are Over," *The New York Times*, July 27, 1989.
45. Author's interview, December 7, 1992.
46. Enid Nemy, "Masters and Johnson: Divorced, Yes, but Not Split," *The New York Times*, March 24, 1994.
47. Essay by Nicholas Hytner, director of the Vivian Beaumont Theater production of *Carousel*, February 1994, Lincoln Center Theater Publication, New York City.

17. MEN: MAKE MY PASSAGE

1. Stuart Fischoff, "Clint Eastwood and the American Psyche: A Rare Interview," *Psychology Today*, January/February 1993, pp. 38–41, 75–79.
2. Bernard Weinraub, "Even Cowboys Get Their Due," *GQ*, March 1993, pp. 213–17.
3. Peter Biskind, "Any Which Way He Can," *Premiere*, April 1993, pp. 53–60.
4. Ibid.
5. Author's interview with Irwin Winkler, March 1994.
6. Survey by Roper Starch Worldwide in New York City, 1993, cited in Paula Mergenhagen, "Rethinking Retirement," *American Demographics*, June 1994, pp. 28–34.
7. According to Mark Hayward, sociologist at Pennsylvania State University, whose team studied a group of retired men over seventeen years, cited in Mergenhagen, p. 30.
8. Evelyn Mann, "Percent with Income from Retirement Benefits by Age, Marital Status and Sex Aged Units 55 or Older, U.S. 1990," unpublished tables, based on "Income of the Population 55 or Older," U.S. Department of Health and Human Services, April 1989, GS Publication, No. 13-11871, data from Table I.1.
9. Mergenhagen, p. 28.
10. George Gallup, Jr., and Frank Newport, "Baby-Boomers Seek More Family Time," *The Gallup Poll Monthly*, April 1991, pp. 31–34.
11. Dr. B. Douglas Bernheim, Stanford University economist, for the updated "Merrill Lynch Baby Boom Retirement Index," July 14, 1994.
12. Ibid.
13. Ibid.
14. "A 1993 Gallup Poll found that 59 percent of 30- to 49-year-olds are afraid they won't be able to afford retirement at a reasonable age." Mergenhagen, p. 34.
15. *Barbara Bush: A Memoir* (New York: Scribner's, 1994), p. 497.
16. Ibid., p. 532.
17. Lois Romano, "Reliable Source: We've Heard That . . . ," *The Washington Post*, February 1, 1994.
18. Barbara Bush, *Larry King Live*, September 14, 1994.
19. Wayne King, "Carter Redux," *The New York Times Magazine*, December 10, 1989, pp. 38–40.
20. Ibid.
21. Maureen Dowd, "Despite Role as Negotiator, Carter Feels Unappreciated," *The New York Times*, September 21, 1994.
22. Rosalynn Carter with Susan K. Golant, *Helping Yourself Help Others: A Book for Caregivers* (New York: Times Books, 1994).
23. According to the U.S. Department of Labor, Bureau of Labor Statistics, in 1989 (the last year for which figures are available), 21 percent of people 55 to 64—and 17 percent of people over 65—were engaged in unpaid volunteer work. See the bureau's press release "38 Million Persons Do Volunteer Work," March 29, 1990 (press release #90-154). Data are from May 1989 Current Population Survey.
24. The phrase is that of Alan Pifer, director of the Southport Institute for Policy Analysis in Westport, Connecticut, quoted in "Forget the Rocking Chairs," *Business Week*, September 25, 1989, pp. 145–48.

25. Marilyn Wellemeyer, "The Class the Dollars Fell On," *Fortune*, May 1974.
26. Sheehy longitudinal study of Harvard Business School class of '49 and their wives in 1974, 1979, and 1989.
27. Evelyn Mann, "Life After 40: Grandparenthood," unpublished report, based on U.S. Bureau of the Census Population Projections of the United States by Age 1993–2050.
28. Ibid., quoting *The New American Grandparent*, February 1994.
29. Mann, "(White-Nonhispanic) Males 65 and over Labor Force Participation Rates and Part-Time Employed."
30. "Remarks of the First Lady at Liz Carpenter's Lectureship Series."
31. Quoted in Kolata, "Study Challenges Longevity Theory."
32. Wallace appeared on ABC News' *Nightline* with Ted Koppel, January 7, 1993.
33. Moyers. See "Emotions and the Immune System," pp. 195–211.
34. New York: Plume, 1990.
35. Exchange was related to me in an author's interview, June 1991.

18. WISEWOMEN IN TRAINING

1. *Søren Kierkegaard's Journals and Papers.*
2. New York: Brunner/Mazel, 1974, p. 112.
3. Author's interview, 1980.
4. Ken Dychtwald and Joe Flower, *Age Wave: The Challenges and Opportunities of an Aging America* (Los Angeles: Jeremy Tarcher, 1989), p. 241. For detailed analysis and social policy suggestions, see Susan Foster and Jack Brizius, "Caring Too Much? American Women and the Nation's Caregiving Crisis," *Women on the Front Lines: Meeting the Challenge of an Aging America*, ed. Jessie Allen and Alan Pifer, pp. 47–73.
5. Ellen McGrath, "New Treatment Strategies for Women in the Middle," *Gender Issues Across the Lifecycle*, ed. Barbara Rubin Wainrib (New York: Springer, 1992), p. 128.
6. Carter with Golant.
7. Allen and Pifer, eds., *Women on the Front Lines.* A prophetic book.
8. Author's interview, May 1993.
9. Evelyn Mann, Table 17, unpublished table, based on the U.S. Department of Education, National Center for Education Statistics, Integrated Postsecondary Education Data System's, "Fall Enrollment, 1991 Survey."
10. For more information about the "College at 60 Program" write to Fordham University, Lincoln Center Campus, 113 West 60th Street, Suite 422, New York, NY 10023. Phone: 212-636-6740.
11. Ruth Harriet Jacobs, "Expanding Social Roles for Older Women," Allen and Pifer, pp. 191–219.
12. Cecilia Hurwich, "Vital Women in Their Eighties and Nineties: A Longitudinal Study," dissertation, University of California, Berkeley. Available through UMI Dissertation Services in Ann Arbor, Mich., order #LD01950.
13. Marija Gimbutas, *The Civilization of the Goddess: The World of Old Europe* (New York: HarperCollins, 1991).

19. TWO SPECIES OF AGING

1. Moyers, "Emotions and the Immune System," in which Moyers interviews Margaret Kemeny, Ph.D.
2. Erik H. Erikson, Joan M. Erikson, and Helen Q. Kivnick, *Vital Involvement in Old Age* (New York: Norton, 1986).

3. According to Dr. Steffi Woolhandler, Harvard Medical School, as reported in *Newlife*, January/February 1995.

4. Dr. James Carey, University of California at Davis, quoted in Gina Kolata, "Study Challenges Longevity Theory."

5. According to Dr. James Vaupel, demographer at Duke University, ibid.

6. Author's interview with Dr. William Haseltine, September 1993.

7. Daniel Goleman, "Mental Decline in Aging Need Not Be Inevitable," *The New York Times*, April 26, 1994.

8. Anthony and Sally Sampson, eds., *Oxford Book of Ages* (New York: Oxford University Press, 1985).

9. Harold C. Schonberg, "Horowitz's Parting Gift: Charming Novelties," *The New York Times*, April 22, 1990; recollections from Thomas Frost, who produced the final recordings.

10. Deepak Chopra, M.D., *Ageless Body, Timeless Mind* (New York: Harmony Books, 1993), p. 201.

11. Associated Press, "Study Finds That Weight Training Can Benefit the Very Old," *The New York Times*, June 23, 1994. The study involved a hundred men and women who lived at the Hebrew Rehabilitation Center for the Aged in Boston; average age was 87, and about a third were in their nineties.

12. Anthony Campolo, *Who Switched the Price Tags?* (Waco, Texas: Word Books, 1986), pp. 28–29.

13. Chopra, p. 196.

14. Ibid., pp. 196–97.

15. Ibid., pp. 198–99.

16. Vivian Gornick's introduction to *O Pioneers!* (New York: Bantam, 1989).

17. Chopra, p. 166.

18. Ibid., p. 172.

Index

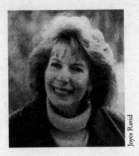

Joyce Ravid

ABOUT THE AUTHOR

GAIL SHEEHY, the author of eleven books, is best known for her landmark work *Passages* and the book that broke the silence about menopause: *The Silent Passage*.

Ms. Sheehy is also a political journalist and contributing editor to *Vanity Fair*. The mother of two daughters, she divides her time between New York City and Berkeley, California, where she lives with her husband, publisher and editor Clay Felker.